Vaccines

Making the Right Choice for Your Child

Fourth Updated and Expanded Edition

DR RICHARD HALVORSEN

For my granddaughters
Sofia, Katie and Miranda

Also by Dr Richard Halvorsen:
Managing Pain and Other Uses of Acupuncture

This expanded and updated fourth edition first published in 2020 by

Gibson Square, London

UK   Tel: +44 (0)20 7096 1100
US   Tel: +1 646 216 9488

rights@gibsonsquare.com
www.gibsonsquare.com

ISBN 9781783340958

Previously published in two editions as *The Truth About Vaccines*.

Printed by Clays St Ives

Contents

Preface to the Fourth Edition

Ever since the first edition I have ended this book with a plea for greater openness in discussions about vaccination. To my dismay the reverse has happened over recent years. When I was writing the first edition of this book, over ten years ago, the debate over the safety of the MMR vaccine was very much in the public domain. Television and newspaper discussions about the pros and cons of the vaccine were commonplace. Not anymore.

Criticism of vaccines or immunisation policy, whether by scientists, doctors or parents, is now condemned. Doctors or scientists who question vaccination are a potential threat to the public perception that all the experts support vaccination policies. Those who dare to question the benefits of vaccination may be subjected to a wide variety of attacks including the spreading of rumours, vilification, harassment, reprimand, demotions, deregulation and dismissal. The case of Dr Andrew Wakefield, who suggested the possibility of a link between the MMR vaccine and autism, is discussed in detail in this book. He was subjected to a 'degradation ceremony' and vilification, and was struck off The Medical Register, a response that was out of all proportion to any mis-demeanours he may have committed. This serves as a warning to others not to follow in his footsteps. No professional supporter of vaccination has ever been submitted to similar sustained campaigns, despite extensive evidence of bias in research published by the pharmaceutical industry.

Researchers have difficulty in obtaining funds and permission for research that looks into contentious side-effects of vaccines. There is evidence of researchers being denied access to research materials and of having unwelcome research censored. If they manage to finish the research, they may not be able to get it published if the findings are unwelcome. This prevents the opportunity for debate, instead of encouraging debate, which is a central tenet of scientific advancement.

Moreover, if all dissenting scientists and doctors can be silenced, it then appears as if all professionals are one and in full support of official vaccination policy.

An Australian mother who set up a group critical of government vaccination policy was subjected to abusive comments, unsupported claims about her belief in conspiracy theories, complaints to the media if she was given space to air her views, and threatening phone calls.

The media is discouraged from writing or talking about side-effects of vaccines. They are told that if they write a 'scare story' which then causes some parents not to vaccinate their children, the result of this is that children are likely to die and it will be the journalists' fault.

Parents are having an equally bad time. Many I have spoken with have been severely criticised by their GP or Practice Nurse for querying vaccination, sometimes being threatened with the involvement of social services or being accused of putting their children's lives at risk. This is happening the world over. In 2015 Pakistani police arrested more than 450 parents who refused to vaccinate their children against polio. In 2016 the Australian government hardened its pro-vaccine agenda by refusing to pay Child Care and Family Tax benefits for any children who are not fully up to date with their vaccines, forcing parents to give their children thirty-three vaccines by 18 months of age.

Anyone who queries an aspect of official government policy is accused of being 'anti-vaccine'. Critics are also often labelled 'anti-science', implying, incorrectly, that all the science fully supports vaccination.[2] Shutting down debate, however, is bad for parents, bad for science, bad for scientific truth and, most importantly, bad for our children.

A further four vaccines have been added to the UK children's immunisation schedule since the previous update.

Over the same period more research has been published that questions the safety of giving so many vaccines to our babies. I have therefore added new chapters on the rotavirus, flu, meningitis B and hepatitis B vaccines that are now given routinely. I have also updated other chapters where new research has provided us with more information on a vaccine's effectiveness or safety.

I approach the issues in this book also from a different research angle: can childhood infections prevent other diseases. In the book, I discuss in further detail the possible protective effect of childhood illnesses against such diseases as asthma, eczema, hay fever and allergies.

But researchers are discovering that many common childhood diseases may prevent cancers in children and in later life.[1,2] The evidence is strongest for cancers of the blood — leukaemia and lymphomas — which are the most common cancers in children.[3,4,5,6]

The childhood diseases that appear to help to prevent these cancers in later life in include chickenpox, measles, mumps, whooping cough, scarlet fever and rubella (German measles). Measles, which we already know can lessen the risk of asthma and allergies in later life, may be especially protective. In fact, nearly all infectious dieses looked at seem to protect against cancer, the only significant exception being glandular fever.

So whilst there is a threat from these diseases, though that threat is very small from infections such as mumps, chickenpox, rotavirus and even — in healthy children — measles, we are now beginning to appreciate the benefits of allowing children to contract these illnesses.

Interestingly it seems that the protective effect may be greatest in febrile infections, that is those associated with a high temperature (this suggests that we shouldn't be rushing for the paracetamol or ibuprofen every time our child develops a high temperature.)

We now have another reason, based on medical research, to consider carefully whether vaccination against relatively mild and harmless diseases is a necessary thing.

I am grateful to Karin Marais for proofreading the fourth edition.

Notes to the Preface of the Fourth Edition

1 Albonico HU, Bräker HU, Hüsler J. Febrile infectious childhood diseases in the history of cancer patients and matched controls. *Medical Hypotheses* 1998 (Elsevier); 51(4): 315-20

2 Hoption Cann SA, van Netten JP, van Netten C. Acute infections as a means of cancer prevention: opposing effects to chronic infections? *Cancer Detection and Prevention* 2006 (Elsevier); 39(1): 83-93

3 Montella M, Maso LD, Crispo A et al. Do childhood diseases affect NHL and HL risk? A case-control study from northern and southern Italy. *Leukemia Research* 2006; (Elsevier); 30(8): 917-22

4. Greaves M. A causal mechanism for childhood acute lymphoblastic leukaemia. *Nature Reviews: Cancer* 2018; https://doi.org/10.1038/s41568-018-0015-6

5. Parodi S, Crosignani P, Miligi L et al. Childhood infectious diseases and risk of leukaemia in an adult population. *International Journal of Cancer* 2013 (Wiley); 133(8): 1892-9

6 Alexander FE, Jarrett RF, Lawrence D et al. Risk factors for Hodgkin's disease by Epstein-Barr virus (EBC) status: prior infections by EBV and other agents. *British Journal of Cancer* 2000; 82(5): 1117-1121

Preface & Acknowledgements

'Experience of the past should teach us how unwise it is ever to introduce a new vaccine without first determining its protective power in man. Once a vaccine has been introduced with apparently good results, it becomes extremely difficult ever to find out its real value'
Graham Wilson, Former Director of the
Public Health Laboratory Service, England and Wales[1]

The overwhelming benefits of childhood vaccinations appear indisputable. They've saved millions of lives and are revered as one of the greatest public health interventions of all time — perhaps even the greatest success story of modern medicine.

Despite this apparent success, the debate over the risks and benefits has been with us for as long as vaccines have existed. There were riots, and jail sentences, in response to compulsory smallpox vaccination in the nineteenth century. A century later, parents, and even the government, shunned the diphtheria vaccine because children who received it were at increased risk of paralysis from the polio outbreaks that were threatening at the time. Later came the bitter whooping cough vaccine controversy of the 1970s, resulting in plummeting take-up rates. More recently, the acrimonious debate over the measles, mumps and rubella vaccine (MMR) continues, and appears no nearer a resolution, even a decade on.

The question is, if vaccines are so obviously good, why are they criticised? It's almost axiomatic that politicians aren't to be believed, but it's hard to imagine they'd mislead the public over such a sensitive issue as children's health. As for doctors — they are amongst the most trusted groups of people in the country, and most staunchly support vaccination.

But, beneath the surface, this support is wavering. Though a few doctors have repeatedly challenged the perceived wisdom, I started my journey of exploration into vaccines with no preconceived ideas. I was simply a family doctor who routinely immunised many children and who wanted to find out for myself whether I was being told the whole truth about vaccination.

This book evolved out of my own research and is the result of seven years of research and writing. It has been made accessible for as many readers as possible so that the information that is contained in the book does not merely reach medical specialists. Medical terminology has been avoided where possible in favour of words in common usage.

I apologise to those who find the reference numbers in the text irritating, but they will prove useful to those who wish to explore the issues contained in this book further, or simply want to check the accuracy of what I have written.

It should be emphasised that the conclusions and advice given in this book are mine alone, and are sometimes in contrast to official policy and advice.

Parents are advised to discuss any vaccine issues of concern with a health professional.

I thank my family — Charlotte, Sam and Rebecca — for putting up with me during the thousands of hours I have spent working on this book. Thanks also go to all those who supported and encouraged me in my research and writing. I am also grateful to everyone who allowed me to interview them, some of whom spoke out bravely. Special thanks go to my agent, Doreen Montgomery, and publisher, Martin Rynja who both believed in this book and worked hard with me to ensure that it reached a wide audience.

I am grateful to Abigail Paskins for help proof reading the third edition.

Introduction

When, as a junior hospital doctor, my son was born in 1983, I felt a slight unease about the whooping cough vaccine, about which there had been much adverse publicity during the 1970s. I took advice from a senior paediatrician who had sat on a committee examining the vaccine; he assured me that, though the vaccine did indeed have an extremely small, but real, risk of brain damage, the chance of my son getting brain damage from catching whooping cough was greater. Feeling caught between the devil and deep blue sea, but nevertheless partially reassured, I allowed my son to have the vaccine. Like every other parent, I only wanted to do what was best for him.

Then, in the spring of 2000 I was asked to write a feature on the MMR vaccine for a Sunday newspaper. My immediate reaction was, 'Why? What's the story? I gave MMR to my children, and give it to my patients every week.' I wasn't aware of any significant problem with the vaccine. I knew there were a few, probably rare, side-effects, but was in little doubt that the benefits of the vaccine far outweighed its risks. I had no reason to question the information provided by the Department of Health and I started to write the article with an open mind.

But, like any conscientious writer, I investigated the MMR vaccine — by researching the scientific literature, and also talking to doctors, parents and others. The more I discovered, the more disturbed I became. Though not overwhelmed by the evidence linking MMR to autism, I felt there might be something in it. I moved on to the government's evidence of safety, expecting — and hoping — to be reassured. I was alarmed to find that its defence of the vaccine was based on virtually no evidence at all. One international vaccine expert has controversially described the evidence demonstrating the safety of the MMR as 'crap'.

The fact that I'd found limited evidence suggesting the vaccine was a problem, but hardly any to demonstrate its safety, worried me and led me to change my practice as a family doctor. I started offering all parents the choice between giving their children the MMR or the three separate vaccines. I felt there were sufficient medical concerns that, at least for some children, giving the vaccines separately might be safer than the MMR. Although I would like to have offered only the separate vaccines on the basis of my concerns, I offered parents the choice because I did not want to incur the wrath of the Department of Health by not offering MMR.

On considering the Department of Health's arguments against using the single vaccines, I found them, to put it bluntly, feeble. I was, I believe, the only doctor in the country going against the government's advice by offering parents a choice. I felt unable to do anything else; my duty was to my patients – not the government. It seemed to me that, though slightly more expensive, the single vaccines were a perfectly safe and effective alternative. With a sufficient measure of uncertainty over the safety of the MMR, parents should, I felt, be allowed to make an informed decision for themselves. There were others who supported my view, but most felt unable to say so in public for reasons I will investigate in this book.

This made me wonder whether the problem with the MMR might not be an isolated case but rather a symptom of a much larger problem. It led me to look critically at other vaccinations as well, and also to the history of vaccines. Were they really ever our silver bullet? More often than not I was uncomfortable with what I found. My research unearthed facts which often challenged, and sometimes contradicted, the established view that I had been taught at medical school, and which is presented to the public as indisputable.

For example, at the turn of the millennium there was considerable controversy in the USA about the use of mercury in vaccines. Mercury is a highly toxic poison that's been used in childhood vaccines for over half a century. Not only is it dangerous, but it serves no purpose in vaccines used in this country. It had always been assumed to be safe because such small amounts were used in vaccines. But no one in Britain had actually checked whether this was the case. It was found that American children were receiving potentially dangerous quantities. I wondered whether this might also be the case in the UK. As no figures were available, I did the calculations myself. I discovered, to my amazement, that UK children were receiving over 100 times the upper limit of safe levels of mercury, quite possibly resulting in cases of autism, hyperactivity and speech disorders.

As a result of this discovery, I stopped giving children any injections containing mercury in 2002. I wrote letters to a leading medical magazine and appeared on national TV and radio arguing for the removal of mercury from children's vaccines. But it was over two years later before it was removed from routine childhood vaccinations in the UK, in October 2004. Mercury-free vaccines were freely available before 2004, but I don't know of any other doctors who offered these rather than the recommended ones. I even checked that the Department of Health was happy with my using mercury-free vaccines – which they were. I didn't want to upset them again if I could help it. But this time I didn't see any point in offering parents a choice: who would choose a vaccine containing an unnecessary toxic metal over one that was equally effective but free of mercury? All these decisions were based on my duty as a doctor to do what is best for my patients.

Including a substance as toxic as mercury in vaccines may have been an honest mistake (even though it beggars belief that this could have gone unnoticed for over half a century). Nonetheless, the mistake was a big one. Instead of investigating how this happened, with the hope of preventing such mistakes in future, governments, drug companies and most doctors merely attempted to sweep the issue under the carpet. During recent years, mercury-free vaccines have replaced mercury-containing vaccines throughout the Western world, but we are told this is entirely coincidental and not because of any concerns over safety. Sadly mercury is still present in some flu vaccines given to children in this country.

Next, I looked at the polio vaccine. The UK had for many years used the oral polio vaccine, given as drops, that contains live polio viruses. As a family doctor, I had been informed by health officials that there was a risk, albeit extremely small, of this vaccine causing polio and paralysis. However, this vaccine was, we were expressly told, more effective than the safer, injected vaccine, which cannot cause polio. However, when I looked at the figures while researching this book, I discovered that, during the previous 20 years, the oral polio vaccine had caused more people to become paralysed from polio than the illness itself. In addition, the evidence did not support the government's assertion that the oral polio vaccine was more effective, though it was certainly cheaper.

I felt that I had been grossly misled by the Department of Health and my trust in what I was being told by officials was being seriously undermined. Here was another example of children being given a less safe vaccine when safer alternatives were available. I started to offer children the safer but more expensive injected polio vaccine that has since been introduced nationally.

In the pages that follow I am investigating what else we — patients and doctors alike — are not being told. I am deeply disturbed by what I have found and how information about our health is increasingly held ransom to vested interests rather than freely available. Government advisers appear to be more interested in statistics of whole populations and financial costs than in individual safety. One vaccine expert told me: 'The government can't bear any suggestion of lack of safety of vaccines. They will not even discuss it. I think they have a policy of suppression of any discussion on safety.' Of equal or even greater worry is that I discovered that the confusion about vaccines is being exploited for profit. Vaccines are becoming big business.

It strengthened my belief that this book had to be written to inform parents, honestly, and without bias, so that they can form their own decisions. Such information is currently not available or not reliable. My interest in vaccines led me to consultations with thousands of parents who simply wanted to have a calm and rational discussion about the arguments for and against immunisation. As a result, I heard repeated stories of parents being patronised, bullied and forced into a corner where they were made to feel they no longer had any choice. Their questions had been dismissed as inconvenient, troublesome and unnecessary. Parents, but also doctors (and researchers), who question the safety — or value — of a particular vaccine are accused of putting children's lives at risk, and dismissed as cranks or scaremongers. Parents who, having deliberated long and hard, decide not to vaccinate their child with a particular vaccine, or even, as in the case of MMR, choose to give their children the vaccines separately, are made to feel like social outcasts or even accused by some of abusing their children.

I realised that parents don't know where to turn in order to get vaccination information they can trust. They don't trust government information any more than they do extreme anti-vaccine websites. Nor do parents believe newspaper scare stories that appear designed to sell newspapers rather than responsibly to inform the reader.

Many look to their doctor for impartial information, but on this issue doctors are, unusually, letting their patients down by feeling forced to follow the party line. A Department of Health survey from 2003 showed that a quarter of all family doctors, and an even greater proportion of Health Visitors, felt that babies were receiving too many immunisations — and now they're receiving many more.[1] Yet most doctors are unwilling, or unable, to enter into a discussion on childhood vaccinations.

Informed consent is the key to all medical decisions. A parent making a decision about vaccinating their child has the right to a truthful and open discussion. But this is all too often being denied, and we are being misled over vaccinations. For this reason, I will cover both the history of vaccines to the extent it tells us something about modern vaccines, as well as the spin and half-truths we're being fed today. Exposing these misapprehensions is what this book seeks to address.

A Quick Reference Guide to Vaccines

Which vaccines should I give my child?
What I have tried to do in this book is share what I found after seven years of research — that the benefits, and risks, of vaccines vary substantially, even if we are told that immunisation is the key to our children's health. Vaccines vary greatly; each new one will be different, and may not be as effective, or indeed as useful, as one that preceded it. Each one — old and new — has to be constantly monitored for it to remain on, or indeed before being added to, the national schedule. The benefit of most individual vaccines — the number of deaths or disabilities prevented — is currently small, so that it doesn't take many side effects to outweigh the benefit. It is an assessment that is not easy to make, but the fact that it is hard is of course no reason not to do it. It is a difficult assessment, partly because of our limited knowledge of the vaccines, but also because most of the vaccines do offer some benefit (though often less than we are led to believe), and have side-effects, some of which may be unknown or, as yet, unproven. The largely known risks of the illness must be weighed against the largely uncertain risks of vaccination. There is also another factor that has become important. The number of vaccines routinely given to every child in the UK has increased dramatically in the last hundred years. In the last twenty years

alone, the number of vaccines given to under five-year-olds has doubled, from sixteen in the 1980s, to thirty eight in 2017. This greatly increases the risk of side-effects that are a result of the manufacturing process from the use of mercury, or, as we have seen, aluminium where previously the risk was considerably lower because fewer vaccinations were given. There is also the added risk of a cumulative effect: whilst the use of one vaccine on its own may pose only minimal risk of harm, the addition of every extra vaccine to the schedule increases the risk of a combined effect on the body. There remains uncertainty whether the growing number of childhood vaccinations is contributing to the rising numbers of children affected by asthma, diabetes and other immune-related disorders. The main points for each vaccine are summarised below. Do bear in mind that there is no one absolutely right way to vaccinate your child. Countries have widely differing vaccine schedules and recommend different vaccines. The UK has the most concentrated vaccine schedule in the world, giving twenty-one vaccines — at eight, twelve and sixteen weeks — by four months of age. Most countries recommend giving vaccines at two, four and six months; all the Scandinavian countries recommend vaccines far more spread out at three, five and twelve months; all give them later than in the UK. Also bear in mind that the earlier a vaccine is given, the less and shorter lasting is the protective effect.[1]

Ultimately, the decision on what vaccines to give should rest with the parents, who should be allowed, and encouraged, to make informed decisions — without pressure or propaganda — in the light of the scientific evidence and their own wishes, and after taking medical advice. The advice that follows may differ from official Department of Health recommendations. Before making any final decisions, you are advised to consult a health professional about the specific needs of your child.

Smallpox
I am including it here because of the claims made about its success. Vaccination didn't rid the world of smallpox, but it played a contributory role. Neither immunisation, nor antibiotics contributed much to the decline in deaths from infectious diseases, by far the largest part of which occurred before the introduction of either. History demonstrates the natural ebb and flow of all infectious diseases, largely independent of any medical interventions.

Diphtheria
Diphtheria is one of the safer immunisations. By far the most common side-effects are redness, pain and swelling at the site of the injection. A painless nodule, that may last weeks or months, can form at the injection site, probably related to the aluminium in the vaccine. Because diphtheria 'poison-made-safe' has been given in combination with other vaccines — whooping cough and tetanus for over fifty years, and more recently Hib and polio as well — side-effects from the diphtheria component are difficult to distinguish from side-effects from the other constituents of the vaccine. The serious side-effects that occurred with the diphtheria-containing DTP triple vaccine are most likely to

be related to the whooping cough component which, until October 2004, also contained mercury. Combination vaccines occasionally cause swelling of the entire limb; this may be related to the strength of the diphtheria toxoid in the vaccine. Guillain-Barré syndrome (GBS), a disorder of the nerves causing, usually temporary, paralysis can probably, though rarely, be caused by the vaccine.

We know immunisation cannot be expected to get rid of diphtheria. We also know at least a third and possibly a half of all UK adults aren't immune to it and so are at much greater risk of becoming ill or even dying should the disease return. The disease is currently extremely rare in the UK, with an average of one case every year, though it is more common in other parts of the world such as India. As it's one of the safest immunisations and there is no longer a single diphtheria vaccine available, it should continue to be used, given with tetanus with or without whooping cough. Those who aren't vaccinated will gain little, if any, protection from others being immunised. In Britain, the diphtheria vaccine is now given as part of the 6-in-1 vaccine; it is available in 2-in-1 and 3-in-1 combination vaccines privately.

Tetanus
Though tetanus is very rare, and the chances of getting it small, the consequences are potentially severe, with 1 in 5 dying despite the best modern treatment. Many people believe — mistakenly — that protection against tetanus is not important because anyone who attends casualty with a serious wound will be given a tetanus-containing vaccine. This is true, but this vaccine will be too late to prevent tetanus occurring from the wound that necessitated the trip to casualty. For children in the UK there is no easily obtainable alternative to the new 6-in-1 tetanus-containing vaccine. On the other hand, it is not a disease that endangers the entire population. With the rising number of vaccinations there may be an argument for dropping, or at least postponing (a baby won't contract tetanus until crawling in the dirt), this vaccine — except for those at risk. In Britain it is only widely available as part of the 6-in-1 vaccine. It is also available singly, or in small combination vaccines, though these are not available through the National Health Service, only privately.

Whooping Cough
The approach to vaccinating against whooping cough has changed much over the years. In the early days, no child who had any sort of neurological reaction, 'however mild' (including any fit or collapse), was given a further dose of vaccine. The vaccine was also not given to any child who had ever had any sort of fit, including a relatively common 'febrile convulsion' (a fit associated with a high temperature).

Many doctors also withheld vaccination in any child who had suffered from any sort of allergy, including eczema, asthma or hay fever. It's likely that some of the children developing brain damage after vaccination did so because the doctor vaccinated despite a 'contra-indication'. Following the 1970s scare, doctors were, at least for a while, more careful. Though children are more likely to suffer serious side-effects from whooping cough in the first few months of life, it's also probable their immature immune and nervous systems are more prone to serious side-effects from vaccines.

A fourth dose was added to the UK schedule in 2001. A teenage booster dose has been introduced in several countries and is now recommended for all countries, and this is under consideration by the Department of Health. However, this will only push the illness into adults in their twenties – a particular worry because it is at this age that many people start to have children, thus posing a risk to newborn babies. The USA now advises ten-yearly boosters up to the age of sixty-five. Adult boosters may be introduced into European countries (already recommended in Austria) if the disease is really to be controlled, though even this is unlikely to eradicate the disease.

The whooping cough vaccine is not very effective, and the whole-cell vaccine has serious side-effects considered by some doctors to be unaccept-able. The whole-cell vaccine, though withdrawn from the UK, is still widely used around the world. It is worrying that those still receiving it – the mal-nourished and impoverished – are the very children who are most likely to suffer from the more serious side-effects such as brain damage. We now have a much safer (though possibly less effective) vaccine. The vaccine has done little, if anything, to eradicate whooping cough, which remains widespread in the community. Though whooping cough is a far less serious illness now than fifty or hundred years ago, vaccination can take little credit for this.

Though it's one of the least effective of the childhood vaccines, providing only short-term protection at best, it is likely to make an attack of whooping cough, which is an unpleasant and distressing illness, less severe. It is available as part of the 6-in-1 vaccine on the NHS, or as part of a 3-in-1 DTaP vaccine privately.

Polio

The chance of catching polio in the UK at present is virtually non-existent. Europe was certified polio free by the WHO in 2002. The risk of catching polio from travelling to developing countries is greater but still very small. As long ago as 1980 the risk to a traveller of contracting polio when visiting a country where polio was still present was less than 1 in 100,000, and even then only one in three million travellers to polio-containing countries would become paralysed. The risk now is clearly a lot less.

So, on an individual basis there may appear to be little point in being immunised against polio as the chances of catching it are so small. Now that the long overdue switch to the safer killed IPV has been made, however, it does make sense to continue vaccinating for a few more years because: a) The IPV is a very safe vaccine; b) The risk of contracting polio may become higher as the effort to eradicate polio hits obstacles; c) There are small but unknown risks of outbreaks of vaccine-polio-virus; d) The goal of global eradication of polio will be supported.

Hib

Hib is an uncommon but potentially serious disease. Despite the initial success of the Hib vaccination campaign, the vaccine is not as effective as was first thought. The three-dose schedule offered good immunity only until the second year of life, when protection fell rapidly. A recently introduced booster dose, given early in the second year of life, prolongs protection until five years of age, when the chance of catching Hib disease becomes much less. It may not be enough to prevent pushing the illness further into the older age group, in whom the disease is more serious. However, invasive Hib is a life-threatening disease which can cause meningitis and blood poisoning and kills 1 in 10 of those who are infected. It is of most importance in socially deprived children, and those with underlying serious medical problems who are more likely to suffer the effects of Hib infection, but worth considering in all children. In practice, choice is not available in Britain, as the vaccine is part of the 6-in-1 vaccine. It can be obtained privately, though not on the National Health Service, as a single or 2-in-1 vaccine.

Hepatitis B

Very few babies have any need to be vaccinated against hepatitis B, a disease that is contracted though blood or sexual contact. Fewer than ten children a year in the UK contract the disease, for which the biggest risk factors are injecting drug use and unprotected sex between men. Unfortunately the vaccine is given as part of the 6-in-1 vaccine and is, therefore, impossible to selectively leave out on the NHS. The only way to avoid this unnecessary vaccine is to seek smaller combinations, such as the DTaP, privately.

The 6-in-1 vaccine

The introduction of the 5-in-1 vaccine marked a big safety improvement in the UK vaccination schedule. Any benefit from this vaccine has now been reversed by its replacement with the 6-in-1 vaccine which includes hepatitis B, a vaccine that is not needed in this country and about which there are serious safety concerns. The big problem is that this vaccine comes as an all or nothing package, making it more difficult for parents to select which vaccines to give to their children – in any case, something the government wishes to avoid. In order to vaccinate a baby against Hib disease parents are obliged to give them a hepatitis B vaccine that is just not needed, a whooping cough vaccine of poor effectiveness and diphtheria, polio and tetanus vaccines earlier than necessary. Abnormal crying, irritability and restlessness are all common reactions as is a fever which is very likely to occur when the vaccine is given at the same time as the pneumococcal and meningitis B vaccines, as it is in the UK schedule. Convulsions can also occur, again more commonly when the vaccine is co-administered with the other vaccines in the UK schedule.

Pneumococcus

Pneumococcal disease can be serious, but is uncommon, especially in healthy children living in good social conditions. It's more likely to affect children who already have other medical problems. What's more, a common and dangerous time to get the illness is in the first weeks of life before vaccination is given. There's no certainty that 'herd immunity' from a successful vaccination campaign would protect these very young children. The pneumococcal bug is already responding to vaccination – perhaps predictably – by mutating into forms untroubled by the vaccine, an increasing proportion of which are resistant to commonly used antibiotics.

The pneumococcal vaccine has been introduced into an already crowded immunisation schedule without proper long-term studies.

The decision on whether to give this vaccine to an individual child should be a personal decision made between the child's parents and their doctor. This vaccine is probably, on balance, worth giving to healthy children, but is most important for high-risk children such as those with serious illnesses.

Rotavirus

Rotavirus is a sickness and diarrhoea bug that does not kill or cause permanent harm to babies in the UK. The vaccine is, rarely, associated with serious side-effects. The main reason for its introduction appears to be to save the NHS money. The vaccine is an unnecessary addition to an already overcrowded immunisation schedule and I do not recommend it.

Meningitis B

Meningitis B is a rare cause of life-threatening meningitis and blood poisoning. Prior to the introduction of the vaccine in 2015, two hundred and fifty children under five years of age contracted meningitis B every year, of which twenty-five died and a further fifty suffered permanent harm such as brain damage or loss of a limb. It is a nasty, but rare, illness. If we knew the vaccine were safe then I would recommend it. The problem is that it causes more side-effects than nearly every other vaccine, particularly a fever. This does not mean that it will necessarily cause more serious problems but at the moment it is simply too early to tell. The UK was the first country to introduce the vaccine in to the national schedule. The vaccine is made in a unique and novel way and until we have considerably more experience of it and evidence of its safety, I am unable to recommend it.

Meningitis C

This is a serious, life-threatening disease though, thankfully, rare. Having started off, in 2000, with three doses by 12 months of age on the NHS, this has now been cut back to a single dose at 12 months of age, with a booster as a teenager. This does leave babies unprotected until 12 months of age. It may be sensible to give a dose earlier, as the NHS did up until 2016. The vaccine is particularly important for children with chronic illness. However, a single dose after 12 months of age is probably sufficient for most children.

Measles

'Even before vaccine was introduced, measles appeared to be becoming a trivial disease in civilised communities,' wrote vaccine expert Professor George Dick in the *British Medical Journal* in 1980. 'There is something to be said,' he continued, 'for allowing a mild 'wild' measles virus to give a natural life-long protection to the healthy children of the community and to offer vaccine selectively to those [who are most vulnerable] or who have escaped a natural infection in the early years of childhood.' The *BMJ* is unlikely to print such wise and cautious words today for fear of being accused of putting children's lives at risk, so fevered and irrational has the debate on children's vaccinations become. However, Professor Dick's argument is sound. Though healthy children have little to fear from measles, the risks from the disease remain greater than the risks from the vaccine. However, the vaccine does have more side-effects than many vaccines. Whether to have this vaccine is a finely balanced judgement, but there is a greater need for it in children with underlying health problems who are more likely to suffer from serious complications form the illness. The single measles vaccine is available from private clinics.

Mumps

Some doctors and the media have been overreacting to outbreaks of mumps, an illness against which we shouldn't be vaccinating in the first place. The predictable consequence of vaccination is that, instead of infecting young children and providing them with life-long immunity, mumps is attacking young adults who are more likely to suffer from serious side-effects.

The vaccine is not only unnecessary, but is making mumps a less trivial disease than it used to be. Whilst there is a case for immunising teenage boys who have not had mumps (ideally after a blood antibody test to ensure they are not already immune, and preferably with a single vaccine which has not been available for many years) routine immunisation of young children is unnecessary. Most people's concern about mumps is that it could make boys infertile. If that can happen, and I write 'if' because no boy or man has ever been proven to have been made infertile from mumps, then it is extremely rare. What's more the only vaccine available that offers any protection against mumps is now the MMR vaccine. Irrespective of any concerns about the safety of this vaccine, it offers inadequate protection anyway. We know this because there are frequent outbreaks of mumps amongst teenagers and young adults who have all, almost without exception, received at least one, if not two, doses of the MMR vaccine. I cannot recommend vaccination against mumps whilst the only option available is the relatively ineffective MMR vaccine of questionable safety.

German Measles (Rubella)

Women need to be immune to German measles before becoming pregnant. All women obtain better immunity from catching the disease naturally, but this is now unlikely because of widespread vaccination. The only option that is readily available is the MMR vaccine, about which there are justified safety concerns. Unfortunately, the Department of Health has stubbornly dug itself into a hole on this one. It may be preferable for German measles still to be circulating in the community, alongside vaccination of susceptible teenage girls (after a blood antibody test); this should be accompanied by a public health campaign to encourage all women to have a blood test for immunity before getting pregnant. Whilst the suffering and tragedy of a baby born disabled because of congenital rubella (CRS) should not be underestimated, it's difficult to justify the vaccination of 35,000 children with the MMR vaccine in order to prevent every case of CRS. The risks of the MMR may be greater than the risks of CRS.

Girls should be offered a rubella-containing vaccine at twelve years, possibly after a blood antibody test to check for immunity, which would ensure that no girl is given the vaccine unless it is needed. Currently there is no single rubella vaccine available, only the 3-in-1 MMR (available on the NHS) and a 2-in-1 MR (measles and rubella, only available privately). Any woman who had one or two rubella-containing vaccines at a young age should have a blood test for immunity before getting pregnant.

MMR

MMR is the first and only vaccine to contain three live viruses. The studies to look in detail at the potential problems that this previously untried combination might cause have never been done. The vaccine causes more side-effects than any other vaccine used in the children's immunisation schedule, apart, perhaps, from the new meningitis B vaccine.

The vaccine serves little purpose.

Mumps is a largely harmless illness that vaccination is pushing into older people who are more likely to suffer complications.

Rubella (German measles) is harmless to all except pregnant women who aren't immune. At the time of the introduction of the MMR in the UK, tragically every year around thirty babies were being born disabled with 'congenital rubella syndrome'. However, this number was falling, probably due to the successful use of the single rubella vaccine in school-age girls. The wisdom of giving over a million MMR jabs a year to prevent a maximum of thirty damaged babies is questionable when we don't know whether the vaccine itself creates the same or a greater number of problems in children.

Measles may be worth vaccinating against; if so, there is a perfectly good single measles vaccine available.

The vast majority of children would be better off catching both mumps and rubella as children, thus receiving lifelong protection. Unfortunately the government's vaccination policy now makes this increasingly difficult.

If there were similar concerns about a food such as baked beans as there were about the MMR, the cans would have been removed immediately from supermarket shelves.

Children don't suddenly lose skills and regress, often over a period of only a few weeks, without a good reason. We are told no one knows what the cause might be, but that it is certainly not the MMR. In some of these children, it is probable that the MMR has triggered their autism.

In my opinion, the MMR vaccine should be withdrawn until adequate safety studies on sufficient children with long-term active follow-up can demonstrate its safety. It should be replaced by the single measles vaccine given at fifteen months.

Girls should be offered rubella vaccination at twelve years after a blood antibody test to check for immunity. This will ensure that no girl is given the vaccine unless it is needed.

Mumps vaccination is unnecessary but could be an option for boys at around twelve years (again, preferably after a blood antibody test to ensure the child is not already immune).

These suggestions will be criticised by some as being large steps 'backwards'. They are, however, steps towards common sense and caution in an era of evangelical and uncritical support for vaccination.

One problem with the immunity derived from vaccination is that it falls away over time far quicker than naturally acquired protection. Immunity after catching measles is usually life-long. After a single vaccine, protection may last twenty-five years, longer in some cases, shorter in others. No-one knows how many vaccinated people will still be protected against measles, mumps or rubella in twenty-five or fifty years' time. But an educated guess can be made by combining the results of studies that have measured antibody levels in children after one or two MMR vaccinations.

It's probable that people's immunity to all three illnesses will steadily fall as they get older, with the likelihood that, by middle age, many will no longer be immune. As it's extremely unlikely that these illnesses will be eradicated, that means that, for the first time in history, older people may be more likely than children to get measles, mumps and rubella — with unknown consequences. Some scientists have made alarming predictions of the consequences of this falling protection.

The period in which we are now — the first generation since the introduction of the MMR — has been described as the 'honeymoon' period. Most people born before the early 1970s will have life-long natural immunity, but those born later have vaccine protection that is likely to fall away. Research published in 2006 found people born before the introduction of immunisation were more likely to have high levels of antibody to measles, mumps and rubella than those born in the vaccine era. After 20, 30 or 40 years a lot of vaccinated people are likely to become susceptible to the illnesses again as their protection from vaccination wears off. This may lead to a resurgence of the diseases. Only this time the diseases could be different from what we knew before vaccination. How different, only time will tell.

On the optimistic side, most people may still have some remaining protection from vaccination and so the illness may generally be mild. On the pessimistic side, there are two things to worry about: the first is that the illnesses will affect older people in whom the side-effects are likely to be more serious. The second is less certain but more concerning: the wild measles virus has been changing, or mutating, so that it's becoming less like the measles vaccine virus. Whilst there is no evidence that this has caused any problems yet, the vaccine may not protect against future mutations. We meddle with nature at our peril. The worst case scenario is that we'll have changed measles, as a direct result of vaccination, from a relatively harmless illness to which we had adapted successfully to a more dangerous illness, with unknown consequences for future generations.

The single measles and 2-in-1 measles and rubella vaccines are available privately, but not on the NHS.

Tuberculosis (BCG)

The rationale for introducing routine BCG vaccination for adolescents in 1953 was sound. At that time fewer than a hundred schoolchildren needed to be vaccinated in order to prevent one case of TB. By 1984, nearly 5,000 children had to be vaccinated to prevent each case. Nationwide vaccination was giving increasingly poor returns, and was eventually stopped in 2005. The current policy of targeting the vaccine at 'high-risk' areas makes more sense, though this still means low risk babies born in Hampstead (in the London Borough of Camden — a 'high risk' area) will be given a vaccine of unproven benefit but with known risks. White children living outside London are at extremely low risk of contracting TB, whilst children from black African, Pakistani, Indian and Bangladeshi groups (especially if born outside the UK) are at greatest risk and should be considered for immunisation. In general, concerted action against factors that fuel TB — poverty, malnutrition and overcrowding — might be money better spent.

HPV

We have only a rough idea how widespread HPV is in the community, and know even less about the distribution of its many types. We have only a partial understanding of the virus' role in cervical cancer. The HPV vaccine has undergone only a few years' trials. Despite our inadequate knowledge, there is much talk of widespread global vaccination of all adolescent girls. It's premature to initiate extensive vaccination before the results of substantive trials of safety and effectiveness are known. The vaccine may be of great benefit, but we won't know for many years yet. The NHS initially offered Cervarix, an HPV vaccine that provides protection against the two types of HPV that cause three quarters of the cases of cervical cancer in the UK. However, there are concerns about the ingredients of this vaccine, particularly the new adjuvant ASO4. In 2012 the NHS switched to Gardasil that offers protection against the same types of HPV as Cervarix, and also an additional two types that cause most cases of genital warts. There have been far too many reports of serious auto-immune reactions to this vaccine — from both doctors and recipients — so that I am very wary of the vaccine as things stand. The HPV vaccine may turn out to be very valuable. However, at this stage too little is known about its long-term effects — both beneficial and harmful — to be able to recommend this vaccine for widespread use.

Mercury

Mercury is extremely toxic and has no place in childhood vaccines. It wasn't even needed in the single-dose vaccines used in the UK. It has almost certainly contributed to the rise in numbers of children with autism, hyperactivity, speech disorders and other developmental problems. Not only is it harmful, it is completely unnecessary. The Department of Health's policy of simply reassuring parents smacks of complacency and irresponsibility. The delay in the introduction of mercury-free vaccines into the UK, long after health concerns were expressed, was unacceptable. The DoH's ongoing complacency is exemplified by continuing to recommend mercury-containing flu vaccines for use in children when mercury-free alternatives are readily available. Sadly, tens of millions of children, many poorly nourished, continue to be vaccinated around the world every year with mercury-containing vaccines. All routine child vaccines used in the UK are now mercury-free. However, one or two flu vaccines still contain mercury. If your child needs a flu jab, request one that is free from mercury.

Aluminium

Aluminium is present in most vaccines. It is highly toxic, is known to cause brain damage and has been implicated in behavioural problems in children. Once aluminium enters the brain it's only excreted very slowly and is liable to accumulate. Very little aluminium is absorbed into the body when eaten because of the gut's 'protective barrier'. However, the gut is bypassed by an injection, so aluminium contained in vaccines passes straight into the bloodstream. The use of aluminium in vaccines has never undergone any safety trials. On the day of vaccination, babies are given doses of aluminium that are the equivalent of up to a thousand times the maximum advised daily safety levels.

The addition of new vaccines to the immunisation schedule is increasing the quantity of aluminium given to babies and young children.

This potential for harm can be reduced by minimising the aluminium load given to your baby wherever possible.

Another way of lessening the amount of aluminium your baby receives at any one time is by spreading out the vaccines. By giving no more than one aluminium-containing vaccine on any one day, the amount of aluminium your baby receives at any one time will be reduced.

None of the MMR, MR the single measles vaccines, or the Hib-Meningitis C booster (Menitorix) contains aluminium. Aluminium-free single polio and Hib and Men ACWY vaccines are available privately.

Vaccination Age

The UK schedule of vaccinating at two, three and four months is one of the earliest and most compact of anywhere in the world. This is in an attempt to get babies protected at the earliest possible age, when the risks of the illnesses are greatest. But it also comes with the risk of greater side-effects, and many parents and doctors are concerned that we may be giving too many vaccines at too early an age. Research also suggests that the immune system may be in a particularly delicate stage of development at two months, and therefore especially susceptible to damaging immune effects from vaccines. If so this supports the argument for starting vaccinations a little later.

But there are alternative options, and I suggest two below. The current UK schedule is not written in tablets of stone; the timing of the vaccines hasn't always been the same as it is now, and varies from country to country around the world. If parents wish to give their baby all, or most of, the vaccines, but not so quickly, the 6-in-1 vaccine could be separated from the other vaccines, at intervals of three to four weeks. That means the baby will not have received all the vaccinations until eight months of age, and thus remain 'unprotected' for longer, but with the possible, if unproven, benefit of spreading the vaccine— and aluminium—load. The vaccines could be further spread out by separating out the components of the 6-in-1 vaccine, but this can only be done privately. Any decision — whether to give a vaccine, delay vaccination or not to vaccinate — involves taking a risk. There is, sadly, no risk-free option. The risks of the individual diseases are reasonably well known. The risks of vaccination are far less certain, especially for uncommon or long-term side-effects.

Availability
The choice of vaccines is also limited by what is currently available. At two, three and four months, babies are given a 6-in-1 vaccine; a few private providers offer these vaccines separately, but there is no alternative on the National Health Service. The separate components of the MMR are not available separately on the NHS and only available to a limited degree privately.

Two alternative vaccination schedules to the NHS
Two alternative immunisation programmes are listed below for those parents who have concerns about the NHS schedule and who wish to spread out the vaccines given to their child. The first uses vaccines readily available on the NHS. This necessitates the use of the 6-in-1 and MMR vaccines, but ensures that only one vaccine is given at any one time. The second uses smaller combination vaccines, some of which are only available privately. Both these schedules are only examples and immunisation plans can be personalized for each individual child. Bear in mind that every country has its own schedule giving different vaccines at different times — there is no gold standard!

Ultimately, parents may wish to formulate a personalised immunisation schedule for their child, taking into account the child's health and any illnesses in the family.

An alternative schedule 1
This alternative schedule uses only those vaccines readily available on the NHS, but spreads out the vaccine load. This also reduces the amount of aluminium given to your baby at any one time. You can request this schedule from your GP. I have omitted the rotavirus vaccine as I consider this unnecessary and also the HPV because of safety concerns and questionable necessity.

Schedule of vaccines available on the NHS

12	weeks	DTaP –IPV-Hib-Hep B (6-in-1)
15	weeks	PCV (Prevenar 13)
18	weeks	meningitis B (Bexsero)
21	weeks	DTaP –IPV-Hib-Hep B (6-in-1)
24	weeks	PCV (Prevenar 13)
27	weeks	meningitis B (Bexsero)
8	months	DTaP –IPV-Hib-Hep B (6-in-1)
12	months	Hib-Men C (Menitorix)
13	months	PCV (Prevenar 13)
14	months	meningitis B (Bexsero)
15	months	MMR
4	years	DTaP-IPV
5	years	MMR
12	years	Men ACWY
15	years	dT-IPV

An alternative schedule II (BabyJabs)

The following schedule is one way in which to give most of the vaccines recommended in the UK, but spreading out the load – and giving aluminium-free vaccines where possible. Not all of these vaccines are available on the NHS, though they are available privately. I have omitted the following vaccines that I do not believe are essential: rotavirus, hepatitis B, mumps, rubella (in boys).

Schedule, including some vaccines that are only available privately

3	months	DTaP (3-in-1)
4	months	Hib-Men C (2-in-1)
5	months	PCV
6	months	Men B
7	months	DTaP

8 months   Hib-Men C

9 months   PCV

10 months Men B

11 months DTaP

13 months Hib-Men C

14 months PCV

15 months measles

18 months polio (IPV)

20 months polio (IPV)

22 months Men B booster

24 months polio (IPV)

2 years   measles (only if negative blood test after first dose)

4 years   dT-IPV (3-in-1)

12 years   Men ACWY

14 years   rubella-containing vaccine if not immune after blood test (only girls)

15 years   dT-IPV (3-in-1)

These two schedules are suggested alternatives for those parents who do not wish to follow the NHS schedule. They are not proscriptive, but merely examples and there are many alternatives. I believe that parents should be able — with appropriate medical advice — to choose a schedule that best suits their child's needs. For example, children with asthma in the family may benefit from delaying the start of immunisation until 5 months.

More information on the vaccines listed above — and other available vaccines — is available at www.babyjabs.co.uk

D	= *diphtheria*	Hib	= *Haemophilus influenzae type b*
d	= *low dose diphtheria*	PCV	= *pneumococcal vaccine*
T	= *tetanus*	IPV	= *inactivated polio vaccine*
MMR	= *measles, mumps, rubella*	P	= *whooping cough*
MenB	= *meningitis B*	MenC	= *meningitis*
HepB	= *hepatitis B*		

1
Autism and Vaccination
Autism, Allergy and Auto-immune Diseases

After the first edition of this book was published, a landmark judgement in the USA changed the debate over a link between vaccines and autism forever. Hannah Poling is the daughter of John S Poling, a doctor from Georgia, and his wife Terry. Both support vaccinations; Dr Poling sees some of the complications of vaccine preventable diseases in his work as a neurologist. Hannah was born a healthy baby girl, and was developing normally. On July 19, 2000, at 19 months of age, she received 9 vaccines in 5 injections. Within 48 hours, she developed a fever, became irritable and cried inconsolably. She refused to walk and, instead, crawled up and down stairs. Over the next three months, Hannah developed classic symptoms of autism: she avoided eye contact with her parents, and lost all language. Four months after her vaccinations she was formally diagnosed with autism.[1]

Hannah Poling's story created a great deal of publicity and debate in the USA. Remarkably, there was a blanket of silence in the UK, where there has been no official acknowledgement of her case, and most remain ignorant of the landmark ruling that vaccines caused Hannah to develop autism.

Though uncommon, Hannah's story is not unique; other children have developed similar problems after receiving vaccines. What makes Hannah's case remarkable is that US Department of Health doctors conceded, in November 2007, that Hannah's autism had been triggered by the vaccines she received. Until that moment, all government doctors, from the US and the UK, had insisted that vaccines do not trigger autism. The admission that they did – in Hannah – was an about turn of immense significance.

Further tests revealed that Hannah had an abnormality called 'mitochondrial dysfunction' (MD). Mitochondria are the powerhouses found inside most cells, and produce most of the body's energy; they are essential for normal function, which is particularly important for parts of the body that require a lot of energy, like the brain or muscles. The government doctors felt that the vaccines aggravated Hannah's MD, and that this resulted in her developing autism. Doctors responsible for vaccination were keen to prevent another vaccine scare – Hannah's story was getting a lot of publicity in the USA – and quickly pointed out that Hannah was a special case, because her condition was rare, and that parents of normal children – without MD – should not worry that their children might also develop autism after receiving multiple vaccines. Subsequent research suggests that this was false reassurance.

It is true that MD was thought to be a rare disorder. However, a study in the UK found that 0.54% (over 1 in 200) children are born with mitochondrial abnormalities – in the form of pathogenic mitochondrial DNA mutations – which may cause some degree of mitochondrial dysfunction or even outright disease.[2] Further research has found that autistic children are much more likely to have MD than other children, with over 4% (1 in 25) of autistic children having the disorder.[3] Researchers believe that MD may be a cause of autism in some children.[4] Autistic children with MD are more likely than other autistic children to have accompanying medical problems, such as stomach or bowel problems and fatigue; they are also more likely to regress, or lose previously acquired skills. These same problems are often present in children who have developed autism following vaccination.[5]

So we now know that MD is not so rare after all: over 3,000 children are born in the UK every year with mitochondrial abnormalities, and some of these children are likely to be at risk of autistic regression following immunisation. The problem is that there is no simple screening test to check for MD, and no way of knowing if a child is at risk. Hannah Poling, remember, was developing completely normally before she received her vaccinations at 19 months.

Dr Poling called for reform of the vaccine schedule, and urged public health doctors to 'heed the writing on the wall (scribbled by my 9-year old daughter).' Sadly his pleas have been ignored as more and more vaccines are added to children's immunisation schedules around the world.

Any number of things in the vaccines could have triggered Hannah's autism. It may have been the mercury present in three of the vaccines that Hannah received; it might have been the four live vaccines – including the MMR; or it may have been the total number – 9 vaccines in one hit; or simply a combination of all of these factors.

A number of constituents of vaccines have been postulated as causing autism.[6] These include:
- DTP vaccine (Using the whole cell pertussis component)
- Mercury (thiomersal) in vaccines
- MMR
- Giving vaccines at two months of age (when the immune system is in a sensitive stage of development)
- Live measles vaccine
- Human DNA in vaccines

In May 2012 an Italian court made the landmark ruling that a child's autism was caused by the triple MMR vaccine. The court, on the advice of independent doctors, ruled that nine year old Valentino's autism had been caused by the MMR vaccine he received in 2004. Valentino's case is the first in which the authorities have acknowledged that the triple vaccine had caused autism.

Whilst much of the medical profession stubbornly refuses to accept any possibly link between vaccines and autism, a survey found that nearly half

(49%) of parents with an autistic child believed that vaccines had contributed (32%) or possibly contributed (17%) to their child's autism. These parents cannot be accused of being poorly informed as those who were better educated were more likely to believe that vaccines caused their child's autism.[7]

Pregnant women are routinely advised to have a flu vaccine during pregnancy. However, recent research has found that children born to mothers given the flu vaccine in pregnancy may be at increased risk of developing autism. In particular, children born to mothers who received a flu jab in the first trimester (first three months) of pregnancy may have a 20% increased risk of developing autism.[52]

There has been much discussion over whether the number of children with autism is really increasing or whether it is simply that more children are being diagnosed. Researchers in Denmark attempted to answer this and concluded that most (60%) of the increase in autism was due to a combination of a change in the way autism is diagnosed and more parents seeking a diagnosis, but that a significant proportion (40%) was due to a real increase.[8]

Autism is, at least in some children, an auto-immune disorder – a disease where the body's immune system attacks its own cells.[9] [10] Autism is one of several immune system disorders, such as diabetes and asthma, that have been linked to vaccines.

Vaccines are designed to stimulate the immune system. That is how they work. So it wouldn't be a complete surprise to think that vaccines can cause immune system related disorders. Indeed, it's widely accepted that vaccines do cause auto-immune disorders in some people; the debate is over how common – or rare – this is. The numbers of children with immune-related disorders have rocketed over the last 20 years. These include allergic diseases – such as asthma and eczema – as well as auto-immune disorders, the most common of which is diabetes. Immune disorders often occur together in the same person or family; for example, family members of autistic children are more likely to suffer from asthma, allergies and other auto-immune disorders.[11] Asthma and eczema are increasing worldwide, especially in younger children.[12] The number of people with diabetes is also increasing in nearly every country in the world, including the UK.[13] The fastest growing age group is children, especially those under five years of age.[14]

So what's happening to cause this?

The most popular theory over recent years is that coming across plenty of bugs in early childhood, and hence getting infections, helps prevent allergic diseases such as asthma and eczema. The reasoning is, in simple terms, that the immune system can, at a very early age, develop in two different ways. The first ('type 1') response is most effective at fighting infections and is stimulated by contact with certain different bugs. The second ('type 2') response is more likely to stimulate allergies and immune disorders. Babies are born with immune systems geared towards 'type 2' (allergic) behaviour but this then shifts towards the preferable 'type 1' behaviour as a result of coming into contact with various infections.[15]

The theory is rather more complicated, as it seems some infections stimulate the immune system more effectively than others. However, certain circumstances in childhood help prevent, or promote, allergic diseases.

Here are some factors that appear to make allergy and asthma less likely to occur:

- Having older brothers and sisters or going to day-care centres at an early age (both of which result in increased contact with infections)
- Living with animals
- Having measles as a child
- Getting repeated colds[16]
- Frequent gut infections[17]
- Catching chickenpox — possibly

In the same way, there are also factors that appear to make allergy and asthma more likely, including:

- Living in a small family
- Living in overly 'hygienic' conditions
- Having antibiotics early in life[18]

The chickenpox vaccine is compulsory in the USA but is not, as I write the 4th edition of this book, part of the UK immunisation schedule. One reason is that chickenpox is usually a mild and harmless illness in children. One might think that chickenpox, with its widespread blistering rash that can sometimes scar, would make a child's eczema worse. Fascinatingly, children who have had chickenpox are much less likely to suffer from eczema, and extremely unlikely to suffer from severe eczema, compared to children who have never had chickenpox.[51] The widespread use of the chickenpox vaccine in the USA may have contributed to the increase in childhood eczema in that country. Contracting chickenpox also appears to protect against the development of asthma.[19]

The role of vaccinations

One of the problems is that most vaccinations stimulate the immune system in an allergic ('type 2') direction, both directly, and via additives in the vaccines such as aluminium.[20] The important question is whether this translates into real disease.

Numerous studies have been done looking at possible associations between vaccinations and allergic diseases and, confusingly, have come to widely differing conclusions.

There's a lot of evidence that vaccinations in general increase the risk of asthma and eczema, though it is often difficult to identify the specific effects of individual vaccines.[21,22,23,24] It has even been suggested that the DTP vaccination caused half of all asthma in children in the USA.[25] Hib and hepatitis B vaccines have been associated with an 18% and 20% increased risk of asthma respectively.[26] The MMR vaccine has been associated with an increased risk of developing eczema.[27]

The authors of one large review expressed concern that vaccines are 'possibly not contributing to optimal stimulation of the immune system in infancy;' they are, in other words, having a detrimental effect on the development of the baby's immune system. Despite this concern, the review concluded that vaccines do not cause allergic disease; this conclusion was criticised on the grounds that inadequate studies had been performed to exonerate vaccines.[28,29,30]

A long-term study followed up over 8,000 children from Tasmania who were all born in 1961, when the only vaccines offered were against diphtheria, tetanus, pertussis, polio and smallpox. The study found all the vaccines, except smallpox, were associated with a 50% increase in eczema and food allergy by age seven. Despite this large and significant increase, the authors concluded, in typical fashion, that 'the fear of their child developing atopic disease [a group of disorders including eczema and asthma] should not deter parents from immunizing their children, especially when weighed against the benefits'.[31]

Different ways to interpret the same research
Most people believe that scientific research is likely to provide clear unequivocal answers. Sadly, in the case of medical research, this is rarely the case. Studying people and diseases is fraught with difficulties; though researchers do try to make allowance for these, all research is inevitably imperfect.

The problem of how to interpret scientific research is exemplified by a study published in 2004 that looked at the medical records of children living in the West Midlands between 1988-1999. The records were searched for information on vaccination, asthma and eczema. The study found that children who'd received the triple DTP vaccination as babies were 14 times more likely to have asthma, and nine times more likely to have eczema, than children who had not been given the vaccine. Children who had received the MMR vaccine were more than three times as likely to develop asthma, and more than four times as likely to develop eczema, than children not given the vaccine. These appear powerful figures–on the face of it. However, they did not stop the researchers from concluding, 'Our data suggest that currently recommended routine vaccinations are not a risk factor for asthma or eczema.'

How did they come to this conclusion, which appears to fly in the face of their own results? By looking at how often the children went to see their GP. The increased risk of developing asthma and eczema was greatest in children who had visited their GP fewer than four times in the previous six months — something that is not particularly unusual. The authors argued that these children would be less likely to be vaccinated, and also less likely to have been diagnosed by their GP with asthma or eczema. That could be so, but it may also be that children who visit the doctor less, who may have fewer risk factors for asthma or eczema, may be most vulnerable to the effects of vaccination. In any event, those children who visited their doctor between four and six times over the previous six months — frequently enough, one would have thought, to make a diagnosis of asthma or eczema — were still four times more likely to suffer from asthma if they had received a DTP vaccination.[32]

Clearly this one study doesn't, and cannot, prove anything. What is, however, extraordinary, is that, despite finding that vaccinated babies were so much more likely to develop asthma than unvaccinated babies, its authors concluded that vaccinations aren't a risk factor for asthma. An equally, and possibly more, plausible explanation is that vaccination does cause an increase in asthma in certain children.[33]

Another Australian study found that 'full immunisation (MMR, OPV and DTP) or influenza vaccination was associated with a significantly increased risk for asthma.' Fully vaccinated children had a 52% increased risk compared to those who had never been immunised. However, the final sentence of the paper reads, 'None the less, we can conclude that it is unlikely early childhood vaccination significantly increases the risk of atopy [a group of allergic disorders including eczema] or asthma in childhood.'[34]

It's not uncommon to read scientific papers in which the authors reach conclusions that are, at best, challengeable and, at worse, a contradiction of their own findings.

Delaying immunisation
While the link between vaccines and immune disease remains unproven, though probable, it seems that delaying — but not omitting — the baby vaccines may reduce allergic disease. The only two studies that have looked at this have found large reductions in the risk of developing allergic disease by delaying vaccinations. The first showed that delaying starting vaccinating until 5 months of age reduced the chances of asthma developing by over half (57%); the second study found that delaying completing the primary course of vaccines until after 12 months, or delaying the MMR until after 2 years, reduced the chances of developing hay fever by nearly half (40%).[35,36] This research suggests that the timing of the vaccines may be more important than whether or not a child actually receives the vaccines. There is, however, a down-side to delaying immunisation, and that is that many of the diseases are more likely to be serious in a young baby; parents will have to weigh up the potential risks and benefits for their child.

Diabetes and other auto-immune disorders
Most of the studies done on vaccinations and diabetes conclude that childhood vaccinations do not increase the risk of diabetes.[37,38,39] But the research has been poor and one influential group felt that the trials done were inadequate 'to shed light on the possible link between onset of IDDM [diabetes] and vaccination.'[40] However, other researchers have found a link

between vaccines and diabetes, particularly in children with a family history of diabetes.[41,42] Overall the research on diabetes and vaccines has been poor, and some of the little research that has been done is open to different interpretations.

Guillain-Barré syndrome (GBS) has been associated with the majority of childhood vaccinations and it is generally accepted that there is a small increased risk of GBS after diphtheria, tetanus, polio and measles vaccines.[43]

Multiple Sclerosis (MS), a serious and progressively disabling condition, has been convincingly associated with the hepatitis B and yellow fever vaccines, at least in adults.[44] Though no conclusive link has been shown in children — partly because MS is so rare in childhood — optic neuritis (an inflammation of the optic nerve at the back of the eye causing loss of vision), which is the most common first sign of MS, has been associated with vaccines given in childhood. Most of the children who got optic neuritis went on to develop MS.[45]

Idiopathic Thrombocytopaenia Purpura (ITP) is a rare auto-immune bleeding disorder. It can be serious though most children make a full recovery within six months. It's widely accepted, even by the Department of Health, that the MMR vaccine causes ITP; the only debate is how common or rare this is, but it probably occurs in one in 25,000 vaccinations.[46,47] It has also been reported in children after receiving the hepatitis B and flu vaccines.[48]

Acute disseminated encephalomyelitis (ADEM) is a rare serious auto-immune disease affecting children which causes symptoms similar to MS (multiple sclerosis) such as headaches, confusion, visual disturbances, coma and paralysis. It has been reported in children after receiving a variety of vaccines including MMR, DTP, hepatitis B and HPV.[50]

There have been many case reports of adults and children developing auto-immune disorders including MS, GBS and rheumatoid arthritis following vaccination. This does not prove, but certainly suggests, a causal relationship. Japanese scientists have recently suggested that auto-immune diseases are 'the inevitable consequence of over-stimulating the immune 'system' by repeated [vaccines]'.[49] If they are correct then we can only expect the numbers of children suffering from auto-immune diseases to rise as a direct result of receiving an ever-increasing number of vaccines. The relationship between vaccines and immune disorders is likely to remain controversial and unresolved for some time. Whilst most children will be unaffected by immunisation, the evidence is sufficient to suggest that vaccines trigger allergic disorders, such as asthma, in some children. Similarly, vaccines will not cause auto-immune disorders in most children. However, vulnerable children, like Hannah Poling, will be damaged by vaccines. The challenge is to detect these children at risk so that they can be protected; this may be by offering them fewer vaccines or safer immunisation schedules, or possibly by delaying the start of immunisation and spreading out the vaccine load.

2
Mercury

One of the Greatest Scandals in Medicine

The doubt sowed in my mind, in 2000, by the MMR scare was intensified by the concern about mercury that started in the USA around the same time. Mercury is a silver-coloured liquid at room temperature and one of the most toxic substances known to man. It is often found in old-fashioned glass thermometers, blood pressure machines, as fillings in our teeth and, also, though we may not know it, in vaccines. Yet formal safety studies have never been done on humans to this date. It is hard to believe that one of the most toxic elements known to man has been injected into babies for over sixty years without anyone ever ensuring that it was safe to do so. In the USA concern about mercury in vaccines has been bigger news than the MMR scare in Britain.

The USA scandal
The type of mercury contained in vaccines is Thiomersal, a preservative. About half of this preservative is made up of ethylmercury, which is harmful to many areas of the body, particularly the brain, nerves, immune system and kidneys. The question of whether the amount in vaccines could be enough to cause any damage to babies has been hotly debated ever since the alarm was raised in the USA.

But the warning signs have been there all along. Thiomersal was first registered in 1929 as an antibacterial and antifungal product by its manufacturer, the drug company Eli Lilly under its trade name, Merthiolate, and it soon became a widely used chemical to prolong the shelf-life of vaccines. As long ago as 1935, there was concern that Thiomersal could be harmful if injected into dogs. Back in 1986 a senior doctor at the UK Department of Health, Dr K Winship, expressed concern about the use of mercury. 'Multidose vaccines... contain a mercurial preservative, usually 0.01% Thiomersal, and may present problems occasionally in practice. It is, therefore, now accepted that multidose injection preparations are undesirable and that preservatives should not be present in unit-dose preparations.'[1] Sadly little attention was paid to his concern by other health officials in Britain.

By 1991, at least one drug company was aware of the concern over mercury in childhood vaccines. An internal memo at Merck (one of the large multinational vaccine manufacturers and one of the largest pharmaceutical companies in the world) from March 1991 noted that regulatory authorities in Scandinavia, the UK, Japan and Switzerland were concerned about mercury in vaccines. The company's immediate priority was to ensure their mercury-free vaccines would be approved for sale in Sweden, Norway and Denmark. The memo calculated that an average sized Swedish baby might be receiving in vaccines 87 times the maximum advisable oral daily allowance. 'When viewed in this way,' it stated, 'the mercury load appears rather large.'2

Six years later, in 1997, the USA Environmental Protection Agency (EPA) reduced its recommended safe levels for the intake of a closely related chemical, methylmercury, which raised the public awareness of the threat from other forms of mercury. The amount of mercury in a vaccine had hitherto been described as a percentage of the total vaccine. As most vaccines contained about 0.01% mercury, this was generally considered to be such a small amount it must be harmless.

But when the USA Food and Drug Administration (FDA) looked at exactly how much mercury children were getting from their vaccines, they concluded that some USA children's average exposure to ethylmercury over several months was greater than the maximum food intake of methylmercury advised by the FDA. The actual amount in one vaccine could exceed the recommended daily intake by up to a hundred times.

When Dr Neal Halsey, a past chairman of the Committee on Infectious Diseases and past Director of the Institute for Vaccine Safety, was informed of the quantities involved, he was shocked. 'My first reaction was simply disbelief, which was the reaction of almost everybody involved in vaccines,' he said. 'In most vaccine containers, thimerosal [the name of Thiomersal in the USA] is listed as a mercury derivative, a hundredth of a percent.... no one did the calculation.'3

By 1999, there was growing concern at the FDA. An internal email sent in June 1999 said: 'Will raise questions about FDA being 'asleep at the switch' for decades, by allowing a potentially hazardous compound to remain in many childhood vaccines, and not forcing manufacturers to exclude it from new products.... What took the FDA so long to do the calculations? Why didn't CDC [Center for Disease Control] and the advisory bodies do these calculations while rapidly expanding the childhood immunisation schedule?'4

Regardless of the answers to those questions, the concerns led to swift action to remove mercury from childhood vaccines in the USA. Vaccine manufacturers were asked in July 1999 to remove it from their vaccines and, within months, approval for the introduction of safer vaccines was agreed. Also in July, the American Academy of Pediatrics called for mercury to be removed from vaccines as soon as possible, despite pressure from WHO to 'tread lightly' because of the 'global ramifications' of demands for the removal of mercury from vaccines.5

Precautions
One might conceivably argue that the health officials in the USA were jumping the gun in 1999, certainly given the advice of the WHO. Since no

safety studies have ever been done since the introduction of Thiomersal in 1929, there are, strictly speaking no known human safety levels for ethylmercury, the type of mercury in the preservative.

Mercury, however, is known to be toxic in all its forms, even in extremely small doses and of no benefit to the body. Eating a low level of mercury naturally occurring in some fish as methylmercury — at levels considered 'safe' — impairs children's speech, attention and memory.[6] The chemical is known to damage the brain, nervous and immune systems. Mercury poisoning causes symptoms remarkably similar to symptoms of autism. Both cause social withdrawal, lack of eye contact and facial expression, heightened sensitivity to noise and touch and repetitive behaviour.[7]

There are, furthermore, known cases of food poisoning of children by ethylmercury. The 1980 *Journal of Neurology, Neurosurgery & Psychiatry* (a sister journal of the *British Medical Journal*) describes in detail a case in Romania. A family had fed a hog seeds that had been treated with the fungicide ethylmercury (exactly the same type of mercury that is used in vaccines). The hog started to behave unusually, becoming unsteady and falling over. It was slaughtered and some of its meat was eaten by the mother and her three children. Ten days later, her fifteen-year-old boy became unable to walk or talk, and died of mercury poisoning. Her ten-year-old boy developed walking and talking difficulties before entering into a coma. He too died. The forty-eight-year-old mother developed walking difficulties, became agitated, confused and delirious, but went on to make a remarkably good recovery. Her fifteen-year-old daughter developed similar symptoms to her brothers as well as vomiting and drowsiness. She didn't die, but still had poor vision and difficulty walking when she was discharged. The doctors who treated the family wrote that this type of mercury 'has a very high toxicity, not only for the brain', but also the nerves, muscles and heart.[8]

It is no great surprise that a 2003 report by the USA Congress summed up the problem in clear terms: 'Mercury is hazardous to humans. Its use in medicinal products is undesirable, unnecessary and should be minimised or eliminated entirely.' The report continues: 'Manufacturers of vaccines and Thimerosal have never conducted adequate testing on the safety of Thimerosal.' The report concludes: 'No amount of mercury is appropriate in any childhood vaccine.'[9] The report's conclusions were supported by subsequent research finding that newborn baby boys given the mercury-containing hepatitis B vaccine at birth were three times more likely to develop autism than those not given the vaccine.[41]

The British response

Mercury, too, was also finally removed from the majority of vaccines given to children in the UK, in 2004. But not, we are told by the Department of Health, because of any concerns about its safety. The furore in the USA driven by official agencies has not elicited an acknowledgment in Britain.

Which vaccines contained Thiomersal? The triple DTP, the diphtheria, tetanus and whooping-cough (pertussis) vaccine, given to babies three times in their first year from 1961 until 2004; the DTP-Hib vaccine, introduced during the 1990s and used until late 2004; the DT preschool booster given routinely to four year olds until 2001 (when it was replaced with a mercury free vaccine); tetanus, or tetanus and diphtheria, boosters; certain 'flu vaccines.

The quantity of Thiomersal in most of the vaccines listed above is 50µg (micrograms), which is equivalent to 25µg of mercury. As a µg is one thousandth of a milligram, this does not sound very much. In fact it sounds like a tiny amount of mercury.

Britain, like the USA, has no guidelines on safety levels for Thiomersal in humans. But such guidelines do exist for methylmercury, the type of mercury found naturally in some fish such as tuna. Unlike mercury in vaccines for children, this is something that the UK government has looked into. The UK Food Standards Agency (FSA) measured the amount of mercury in fish and in 2003 issued safety guidelines on the maximum amount that should be eaten.

The guidelines stated, 'The critical effect of methylmercury is on the developing central nervous system and therefore pregnant women are considered to be the most susceptible population because of the risk to the fetus'. The FSA went on to advise pregnant or breast-feeding mothers to be especially cautious with their intake of mercury. The FSA explained why: 'This is due to the potential risk to the developing fetus or neonate.'[10] The baby in the womb, or a *new-born baby* is especially at risk from the harmful effects of mercury. For these vulnerable groups the FSA recommended a maximum safe daily intake of methylmercury of 0.0001 mg/kg (milligrammes of mercury per kilogram body weight). These conclusions and recommendations were confirmed in a subsequent statement issued in 2004.[11]

I was alarmed that no one appeared to have done the calculations for British babies, so I researched the issue.[12] In the first jab at two months, an average sized baby received 49 times the maximum safe daily dose if one adopts the safety levels of the FSA for methylmercury found in fish. A small baby would have received over 60 times the maximum recommended daily intake. A baby born prematurely, being particularly small, may have received up to 100 times the maximum recommended safe daily intake in a single injection. It is also probable that intermittent large exposures pose more risk than small daily doses.[13]

Though the total quantity of mercury may have remained unchanged for 35 years, there was an important change to the vaccination schedule in 1990 that is likely to have increased the toxic effect of the mercury in Britain. Before 1990, babies were immunised at three, five and ten months. In 1990 this schedule was changed so that babies were immunised at two, three and four months.

This increased the amount of mercury received by babies compared to their body weight, because they would have been smaller when they received the vaccines. More importantly, the babies' immature brain and immune systems are more vulnerable to damage at an earlier age.

The long-term consequences will be with us for some time, and there are important research questions. There has been a large increase in the number of children with neurodevelopmental disorders over recent years. These include speech disorders, hyperactivity (attention deficit disorder) and autism. Could it be more than coincidence that the rate of autism was rising rapidly in the early 1990s? Could giving babies mercury-containing vaccines at an earlier and more crucial stage of development followed by the introduction of the MMR in 1998 have constituted a 'double whammy' which was just too much for some susceptible children?

The mystery

The Department of Health, however, argues these calculations are invalid because the FSA advice was given for methylmercury and not ethylmercury. It has consistently sought to reassure parents about mercury in childhood vaccines. In response to mounting public concern, the Department of Health issued a 'Factsheet' on mercury in vaccines in 2003, which argued:[14]

Government factsheet: 'There are very large safety factors built into the estimated levels recommended, and the mercury in UK vaccines does not exceed these safety levels.'
   Fact: there are no safety levels for the mercury in vaccines and never have been. The only safety levels, which have already been discussed, relate to mercury in foods. The dose in a single vaccine exceeds the recommended maximum daily level for food by up to 100 times. The safety levels are for swallowed mercury, whereas the mercury in vaccines is injected, which bypasses the body's natural defences and may be dangerous at even lower doses.
Government factsheet: 'Vaccines with Thiomersal have ethylmercury in them. The mercury that may be toxic in the diet or the environment is methylmercury. Ethyl- and methylmercury are handled quite differently by the body. Ethylmercury is excreted quickly and does not accumulate.'
   Fact: it is true that the body excretes about half the ethylmercury in vaccines in a week or so, whereas it takes seven to eight weeks to get rid of half of the methylmercury eaten in fish. But this has no bearing on the maximum blood levels of mercury which are likely to cause the harm.
Government factsheet: 'Ethylmercury that is in Thiomersal is not the same [as methylmercury], and has not been linked to harm in levels present in vaccines'
   Fact: most experts agree they are similarly toxic.[15] Ethylmercury (in Thiomersal) in vaccines has been linked to autism and other developmental disorders in scientific studies and by doctors.[7,16,17,18,19]
Government factsheet: 'Studies on babies in the UK found no link between the Thiomersal they received and their subsequent development, including autism. USA and Danish studies have found the same.'
   Fact: the studies referred to have all been criticised and have had flaws, or conflicts of interest, exposed.[20,21,22] Other epidemiological studies

that the Department of Health doesn't mention have found a link between mercury in vaccines and developmental problems including autism.[18,19] Both the UK studies the Department of Health refers to found that mercury in the vaccines was actually good for the babies, and protected them against developing autism, hyperactivity and other developmental problems.[23,24] It's difficult to have confidence in studies that reach such a conclusion. The problem with 'epidemiological' studies, furthermore, is that they look at statistics; they look at large populations. As is so often the case with vaccine-related problems, it appears to be a minority of susceptible children who are most affected. Many autistic children seem unable to get rid of mercury from the body as efficiently as most children.[16] This probably leads to a build-up of mercury in the brain and causes, in effect, mercury poisoning in these children.[17] The studies don't distinguish between those children who are vulnerable to the effects of mercury and those who aren't. They were not given a brief to detect a subgroup of susceptible children who may have been adversely affected by Thiomersal. (See also below USA epidemiological research.)

Government factsheet: 'The European Medicines Evaluation Agency has looked at Thiomersal in vaccines [in 1999] and has found no evidence of harm. However, on the basis of good practice of reducing any exposure to mercury, they have advised vaccine manufacturers to try to find ways to reduce or remove Thiomersal wherever this is possible'

Fact: the economy of the truth, here, runs very close to deception. The agency could find no evidence of harm because the research hadn't been done. As for removing Thiomersal (mercury) from vaccines, the Agency said that 'this should be done within the shortest possible time frame', words which suggest concern.[25] It took Britain five years to follow the recommendation they are quoting.

Paradoxically — and despite their swift response — even American health officials in charge of immunisation vehemently contest the risks of ethylmercury in vaccines. After the alert in 1999 an Institute of Medicine Immunization Safety Review recommended, in 2001, 'the use of Thiomersal-free…vaccines in the United States, despite the fact that there might be remaining supplies of thimerosal-containing vaccines available.'[26] By 2002, no mercury-containing vaccines were being routinely given to children in the USA. Yet the official stance remains denial of any actual problem. Dr Stephen Cochi, head of the USA National Immunisation Programme at the CDC argued as recently as 2004 that only 'junk scientists and charlatans' supported any link between mercury in vaccines and autism.[27]

Why? Only in America is it possible to get a sense of the answer due to their greater freedom of information.

Five years before Dr Cochi's denunciation, in 1999, a researcher at the USA Epidemic Intelligence Service Office of the National Immunization Programme was given the task of looking into a possible relationship between mercury in vaccines and neurodevelopmental disorders such as autism, hyperactivity and speech disorders. He searched the computerised databases of two (later three) private insurance companies (HMOs) providing comprehensive medical care to communities to see which children had been given mercury-containing vaccines, and which had developed any of a large number of illnesses including autism and other developmental disorders. The results of this research went through several changes before finally being published in a medical journal in November 2003.28

Most of the versions were not made publicly available and what I describe below is information obtained through the use of the (USA) Freedom of Information Act.

In the researcher's first version of November/ December 1999, preliminary figures suggested babies who had received a relatively high dose of mercury by one month of age were between eight and eleven times more likely to develop autism than babies who had received no mercury by one month. These same babies were between three and four times more likely to suffer from attention deficit disorder (ADD), and four to five times more likely to suffer from a sleep disorder. These results were provisional and sometimes based on small numbers of children, but alarm bells started ringing.

On 29 November 1999, the researcher sent an email to his collaborators saying: 'After running, re-thinking, re-running, re-thinking....for about two weeks now I should touch base with you, I think, to see whether you agree with what I came up with so far. I'll attach the SAS [statistical software] programs hoping you or one of your statisticians can detect major flaws before I jump to conclusions.'29

By February 2000, some children had now been excluded from the second version of the research, ostensibly in an attempt to make the findings more accurate. This version suggested children receiving the maximum dose of mercury at three months were two and a half times more likely to be autistic or to suffer from ADD than those children who, by three months of age, had received the smallest amount of mercury.30

Then on 7 and 8 June 2000 a secret meeting was arranged at the Simpsonwood Retreat Center in Georgia to look at the latest figures contained in the third version of the research. This meeting was attended by over 50 people: vaccine experts, public health doctors, paediatricians, neurologists and others, including representatives from all the major vaccine manufacturers.

Here the researcher said 'what I will present you is the study that nobody thought we should do.' He continued, 'We have found statistically significant relationships between the exposure [to mercury in vaccines] and the outcome for these different exposures and outcomes. First, for two months of age, an unspecified developmental delay. Exposure at three months of age, tics. Exposure at six months of age, an attention deficit disorder.'

He continued, 'Exposure at one, three and six months of age, the entire category of neurodevelopmental delays.' As if this were not worrying enough, he went on to add, 'But one thing is for sure, there is certainly under-ascertainment of all of these because some of the children are just not old enough to be diagnosed.' So his research had found relationships between mercury and all these disorders and even this, he is saying, is likely to be an underestimate of the problem.

One participating doctor was worried. His first grandson had just been born. 'I do not want that grandson to get a Thiomersal [mercury] containing vaccine until we know better what is going on,' he told fellow delegates. Some of the participants attempted to downplay the findings, or to play around with the figures to make them appear less damaging: 'So you can push, I can pull,' said a government statistician. But another participant countered that 'The number of dose-related relationships [between mercury and various neurodevelopmental disorders] are linear and statistically significant. You can play with this all you want. They are linear,' he repeated, 'they are statistically significant.'

A representative of the WHO immunisation programme in Geneva, at the meeting argued: 'I am really concerned that we have taken off like a boat going down one arm of the mangrove swamp at high speed, when in fact there was not enough discussion really early on about which way the boat should go at all. And I really don't want to risk offending everyone by saying that perhaps this study should not have been done at all, because the outcome of it could have, to some extent, been predicted... I know how we handle it from here is extremely problematic.'

Finally there was a call for secrecy from the USA's National Immunization Program, 'Just let me reemphasize, if I could, the importance of trying to protect the information that we have been talking about. As many of you know, we are invited here. We have asked you to keep this information confidential... so basically consider this embargoed information.'[31]

The final published study (the fourth version) involved a great deal of statistical juggling and the addition of children from a third health provider. It was sensible to recruit a third HMO in order to increase the numbers of children in the study. But the HMO selected was the Harvard Pilgrim in Massachusetts, a puzzling choice. This HMO had undergone aggressive expansion in the mid-1990s and was chaotic (it went into receivership in 2000). It had failed to unify its IT systems with the result that its different computer systems with little ability to communicate effectively with one another were simply incapable of consolidating the data.[32] It was also based in Massachusetts, a state that had a unique pattern of autism statistics. Whereas every other USA state was reporting progressively increasing numbers of children with autism from the early 1990s, the number of children with autism in Massachusetts was static, and low, throughout the study period and did not start to increase significantly until 2001.[33]

When the study was eventually published, it concluded that 'no consistent significant associations were found between TCVs [Thiomersal Containing Vaccines] and neurodevelopmental outcomes.' Allegations that this conclusion was pure fudge were hotly denied by the authors. The lead researcher, who was by then working for the British vaccine manufacturer GlaxoSmithKline

(GSK), wrote, 'the bottom line is, and always has been the same: an association between Thiomersal and neurological outcomes could neither be confirmed, nor refuted, and therefore more study is required.' Furthermore, 'any suggestion that GSK intended to have me manipulate this data is nothing short of an insult to both me and my company's integrity.'[34]

Whilst research published in 2006 suggests the number of new cases of autism and speech disorders in the USA, following a long period of increase, has started to decline following the switch to mercury-free vaccines, other research suggests that autism is continuing to increase.[35,38] This means that it is unlikely that mercury in vaccines is causing most cases of autism, but may still have caused autism in a susceptible minority. More recent research has shown that monkeys injected with (mercury-containing) vaccines equivalent to the USA schedule had abnormal brain development, supporting the possibility that early immunization, at least with mercury-containing vaccines, could be linked to autism. Finally, research published in 2014 shows a 'dose-response relationship' between mercury in vaccines and neurodevelopmental disorders such as autism and other disorders causing developmental delay, speech disorders and hyperactivity. [39] That means that the more mercury a child received in vaccines, the more likely he or she is to suffer developmental delay.

'Cool'

Sweden stopped using mercury-containing vaccines for children in 1989, with Denmark following suit in 1992. Marta Granstrom represented Sweden on the Vaccine Expert Committee of the European Pharmacopoeia (a listing of substances used to prepare pharmaceuticals), and had been trying in vain to get mercury banned from childhood vaccines in Europe.[36] The risk from mercury was felt to be very small in Greece, where, 'the national immunisation committee, under the Ministry of Health, kept Thiomersal a 'cool issue' because the [Greek] government did not want to be placed in a position of having to purchase a new, and potentially more expensive, vaccine product.'[37]

'Cool' was also the UK response. As mentioned, not until October 2004 was mercury finally removed, with the introduction of three new childhood vaccines replacing ones containing mercury. The vaccines were not, we were told, introduced for this reason.

There are indeed still vaccines given to some children that contain mercury. These include some brands of the flu jab that is recommended for children with asthma and diabetes. Mercury-containing vaccines are still widely used around the world, mainly in poorer countries that cannot afford the more expensive mercury-free alternatives.

Mercury, even in very small amounts and in the quantity used in vaccines, is extremely poisonous and can cause numerous adverse effects. It should not be, and should never have been, a constituent of vaccine given to babies and young children.[40]

3
Aluminium
'Mix It with Orange'

When the people of Camelford, in North Cornwall, woke up on the morning of the 6th July 1988 to find thousands of dead fish floating in the river they were told by the local water authority not to be alarmed. They were assured that, though the water was 'slightly acidic', it was perfectly safe to drink; if they didn't like the strange taste they could always mix it with orange juice. Over the next few days many people suffered stomach upsets, rashes and mouth ulcers followed by muscle pains, malaise, loss of memory and difficulty concentrating.

What they hadn't been told was that twenty tonnes of aluminium sulphate solution had been discharged into the wrong tank at a water treatment works at Lowermoor, near Camelford. This resulted in the supply of contaminated water to twenty thousand people over a large area of North Cornwall. Over the following eighteen months, four hundred people reported symptoms they felt were caused by the contamination. Those who complained of symptoms were accused of making them up or that, if real, they were caused by worry — not the aluminium. Three government enquiries have found no conclusive link between the incident and the chronic symptoms and diseases reported by the local residents, though concern was raised about possible effects on the brains of bottle-fed infants, because of the relative greater proportion of tap water in their diet.[1]

The local MP, Paul Tyrer, referred to 'thirteen years of cover-up,' and the conclusions of other research are more disturbing.[2] One found an increase in hospital admissions in the area of Cornwall affected.[3] Another study, published in the *British Medical Journal*, concluded, 'People who were exposed to the contaminated water at Camelford suffered considerable damage to their cerebral [mental] function, which was not related to anxiety.'[4] In some people, the aluminium contamination caused long-term brain damage. Those allegedly affected included five children who suffered memory loss, fatigue, depression, behavioural changes and learning difficulties. Carole Cross, a Camelford resident, died aged 59 from a rare form of dementia 16 years after the disaster: at post-mortem examination, she was found to have exceptionally high levels of aluminium in her brain.[5] In a subsequent inquest the coroner accused the water company of 'gambling' with the lives of twenty thousand people by not telling them about the poisoning for over two weeks. He said there was a 'real possibility' that the accident had contributed to her premature death.

Déjà vu

There is a sense of déjà vu here with regards to vaccines. Like mercury, aluminium has also been used in vaccines for eighty years, yet there is remarkable complacency surrounding its use. The most common argument to defend its use is that, as it has been used for so long, it must be safe. But, while we can map the human genetic code, we know little about what happens to aluminium after it is injected into the body, or what it does while it's there.

A recent, comprehensive review of adverse effects after immunisation with aluminium-containing DTP (diphtheria, tetanus, polio) vaccines, published in 2004 in the authoritative medical journal *Lancet*, confirmed only that aluminium-containing vaccines caused more redness and swelling at the injection site than vaccines without aluminium. The authors commented on how little research had been done on aluminium safety in vaccines. Nonetheless, they concluded, 'we found no evidence that aluminium salts in vaccines cause any serious adverse effects' – an inevitable conclusion since so little research had been done.[6]

Billions of children worldwide have received, are, or will be, receiving, shots containing aluminium. One might have expected the comprehensive review to have recommended further research, especially as, in the past, aluminium has never had to pass any of the safety trials that any standard drug would today. Instead, the authors concluded, 'Despite a lack of good-quality evidence we do not recommend that any further research on this topic is undertaken.' The report's attitude was criticised, and the opinion voiced that 'substantially increased use of aluminium-adsorbed vaccines should be put on hold until research has demonstrated their safety.'[7,8] But that is as far as it got.

If there has been no research on the safety of aluminium in vaccines, what are the health implications of aluminium in general?

Aluminium is the most abundant metal in the earth's crust. It has many uses, such as in aeroplanes, without which modern life would not be possible. However, the metal is of no use to the body and is very toxic to the brain and to bones. The central nervous system is particularly susceptible to its effects.[9]

It is well known that aluminium is particularly dangerous to certain groups of vulnerable people. It can cause brain damage in people on long-term dialysis for kidney failure – so-called 'dialysis dementia'. Aluminium can cause brain damage in children with failing kidney function.[34] It probably contributes to Alzheimer's disease (another form of dementia) in some people.[10] Once aluminium enters the brain it is only excreted very slowly and is therefore liable to accumulate.[9,11] Here our knowledge stops as there is no funded research of any sort on the effects of aluminium on health in the UK at present, nor has there been for over twenty years.

Crucially, little is known for certain about how aluminium can affect children's health. But it may cause hyperactivity and learning disorders in some children;[12] high aluminium levels have been found in some children with hyperactivity, autism and behavioural problems.[13,14] Although such behavioural disorders are frequently headlined in the papers, on this subject, too, there is little research into the effects of the metal.

Aluminium gets into our bodies through water, food, medicines and vaccines, and can also be absorbed through the skin and lungs. Foods with the highest concentrations of aluminium include bread, cereals and baked processed foods, because aluminium-containing additives are used during processing. Tea contains a high concentration of aluminium. Aluminium sulphate is added to water as part of the purification process, but most is removed before it reaches our taps. It is also a common ingredient in many indigestion (antacid) remedies that are widely available over the counter in pharmacies and supermarkets. Another source is deodorants and certain sunscreens.

Both the WHO and the European Food Safety Authority (EFSA) recommend the same Tolerable Weekly Intake (TWI) of 1mg/kg, noting that 'aluminium distributes to all tissues in animals and humans and…can enter the brain.'[38] These maximum safe amounts of aluminium depend on body weight, because a baby is only able to tolerate a fraction of that handled by an adult.

Effect on the immune system

The function of aluminium in vaccines is different from that of mercury. It has been used as an 'adjuvant' in vaccines for eighty years. It was discovered that adding aluminium to a vaccine activated the immune system more than the vaccine on its own. (The word 'adjuvant' comes from the Latin 'adjuvare', meaning 'to help'.) The stronger stimulation of the body's immune system results in a more powerful immune response, though the mechanism by which the addition of aluminium boosts the body's immune response is still not known.

Many of today's childhood vaccines contain aluminium, which is by far the most widely used adjuvant currently permitted for use in vaccines. Nonetheless, there are no 'safety levels' for injected aluminium because no one has looked to see how much might be too much.

The big difference between the ingested aluminium (as water, food or medicine), and that contained in vaccines, is the proportion that actually gets into our bodies. The gut acts as barrier to the absorption of aluminium, preventing nearly all of it from entering the body.

About nine hundred and ninety nine parts in a thousand of the aluminium that we swallow into our stomachs is excreted in the faeces. Only a tiny fraction, between 0.01% and 1%, gets absorbed into the body.[15,16,17,18] That means that the amount of aluminium that is believed to be safe to consume in water, food or medicine is much greater than the amount it is safe to inject into the body, a process that bypasses the stomach's 'protective barrier'.

Looking, for example, at the food babies receive there are some noticeable differences. Breast-fed babies get hardly any aluminium at all. Babies fed soy milk get rather a lot of aluminium compared to the other babies. Babies who are bottle (formula) fed are somewhere in the middle. Though most babies will receive well below either safety guideline, those who are fed soy milk may breach the EFSA and WHO safety level.

The aluminium in vaccines, however, bypasses the gut, meaning that all of the aluminium in vaccines gets into the body. No one, it appears, has ever calculated whether the amount of aluminium received by British babies might exceed the maximum recommended safety levels. Based on food absorption studies, and assuming that only one thousandth of ingested aluminium in food is absorbed by the body, one can establish a weekly safety level for injected aluminium. Thus, injected aluminium is only safe at levels of a thousandth of aluminium that is eaten. The maximum amount of aluminium that can be ingested, within safety levels, is 1mg per kg body weight per week.

Oral safety level (weekly)	Absorbed/injected safety level (weekly)
1mg per kg	0.001mg per kg

Whether this safety level is exceeded during immunisation depends on the amount of aluminium added as an adjuvant to the vaccines given to babies. In Britain, most of the vaccines given to babies at two, three and four months contain aluminium.

Vaccine	Aluminium content
Infanrix-IPV-Hib-Hep B (6 in 1)	0.82mg
Meningitis B	0.5mg
Prevenar (Pneumococcal)	0.125mg
Rotavirus	Nil

The UK schedule is complicated but, at the time of writing in 2017, all children will receive between 0.5mg and 1.125mg at each visit between two and four months. Compared to the aluminium load from any of the baby feeds that enter the body this is very high — many times the EFSA and WHO limits — even if it were spread out over the whole month.

But this does not tell the whole story, because the aluminium in vaccines is not given gradually spread over a month; it is given instantaneously on a single day. So I calculated an average baby's intake of aluminium on vaccination day. This revealed a big problem: the intake of aluminium that an average sized baby receives from the 8-week vaccines is over two hundred times the recommended maximum weekly intake. For a small or premature baby the figures are even more alarming: the intake of aluminium that a small baby born at 36 weeks gestation receives from the 8-week vaccines is over three hundred and fifty times the recommended maximum weekly intake.

The expert committee that sets these safety levels did this because 'aluminium compounds have the potential to affect...the developing nervous system at lower doses than those used in establishing the previous [safety level]'.[19] It is precisely babies' developing nervous systems that we are concerned about.

I have made a number of assumptions in these calculations. But even if I assume the lowest absorption rate of aluminium from the gut (1%), the aluminium a baby receives far exceeds the maximum recommended safe level.

It is also likely that aluminium can interact with mercury, another common component of vaccines, to increase its toxicity. This is no longer of great relevance to British babies, but of potential importance to babies in much of the world.[20]

It does not mean that all babies are being poisoned with aluminium every time they get a jab. But it does mean that susceptible babies, perhaps premature babies with poorly developed kidneys (which are essential to get rid of the aluminium), or those with a genetic susceptibility, may be harmed by the aluminium in vaccines. Doctors in Cambridge were concerned that very premature babies, born at fewer than thirty-four weeks, might suffer long-term developmental problems from the standard aluminium-containing intravenous feeding solutions that they were given. So they measured the development of these babies at 18 months compared with other very premature babies, to whom they gave feeding solutions in which the aluminium content had been specially reduced. They discovered that the babies fed the aluminium-containing solutions suffered impaired development of the brain.[21] To put this in context, the quantity of aluminium an average sized infant receives from vaccines at eight weeks of age is the equivalent to the quantity of aluminium that would have been fed to the premature babies in this study over 20 years (0.045mg per kg body weight per day).

Warning signs

There has been concern about aluminium in vaccines in the past. In 1957, at the height of the polio epidemics, the UK Department of Health was so worried at the higher rates of polio paralysis that were occurring in children after receiving aluminium-containing vaccines that they were banned completely for a time. Children were then immunised against diphtheria and whooping cough with aluminium-free vaccines.

Certain side-effects of aluminium in vaccines have recently become known. They commonly cause itchy red painful bumps, or 'nodules', at the site of the injection. Up to one in every hundred children may be affected by this. It may not sound very serious and, in medical terms, it isn't. But many affected babies itch so intensely that they scratch their skin until it bleeds. Three quarters are still affected four years after vaccination, and some children are still suffering after seven years.[22,23] The risk of developing these nodules increases with the number of aluminium-containing vaccines given.[40]

The extent of the problem has only recently come to light, because many of these lumps do not develop until weeks after the injection, and so have not been associated, by doctors or parents, with vaccination. The risk of a child developing an itchy nodule increases after repeated aluminium-containing vaccines — which is particularly worrying as more and more vaccinations are added to the immunisation schedule.

Macrophagic myofasciitis (MMF) is a newly discovered disease caused by aluminium in vaccines. During the 1990s, a group of French doctors, specialising in muscle disorders, came across an increasing number of people with aching weak muscles, painful joints and, in some cases, severe generalised fatigue. The doctors took muscle biopsies (small samples) to help them make a diagnosis. What they found did not fit the pattern of any known disorder, and they named it macrophagic myofasciitis (MMF).[24,25]

As time went on, they found an increasing number of affected people, and the doctors discovered evidence of persistent aluminium at injection sites; a high proportion of patients developed auto-immune diseases such as multiple sclerosis (MS).[26] The symptoms of most patients were identical to that of chronic fatigue syndrome (CFS) or ME (myalgic encephalomyelitis); and most people did not start to become ill until several months after vaccination, making the connection difficult to establish.

The French doctors have proposed that, in susceptible people, the aluminium in vaccines is not efficiently eliminated from the body, but instead remains at the site of vaccination for years. It is known that aluminium is a powerful stimulant of the immune system and, in particular, appears to push it in an 'allergic' or auto-immune direction.[27,28] They believe that the aluminium may be directly responsible for triggering MS or other immune disorders in these people.

This theory is inevitably controversial. Many vaccine experts dispute the findings and interpretations of the French team of doctors. They point out that it has only been found in France and that very few people have been affected in this way. It is true that most, but not all, the patients so far discovered have been in France. One possible explanation for this is that the French commonly take muscle biopsies from exactly the same part of the arm as injections are commonly given. Other countries use different areas of the body to obtain muscle biopsies. The injection site has to be examined to find the aluminium. But a few cases have been found outside France — in Italy, the USA, Spain, Portugal, the UK and Australia.

Some research supports the proposition of a link between aluminium and disorders such as MS and CFS. One group has found concentrations of aluminium in the urine of sufferers of MS to be up to 40 times that of normal people, and has suggested that aluminium could be 'the unidentified environmental factor' in MS.[29] Another group has found twice the normal levels of aluminium in the blood of chronic fatigue sufferers, adding weight to the argument that aluminium may be a cause of CFS and ME.[30] A man from Northumberland was the first to have CFS, MMF and aluminium overload. The doctors investigating him are concerned about 'the potential dangers associated with aluminium-containing adjuvants.' They are concerned that up to 1 in 100 people may be hypersensitive to the aluminium in vaccines; the vaccines they receive in early life, while causing no apparent harm, may sensitise their immune systems, so that they overreact to aluminium-containing vaccines received in later life.[35]

MMF may be a rare problem but, because nobody has ever looked for it until very recently, no-one knows. The finding of MMF in identical twins suggests that susceptible people may have a genetic predisposition to the illness, probably triggered by the aluminium in vaccines.[31] Though it is most often reported in adults, the condition has been seen in children as young as seven months.[32] The existence of MMF is slowly but surely being accepted by an increasing number of doctors around the world. It is now believed to be one manifestation of wider group of vaccine related disorders called ASIA (auto-immune syndrome induced by adjuvants).[39] In susceptible children, aluminium from vaccines may accumulate in the brain and research suggests that the metal could be implicated in a number of auto-immune diseases including multiple sclerosis (MS) and also autism.[36,37] In 2009 the first case of vaccine-associated chronic fatigue syndrome (CFS) was described by doctors in a man with aluminium overload. He had received 5 aluminium-containing vaccines over a period of four weeks.[35] It is sobering to remind ourselves that babies in the UK receive 7 aluminium-containing vaccines over an eight week period between 2 and 4 months of age.

Conspiracy of silence

The WHO is one of the staunchest supporters of vaccines. Yet even it acknowledges the possibility, and plausibility, that aluminium could cause more serious disease and strongly recommends further research. At the same time it says there is no reason to conclude that a health risk exists, and does not recommend any change in the use of aluminium-containing vaccines.

This may be because there are no practical alternatives to aluminium, and that advising its removal would derail the global vaccination programme. Some vaccines are already aluminium-free, such as measles, MMR, BCG and rotavirus. Vaccine experts believe that some form of adjuvant is necessary for effective vaccination, and the only one in widespread use is aluminium, with no readily available replacement. Research is underway to look for suitable alternatives to aluminium to act as adjuvants in vaccines, though whether safe and effective replacements can be found remains to be seen.

Though we know aluminium is highly toxic (and babies are receiving over a thousand times the upper safety limits), there seems to be a conspiracy of silence on further investigation. Perhaps more deeply worrying is that there may be real obstacles to actually doing the research the WHO asks for. A group of Swedish doctors who investigated MMF were sufficiently concerned to call for vaccine manufacturers to look for alternatives to aluminium in their vaccines.[22] The same group of doctors was subsequently unable to obtain funding to continue their investigations into the high rate of children affected after receiving one particular vaccine.[23]

4
Smallpox & Scarlet Fever
Vaccination Riots

In order to understand medical thinking about vaccination, it helps to look back at the vaccines that are always put forward as the typical success story of vaccination as I was taught when I trained as a doctor. It tells us much we need to know about the problems we face today with vaccination against other diseases.

Infectious diseases aren't new to our modern age. They've been the scourge of mankind for centuries, during which governments have tried to control the worst epidemics. Back in 1346, Edward II attempted to expel all lepers from the City of London to halt the spread of leprosy. Elizabeth I took rather more drastic measures during an epidemic of the plague in London in 1564. She took refuge in Windsor, where anyone arriving from London was hanged in specially erected gallows in the market square. Another three hundred years later, in 1876, the average life expectancy from birth in England and Wales was forty-one years for a man and forty-three for a woman. A third of all deaths were caused by infection. The biggest killers were tuberculosis, scarlet fever, whooping cough and measles. It's no wonder that control of infectious diseases was seen as one of the most desirable goals in medicine.

It was smallpox that eventually triggered the development of the first vaccine. Smallpox was caught from close contact with an infected person, causing a fever and characteristic blistering rash, which left permanently disfiguring pockmarks on those who recovered. Up to a quarter of those who caught smallpox died. It had grown from a common, but relatively mild, illness in the sixteenth century to become a major killer during the seventeenth century when it replaced bubonic plague as Europe's most feared pestilence. In 1694, Queen Mary of England died of smallpox, one of many European royals to be carried off by the 'pox'. Over a period of forty years in the early eighteenth century, nearly a quarter of the population of London succumbed to smallpox.

After the first English epidemic of 1628, it became apparent that anyone who successfully recovered from the illness was extremely unlikely to catch it again. But there was no effective treatment.

Then Edward Jenner, a country doctor from Gloucestershire, brought vaccination to the notice of the world. In rural areas it was well known that farmers who worked with cows and caught cowpox never caught smallpox. On

14 May 1796, Jenner performed a famous experiment. He took pus from the hand of a milkmaid named Sarah Nelmes who had caught cowpox from milking infected cows. The doctor inoculated the pus into the arm of an eight-year-old boy called James Phipps. Seven weeks later Jenner inoculated James with real smallpox pus. Instead of succumbing to the disease, the child remained well. After repeating the experiment successfully on several other people, Jenner wrote up his results.

News of his experiment soon spread around the world. The possibility of preventing a disease that was widespread, and which killed around a quarter of those who contracted the more serious forms, was enthusiastically welcomed.

In 1841, the English Parliament made (cowpox) vaccination available free to those who couldn't afford it. Lobbying by the medical profession resulted in the act of 1853, which made vaccination compulsory for all children born in England and Wales. Parents who refused were fined 20 shillings, equivalent to around £50 today.[1]

The birth of the 'anti-compulsory vaccination' movement
Nonetheless, at exactly the same time, there was increasing distrust of vaccination, not least because more and more people were succumbing to smallpox despite having been vaccinated. It was the onset of compulsory vaccination that kick-started the doubts about its effectiveness on a large scale. A pivotal moment was the publication, in 1854 by John Gibbs, of a 64-page booklet entitled 'Our Medical Liberties.' Riots followed in several towns. Increasingly harsh laws were passed, including the 'cat and mouse' Act of 1867, sanctioning punishments, by fines or imprisonment, to be inflicted indefinitely until parents complied with law.[2] On 15 January 1869, William Johnson from Leicester was the first of many to be imprisoned for two weeks, for refusing to allow his child to be vaccinated.

Much like today, followers of the anti-vaccine movement argued a right to freedom of choice, were against political interference in family matters and believed (correctly as it turned out) that there were alternative methods to prevent the spread of smallpox.

As the penalties for refusing vaccination became increasingly severe, the National Anti-Compulsory Vaccination League grew with support from prominent MPs and doctors.

Following a large anti-vaccine demonstration in Leicester on 23 March 1885 that attracted 100,000 people, the government set up a Royal Commission. After sitting for seven years, it concluded, in 1896, that smallpox vaccination was effective, but recommended the abolition of ever-increasing penalties for refusal. A new Vaccination Act was passed in 1898, allowing exemption for the 'conscientious objector.' This resulted in a sharp drop in the number of children being vaccinated.[3]

Was smallpox vaccination effective?
Jenner was convinced vaccination provided lifelong protection. It became

increasingly clear over time that he was wrong, and that six or seven repeated vaccinations were required to maintain protection – a lesson doctors continue to learn today. It was also clear that vaccination was only partially effective as was demonstrated in the Middlesbrough outbreak of 1897: in a 98% vaccinated population, 1,411 people caught smallpox, 86% of whom had been vaccinated.[4] Similar outbreaks occurred in Sheffield and London[5] and, in the twentieth century, outbreaks continued but bore no relation to the proportion of the population vaccinated.

The important thing for us today is to see that the success of vaccination was really rather a modest phenomenon. Deaths from smallpox certainly fell after the introduction of vaccination, but then so did deaths from many other scourges, such as measles and scarlet fever, making it difficult to determine the contribution of vaccination to the fall.

Whilst smallpox vaccination does offer some protection, those opposed to compulsory vaccination were persuasively arguing that improvements in sanitation were the true cause of the decline. They also argued that deaths from smallpox were decreasing despite falling vaccination rates – something you would not be expecting to happen if vaccination were causing the fall. In addition, there were the risks of side-effects to consider. The early smallpox vaccine was dirty and unsafe and could transmit infections. In fact, syphilis was spread through Europe by the vaccine.

Despite the development of a safer (cleaner) vaccine at the end of the nineteenth century, other side-effects grew in importance as the disease became less common. The most serious complications were inflammation of the brain (encephalitis) and a severe skin disease ('eczema vaccinatum'). Both could kill. From 1948-1957, there were 26 deaths from smallpox in England and Wales and 34 deaths caused by vaccination.[6] There was, by then, a greater risk of dying from the vaccine than from the disease.

What about smallpox vaccination today?
The number of deaths from smallpox fell sharply during the late nineteenth century and remained low despite falling vaccination figures. As the disease became increasingly rare – and the relative risks of vaccination greater – a growing number of doctors called for the end of vaccination against smallpox.

By the mid-twentieth century, it had become clear that the most important aspect of managing the disease was not universal vaccination, but isolating cases and vaccinating close contacts to stop the chain of infection. Some doctors were calling for the abandonment of 'indiscriminate infant vaccination,'[7] which, they argued, was 'of little value and dangerous.'[8] When compulsory vaccination finally stopped in 1948, the proportion of infants being vaccinated immediately dropped from 37% to 18%. During the 1950s and 1960s, 21 died as a result of smallpox vaccination, but there was only one death from smallpox.

The government abandoned smallpox vaccination in 1971, when it was acknowledged to be a greater threat than the disease. The last cases of smallpox in the UK occurred in 1973 and 1978, both from laboratory accidents. In 1978 there was a small outbreak in Birmingham and one person died. These were the last cases anywhere in the world.

Significantly, mass vaccination had little effect on smallpox worldwide. Smallpox disappeared in countries with little or no vaccination, such as Australia and New Zealand, as well as countries with widespread vaccination.[9] When the WHO launched its Intensified Smallpox Eradication Programme in 1967, its strategy involved mass vaccination of 100% of the populations of countries where smallpox still existed. Soon it learnt Britain's lesson that mass vaccination in the UK was both ineffective and dangerous. A different approach was found to be more successful: the 'surveillance-containment strategy'. Instead of mass vaccination, it depended on quickly finding new cases and isolating them to prevent spread. It was accompanied by selective vaccination of close contacts. This approach proved far more effective, and the last case of wild smallpox was diagnosed in Somalia in 1977. Two years later, WHO declared the world free of smallpox.[10,11,12]

Would smallpox have disappeared on its own like the plague? We'll never know. Mass vaccination alone failed to eradicate smallpox, though it played a supporting role in its elimination. Vaccination certainly isn't entitled to take all the glory when the 'surveillance-containment strategy' played the main role. Leading players have admitted eradication was a close shave, and only just achieved.[13]

Scarlet Fever
To see how the deadliness of a disease changes without human intervention, we only have to look at scarlet fever. Scarlet fever was a mild illness when it was first recognised during the second half of the seventeenth century. Scarlet fever then caused many deaths during the middle of the eighteenth century, before becoming mild again. By the middle of the nineteenth century it had returned as the leading cause of death in children. The disease caused at least 40,000 deaths in England in 1870, since when the death rate has steadily fallen.

The steep decline in severity of the illness from the late nineteenth century remains unexplained. There has never been an immunisation for the disease, and effective antibiotics – primarily penicillin – weren't available until the 1940s. The main reason for the decline in deaths caused by scarlet fever, in common with measles, whooping cough and tuberculosis, is probably better nutrition. Its final demise may have been assisted by the introduction of antibiotics.

But scarlet fever is not the only example. At the dawn of the twentieth century, scarlet fever, along with measles, whooping cough and diphtheria were four of the biggest UK child killers. But deaths from all four fell in an impressive fashion during the first half of the century, before the availability of either vaccination or antibiotics. An even more ancient example is the bubonic plague which killed twenty-five million Europeans (a third of Europe's population) in five devastating years during the fourteenth century, only to vanish without a trace.

Though the smallpox vaccine was a momentous discovery, its use in the first mass vaccination in history does not deserve the same credit. The 1897 Middlesbrough outbreak showed, for example, that the huge majority of patients had actually been vaccinated. As smallpox neared extinction, compulsory vaccination proved to be more lethal than the disease it sought to prevent. Diseases wax and wane naturally, no matter the medical advances of the time. Our most recent 'plague' is AIDS. This disease, unheard of only a generation ago, is now predicted to kill more people than the plague: over half a million children died from AIDS worldwide in 2005 at its most lethal peak. Smallpox grew from a relatively mild illness in the sixteenth century to become a serious threat. Polio is another disease that changed from being comparatively harmless to a dreaded disease over the course of a few decades. The thing to be truly wary of is the dishonest claim that the natural decline of a disease is the result of medical intervention, particularly where that intervention is compulsory.

5
Diphtheria

The Strangler

Another great vaccination success story often quoted is the vaccination against diphtheria. It was the onset of national vaccination against diphtheria in 1941 that heralded the dawn of the UK childhood immunisation programme as we know it.

Its history more or less follows the same pattern as with measles and whooping cough. In 1859, a large epidemic of diphtheria caused over 10,000 deaths and diphtheria became the most important cause of death in children in the UK and much of Europe.

But from the late nineteenth century something strange started happening. Diphtheria was no less common, but it was becoming a less serious disease. Death rates fell steadily even though there hadn't been any major medical advances in treatment or prevention.

Diphtheria is an infection caused by a bacterium* (or bug) that settles in the back of the mouth, initially causing a sore throat, malaise and high temperature. A membrane forms in the throat that may spread and cause breathing difficulties and obstruction (hence 'the strangler'). Sometimes it's serious enough to require a hole to be surgically made in the windpipe so the sufferer can breathe. The main danger, however, is the poison that is produced by the bug. It can spread to the heart and nerves, causing serious illness or even death — the outcome in 5-10% of those getting the disease.

Anti-poison
The first effective treatment for diphtheria was the development of an antidote. If given early enough, it could prevent serious disease by inactivating the diphtheria poison that does most of the damage. Despite an early setback when ten children died in the USA as a result of being given anti-poison (medical term antitoxin) contaminated with live tetanus bacteria, this became a valuable and potentially life-saving treatment and was used, to a small extent, from around the turn of the century. However, in order for it to work, this treatment had to be given very early, making it impractical for widespread use.

True vaccination was developed early in the twentieth century. This works by injecting a safe diphtheria poison into the body to activate its immune system. The safe poison is near enough to the real thing to encourage the body to produce its own antidote that, when required, inactivates the diphtheria poison. This 'poison-made-safe' is called a 'toxoid'.

There was a great deal of debate amongst doctors in the UK about the value of immunisation with diphtheria toxoid. Many doctors didn't trust immunisation, and there was still a strong anti-vaccination backlash following the laws forcing parents to have their children vaccinated against smallpox. Moreover, doctors were aware that diphtheria was already becoming a less serious disease without vaccination. Selective immunisation by some local authorities in some parts of the country began in the 1920s. But it wasn't until the late 1930s that the tide of medical opinion finally turned in favour of widespread immunisation. The government launched a national immunisation campaign in 1941 using films and posters to persuade parents to have their children vaccinated.

The vaccination campaign was hugely successful. By 1943, half of all children in the UK had been immunised. Though the death rate from diphtheria was already falling, immunisation appears to have hastened the decline.

The Department of Health itself admitted the decline in the death rate of children from diphtheria couldn't be attributed solely to immunisation. After all, this had fallen from 888 deaths for every million children in 1901 to 301 deaths per million in 1938 (a 66% reduction), and all this happened before the introduction of widespread immunisation. But there was little doubt that immunisation helped, and it was estimated that the death rate in 1946 was one fifth of what could have been expected had the death rate continued to have fallen at the pre-immunisation rate.[1]

The first vaccine scare

But then disaster struck. It was soon discovered that giving any injection to someone developing polio could trigger an attack causing paralysis that could be permanent. This was called 'injection provocation' and it happens when there is a polio epidemic. As diphtheria immunisation was by far the most widely used injection at this time it became the leading culprit, and is likely to have contributed to the unprecedented polio epidemic of 1947. By the early 1950s, experts calculated that vaccinations (which at that time were mainly diphtheria with some whooping cough) were causing 13% of all cases of paralysis from polio in young children.[2,3,4] The Department of Health was so concerned it advised diphtheria immunisation be suspended whenever there was a local outbreak of polio.[5] This entirely justifiable 'vaccine scare' contributed to a fall in uptake of immunisation by 25% over a one-year period from 1949 to 1950. The introduction of one successful intervention (diphtheria immunisation) had contributed to an entirely different problem − the worst polio epidemic the UK had ever seen.

The steep fall in diphtheria cases led the Department of Health to declare in 1952: 'From being one of the most serious causes of death of children in this country, diphtheria has now fallen to a position of numerical insignificance.'[6] It further claimed immunisation had caused the lion's share of this fall. But the Ministry clearly had a short memory, as only four years earlier it had conceded that the death rate from diphtheria had already fallen by two thirds between 1901 and 1938 before widespread immunisation.[7] It was a forerunner of the many exaggerated claims for the effectiveness of immunisation that would appear later.

By 1955 diphtheria was described in the UK as a 'rare disease', and in the same year the Department of Health thought it 'reasonable to hope the disease might be eliminated altogether.'[8,9] This reference to 'elimination' was surprising if not somewhat misleading. Diphtheria immunisation is based on a toxoid that is only active against the bacterium's poison and not against the bacterium itself. Immunisation would be expected to inactivate the deadly poison that causes the disease, but not to eliminate the organism that produced it.

However, what the government was hoping for may have not been so far off the mark, because the poison-producing diphtheria bacterium appears to have more or less vanished since widespread immunisation was introduced. By the late 1970s diphtheria appeared to have disappeared from the UK. During the past 20 years there have been, on average, one or two cases of diphtheria a year in this country and virtually no deaths. By the 1980s many countries were experiencing the same trend and there was optimism that the disease would indeed be extinguished – until the Russian crisis.

The Russian resurgence – are we safe from diphtheria?
During the early 1990s, the western world was shaken by a huge epidemic of diphtheria that started in Russia and spread to all the countries of the former USSR. The outbreak shouldn't have been totally unexpected, as most European countries, including Russia, were aware of large numbers of adults with little or no immunity to diphtheria.[10] Nevertheless, the epidemic was both unexpectedly large, and different in appearance from those that had occurred earlier in the century. Whereas previous outbreaks had affected mainly children, this affected far more adolescents and adults. Between 1990 and 1998 there were over 157,000 cases reported in the former USSR and 5,000 deaths.[11]

But why did this large epidemic occur? There are several contributing factors that can be listed: massive socio-economic instability following the collapse of the iron curtain; large-scale population movements, possibly introducing diphtheria into populations with poor immunity; temporary collapse of health care systems; delay in putting in place measures to control the epidemic; a recent fall in childhood immunisation coverage; lots of unprotected adults.

A combination of factors, as is so often the case, contributed to this outbreak. The death rate was as high as 20% because of inadequate medical treatment, though the average death rate was 5-10% of cases. The world was reminded that diphtheria could still be deadly. Though the majority of people getting diphtheria had been immunised, those who hadn't were more likely to become seriously ill and die. The main method used to halt the epidemic was repeated mass vaccination campaigns. Diphtheria immunisation, however, can only prevent someone becoming ill from the diphtheria poison, but it cannot prevent the spread of the disease, as it inactivates the poison without harming the bacterium. The mass vaccinations probably contributed to ending the epidemic, but by how much we will never know.

As the Russian epidemic taught us, diphtheria can still be a serious illness. Though full recovery is normal, and outbreaks appear more likely to occur amongst those living in poverty and overcrowding, the chances of healthy victims dying are probably between one in 10 and one in 20. Whilst the disease has been very rare in the UK over recent years — there were only 20 cases in England between 2007 and 2014, of which only one was a child — it's more likely than other rare diseases to make a comeback.

Harmless diphtheria bacteria that don't produce the disease-causing poison probably exist widely in the community — usually in our noses or throats.[12] These could become dangerous if they acquired the disease-causing poison which could happen either by coming into contact with the dangerous poison-containing bacteria or, possibly, by spontaneous mutation.[13]

So, though the illness is rare, its seriousness warrants national immunisation to shield against the poison. Outbreaks have occurred in western (affluent) communities, including England, with over 90%, and up to 99%, of children fully immunised.[14,15] The effectiveness of the vaccine has more recently come into question after an outbreak in Brazil. Nearly all those who contracted diphtheria had been either fully or partially immunised, and two of the three deaths occurred in fully immunised children.[16] Vaccinating against diphtheria doesn't prevent anyone from catching and spreading it to someone else, but it does make serious illness or death much less likely — but not for very long. Research suggests immunity is likely to last fifteen years or more in most people.

Numerous studies show that at least a third, and quite possibly over half, of UK adults are currently susceptible to diphtheria and, therefore, more likely to become ill, possibly seriously, if infected.[17,18,19]

When diphtheria was widespread in the community before the start of immunisation, some got ill and even died, but most people became immune and kept that immunity going by continuously coming into contact with the diphtheria bacterium. As this can no longer happen, the only way that someone's immunity can be boosted is by further immunisation. The Department of Health reacted to this potential gap in immunity by adding a fifth dose of diphtheria to the childhood schedule in 1994, and in 2004 by making only combined tetanus, diphtheria (and polio) vaccine available for any adult requiring a tetanus booster, so that they would receive top-ups against diphtheria.

The important point is that the vaccine certainly makes serious disease less likely, but without giving complete protection. The full course of five doses lasts well into adult life for some people, but one or more boosters in adult life may still be needed to give lifelong protection. The French advise a total of seven doses. Nonetheless, the Department of Health claims that five doses of the vaccine provide 'satisfactory long-term protection' which is not supported by medical knowledge. If this misplaced enthusiasm only applied to the essentially safe diphtheria vaccination it would be a minor transgression. But, as I discovered, the misinformation is much graver in other cases.

6
Tuberculosis

The Captain of Death

The middle of the twentieth century was a golden period for modern medicine. Barely a month passed without a new discovery, or the promise that a cure for some disease was just over the horizon. During the 1950s, 1960s and 1970s there was boundless hope that these advances would result in our living healthier and longer lives. Nothing seemed impossible. Man could walk on the moon, and surely he would conquer disease, too. The list of successes is impressive and instantly recognisable:

1941	Discovery of penicillin
1949	Discovery of cortisone (steroids)
1960	Introduction of the contraceptive pill
1961	First modern-style hip replacement
1963	First kidney transplant
1967	First heart transplant
1978	First test tube baby

Sadly, half a century later, many of the promises of that era have failed to materialise, and the limitless optimism now seems woefully misplaced. The last enthusiasm of that era, gene therapy, along with genetic engineering, has been promising much for several decades but has, so far, delivered disappointingly little apart from inspiration for headlines and sci-fi writers.

Looking back, the killer infectious diseases of a century ago have all but disappeared. But in their place we have chronic diseases such as arthritis, diabetes, asthma and eczema for which medicine has no cure, other than treatment that often does little more than relieve symptoms. In fact, after the optimism in scientific progress, the boundaries of human intervention are becoming very clear indeed. Modern medicine itself causes illness — over 6% of UK hospital admissions are directly caused by side-effects of prescribed drugs.[1] Doctors — and medical treatments — are the third largest cause of death in the USA.[2] Doctors are becoming disillusioned with the direction of modern healthcare, patients are deserting orthodox medicine for complementary therapies, and all the while National Health Service costs are soaring astronomically.

In this modern climate of realism, health officials seemingly cling to one last hope for a silver bullet — vaccines. The eradication of smallpox seemed to offer all the evidence that was needed. Doctors desperately want to believe health officials for the sake of their profession, and parents do so for the sake of their children. But as we see from the previous chapters, it is not at all clear that mass vaccination is the successful, effective or indeed harmless medical intervention it claims to be. Infectious diseases were already growing less dangerous. As a rule they attacked the less well-off more, and the rising standard of sanitation and living during the twentieth century meant that the vast majority, and not just the privileged few, was better able to fend off their risks. Vaccines played, at most, a supporting part in the decline of these diseases but certainly not the lead role.

If one wants to understand the real effect of vaccines, without the propaganda or spin, one would do well to consider the case of tuberculosis. It was probably present in animals before the existence of humans and has certainly plagued mankind from prehistory unto the present day — evidence of TB of the spine has been found in fossil bones dating back to around 8000 BC. Apart from its longevity (it affected the upper classes in Egypt as evidenced by mummies from 2400 BC which had signs of TB infection), it is distinguished from the other diseases in that it was romanticised, at least during the nineteenth century, and earlier. During the seventeenth and eighteenth centuries, TB was associated with an artistic temperament. Frédéric Chopin, for example, caught and subsequently died from tuberculosis. Lord Byron, the romantic poet and serial lover, is quoted as saying, 'I should like to die of a consumption, because the ladies would all say, 'Look at poor Byron. How interesting he looks in dying!'[3] More recently, Thomas Mann wrote *The Magic Mountain*, published in 1924, in which rich TB sufferers die one after another, despite the healthy air, exercise and food, in an opulent sanatorium in the Swiss Alpine town of Davos.

During much of the nineteenth century there was debate as to whether 'consumption', as TB was also called because of the way that it slowly but surely consumed sufferers, was an infection or a cancer. The matter was not settled until 1881 when Robert Koch, a German physician, discovered the tubercle bacillus*, the micro-organism responsible for the disease. It was considered to be incurable. During the nineteenth century, at a time when the disease was the largest cause of death in the UK, sanatoria like the one in Davos were established in the mountain valleys of Europe, or by the sea. Here, those with sufficient finances spent periods of up to many months undergoing regimes of strict rest. Although patients recovered remarkably well during sanatorium treatments, the longer-term results were less impressive with over three people out of five dying within six years of their stay.

Additional treatments included bleeding, purging, poultices, electricity and more or less poisonous drugs, sending many patients to an earlier death than the disease itself would have. During the 1920s, modern medicine struggled to come up with an effective answer. Surgical collapse of the lung became a favoured treatment, and for a quarter of a century, pneumothorax therapy as it was called, was the most frequently used active treatment. An alternative, should lung collapse fail, involved the surgical removal of a rib to reduce the chest volume, or a risky operation in which part of the lung is removed.

The big breakthrough in the treatment of TB came in 1944 with the introduction of mass x-rays used to detect early cases of the disease and, importantly, the arrival of streptomycin, an antibiotic. It was the first successful anti-TB drug, soon followed by others without streptomycin's frequent side effect of hearing loss.

Though it is an infectious disease and is spread through close contact with someone who has the illness, it is actually surprisingly difficult to catch. Only a third of people who are in prolonged close contact with a person with TB become infected. This compares with the four out of five people who will catch measles or chickenpox from an infected person. It is one of the reasons why the practice of isolating the most seriously ill and infectious, initially in workhouses, workhouse infirmaries, and later in sanatoria, helped prevent the spread.[4]

Once infected with TB, just one in twenty-five people will develop the disease within a year and another one in twenty-five will develop TB within their lifetime. The remainder – and vast majority – are able to keep the disease under control and generally remain healthy.

Tuberculosis can affect virtually any part of the body, though the lungs are most commonly affected, typically causing a cough, fever and weight loss. In contrast to most of the illnesses described in this book, the disease occasionally manifests itself years after infection. Like the others, TB is far more common in inner cities, areas of poverty and homelessness, and in families originating from areas with high rates of TB such as the Indian subcontinent.

The fall in cases and deaths from TB applies only to the prosperous countries of the world. One third of the world's population, or 2 billion people, is believed to be infected with TB. There are nine million new cases annually, and up to two million people die from TB every year. The bulk of infections and deaths occur in Southeast Asia, the Western Pacific (including China) and Africa. Global TB notifications have finally started to fall after years of increase fuelled by HIV/AIDS. One billion people live in urban slums, and this number is expected to rise to two billion in the next thirty years. Slums mean overcrowding, malnutrition and inadequate ventilation – the very ingredients on which TB thrives. Further fuel for TB comes from HIV. People suffering from AIDS (the disease caused by HIV) are particularly susceptible to TB. All this is compounded by the increasing emergence of strains of TB that have become resistant to the commonly used anti-TB drugs.

The rise and fall of TB in the UK

Though TB has been ever present in Britain, it has, like all infectious diseases, had its ups and downs. The death rate from TB in London peaked in the mid-eighteenth century, since which it has been steadily falling. During the eighteenth and early nineteenth centuries the spread of TB was probably encouraged by the squalid, overcrowded and insanitary conditions in which people were living in towns and cities as a result of the industrial revolution. During the nineteenth century, cleanliness improved and all infections, including TB, started to fall. The long-term nature of the illness means that looking at deaths (as has been done with most other illnesses described in this book) is less helpful because of the long time-lag between infection and death, should it occur. But reports of new cases, compulsory in Britain since 1914, show how the number of TB cases in England and Wales declined steadily over the last hundred years.

The TB vaccine of choice around the world is the BCG vaccine, 'Bacille Calmette Guérin', named after its French discoverers. Since the 1970s, it has become the most widely used vaccine against any disease, and, paradoxically, one of the least effective. It is a live version of TB (like the measles, mumps and rubella vaccines) that has been altered or 'attenuated' to be made relatively safe.

Dr Albert Calmette and his colleague, Jean Camille Guérin, a vet, started work together on the vaccine in 1908, began human trials in 1921 and announced in 1923 they had a safe vaccine. Though widely taken up in France, it was not received so enthusiastically in other countries. British antipathy towards the vaccine was reinforced by the 'Lübeck disaster' in 1930, when the vaccine caused the deaths of 73 children in Germany, probably as a result of contamination of the vaccine with a dangerous, wild strain of TB. Numerous trials of the vaccine yielded inconsistent results, despite which the WHO (during the 1950s) encouraged its use partly, it is alleged, because of a bribe from UNICEF. One UNICEF health official was the brother of an influential French politician who was in need of reconstruction money, and wanted to be a national hero for France, a country that had suffered so much in the recent war.[5]

During the 1940s there was discussion in Britain whether the vaccine should be introduced in the UK. On the one hand, the numbers of people getting and dying from TB had been decreasing steadily without the use of a vaccine; on the other hand, it was claimed that the vaccine was being used with apparent success in the Scandinavian countries. But countries such as Norway were also using other methods to help combat TB, such as the isolation of infectious sufferers in sanatoria, so it was uncertain how much the vaccine was itself contributing to the fall in TB. The Department of Health, casting a long shadow into the future, was aware in 1947 that 'propaganda' would be necessary to ensure the 'confidence and co-operation of the public.' In its 1947 report the Department of Health concluded, 'Whoever is responsible for the propaganda work, it is most important that the public is not misled into believing that BCG is a complete protection from tuberculosis.'[6]

But there were strong reasons for introducing the vaccine. In 1955 TB still caused two thirds of deaths from all infectious diseases (and that includes measles, whooping cough and the other common childhood infectious diseases). BCG vaccination was introduced into the UK in 1949, first for those at special risk only, and from 1953 it was offered to all thirteen-year-old schoolchildren. The vaccine was given at this age in the hope that it would reduce the disease in young adults in whom tuberculosis was most common. In 1951, vaccination of sixty-seven children was likely to lead to the prevention of one case of TB (in the 1980s, by which time the disease had become much less common, 4,600 had to be vaccinated to prevent a single case). In addition to schoolchildren, some newborn babies were also given the BCG vaccination. Those in certain inner city areas or born into families with a high risk of TB were given the BCG within a few weeks of birth.

There was initial scepticism about the French vaccine, but both doctors and the public were reassured by the results of a Medical Research Council trial in 1956 which showed that the vaccine protected four out of five children who received it – one of the most positive results achieved for the BCG vaccine anywhere in the world.[7] Nevertheless, uptake was low for some time, with only a little more than one in three of thirteen year olds receiving the vaccine by 1958, rising to three in five by 1962.

Did the vaccine do the job? There were two pauses in the steady decline in cases of TB during the twentieth century, both occurring immediately after the two world wars. Because TB may take some years to manifest itself, the effect of the wars did not appear immediately, but only after a period of a few years. There was another slow-down in the decline of TB during the late 1960s and 1970s, which may have been caused by high immigration levels from countries where TB was far more common, such as India, Pakistan and Bangladesh.

The introduction of antibiotics against TB, and BCG vaccination, both occurred over a brief period in the late 1940s and early 1950s. It is difficult to judge the effect of each because, although the notification rate did start to fall more rapidly after their introduction, it did so at no greater a rate than after the First World War when there had been no comparable medical interventions. So the fall in the 1950s may have been simply the resumption of the natural decline following the temporary halt caused by the Second World War. Countries that never used the vaccine had similar falls in TB cases.[5] Holland has never routinely used BCG vaccination but had the lowest death rates for respiratory tuberculosis for any country in Europe.[8] The most notable exception is the USA where the BCG vaccine has never been routinely used in any age group. A UK study concluded that 90% of the fall between 1953 and 1990 was a result of drug prevention (such as treating close contacts of people with TB) and drug treatment, whereas BCG vaccination only contributed to 10% of the fall.[4]

Today, the numbers of people getting TB have fallen over recent years in most western European countries, but the UK is one of the exceptions. Around 7,000 people a year get TB in the UK today. Numbers were rising slowly and peaked in 2011 since when they have been falling. The majority of new cases are in young adults who were not born in the UK. Only a few hundred under the age of fifteen – mainly from Black African and South Asian ethnic groups – are diagnosed with the disease every year. Of the 7,000 who catch the disease, a little under 400 die every year as a result of it (one in twenty). The deaths occur overwhelmingly in older people (over 65 years of age), though, as TB rarely causes a speedy death, many of those will have caught the disease earlier in their lives. The vast majority of people catching

TB can be successfully treated with a six to nine month course of antibiotics.

These (serious) figures, however, distort the real picture. Whether TB can be called common depends exactly on where one lives. TB is concentrated in large urban centres such as London, Leicester, Birmingham, Luton, Manchester and Coventry and in much of the country there is little or no TB at all.

But even overall figures for London are deceptive, as they hide the huge discrepancies between different London boroughs. The boroughs of Newham and Brent have the greatest numbers of cases of TB whereas the disease is very rare in other boroughs such as Richmond or Bromley. People most at risk from TB in London have been those who are HIV positive, the homeless, prisoners and drug addicts. Three quarters of new cases are in people who were born outside the UK. There is also a direct relationship between the degree of social deprivation in which someone lives and their likelihood of contracting TB.

So, for the few who live in certain poorer inner city areas, TB remains relatively common, while for the large majority in Britain it is a disease unlikely to be encountered. To quote a review of tuberculosis which looked at TB in children in England and Wales between 1999 and 2006, 'Tuberculosis among children remains largely a disease of those born to parents belonging to an ethnic minority'.[26] There is nothing to suggest anything has changed since then.

What does this say about the effectiveness of the TB vaccine?

The Department of Health had to act on the changing situation at last. It has suffered repeated problems with its BCG vaccination policy. In September 1999 it was forced to suspend the school BCG vaccination programme for over a year because of difficulties obtaining the vaccine. The policy for vaccinating at-risk babies was also in a mess: the advice on who to vaccinate was unclear, policies varied around the country, and monitoring was inadequate. The only bright light of the policy was that parents were able to request the vaccine for their babies if they wished. It is the only example of a vaccination choice being made available to parents.

The largest outbreak of TB in the UK of recent years occurred at a school in Leicester in 2001. The first pupil was diagnosed with TB in August 2000, and a second in October of the same year. By April 2001 24 students had confirmed TB, twice as many in this age group as Leicester would normally see in a whole year. By then public health doctors were describing the situation as a 'major outbreak' and a 'race against time.' The final count of those who caught TB was at least 62, mainly students at the school, but also a few teachers and relatives. Another 100 showed signs of TB and were started on long courses of antibiotic treatment, lasting three to six months. Many of the children were from families originally from south Asia who are more susceptible to TB. What is of most concern is that 80% of children at the school, including most of those with the disease, had been vaccinated against TB.[9] The powerful Joint Committee on Vaccination and Immunisation (JCVI) of experts that advises the Department of Health acknowledged that the effectiveness of the BCG vaccine had been 'disappointingly low.'[10]

The JCVI knew that the value of school-age vaccination was questionable, but felt that 'a secure neonatal programme needed to be in place' before abandoning teenage vaccination.[11] Then, in 2001, Evans, one of the manufacturers of the BCG, withdrew all their vaccine from the market because of concerns about effectiveness.[12] The replacement vaccine caused increased side-effects, especially abscesses and fainting.[13] As if these problems were not enough, it was discovered that a Liverpool factory, had, between 1989 and 2002, manufactured nine batches of BCG vaccine, comprising as many as 900,000 doses, that may have been under-strength.[14]

In 2005 government experts finally decided, after twenty years of deliberation, that it was time for the faltering school programme to be stopped, and that the focus should be on immunising high-risk babies shortly after birth in high-risk areas. However, they were, for once, uncharacteristically clear about the modest benefit offered by the vaccine, emphasizing that 'BCG does not prevent tuberculosis infection, but does help prevent the development of early serious disease, especially in young children.'[15] A new TB vaccination policy was put into place in 2005. This concentrates on vaccinating new born babies in areas with a high rate of TB. However, it still means that low-risk babies born in Hampstead (in the London Borough of Camden — a 'high-risk' area) will be given a vaccine of unproven benefit but with known risks. The problem is that there is very little direct evidence that the vaccine prevents tuberculosis in infants;[16] studies done on babies of Asian ethnic origin born in the UK suggest an effectiveness of between 49% and 64%.[17,18] Whilst the BCG is relatively ineffective (only 19%) at preventing TB infection, it is considerably better (60-80%) at preventing severe forms of TB in children.[26]

So is the BCG vaccine safe?

Because the BCG vaccine is injected just under the skin (intradermally) side-effects at the site of the injection are common. A lump will normally develop at the injection site (usually on the upper outer arm). This can become ulcerated and may bleed, or ooze pus, requiring a dressing to be applied. A small permanent scar, which is occasionally unsightly, is normal.

BCG is a 'live' vaccine, and so can cause all the same complications as TB. Up to 1 in 50 vaccine recipients get swollen and painful lymph nodes (glands) in the neck or armpit; if severe, they may become infected with pus, leading to an abscess requiring surgical draining. A report from East London suggests that abscesses in the armpits of babies recently vaccinated with BCG are more common than previously realised, with 1 in 320 vaccinated babies being so severely affected that they had to attend hospital to obtain treatment.[19]

The most serious side-effect of BCG vaccination is to get a widespread TB-like infection. This very rare, though occasionally fatal, complication occurs in around 1 in 200,000.[20] It is more common in babies with impaired immune systems, which is often impossible to detect in the newborn, but also occurs in those who are healthy.[21] It is probably much more common than is generally realised for the live BCG vaccine to spread throughout the body. At autopsy (post-mortem examination) in Canada, twenty-six out of thirty-six (72%) of children who had been given BCG vaccination as newborn babies showed signs of widespread TB-like infection in their bodies, despite dying of conditions unrelated to TB. It may well be that this is a normal occurrence in many healthy children who are generally able to deal with the widespread vaccine-induced 'infection' and not become unwell.[22] However, it has been suggested that the vaccine may do more harm than good in populations with a high risk of congenital immunity problems.[23] Various hypersensitivity and skin reactions can also occur.

A BCG vaccination session was held at Penweddig School in Aberystwyth on 16th November 2004. During the morning a team of four doctors and three nurses vaccinated 118 pupils, including thirteen-year-old Dominic Hamer. Shortly after receiving the vaccine Dominic felt unwell and unable to breathe. He collapsed in the school toilets where he was discovered by a friend. The medical team was alerted and gave him emergency treatment before he was taken by ambulance to hospital. Dominic, very ill and requiring help with his breathing, was admitted to the hospital's intensive care unit. There, to the relief of his family, he regained consciousness and went on to make a full recovery.

Dominic had suffered from anaphylaxis, the most severe type of allergic reaction, which can occur as a very rare reaction to any vaccination or drug and even some foods (severe peanut allergy is well known). An anaphylactic reaction can kill and requires urgent injection of a drug called adrenaline, which Dominic was given by the doctors at the school. It is not known how commonly anaphylaxis occurs after immunisations, but it is very rare, perhaps one in a million vaccinations. Because anaphylaxis is life threatening, it is very important that there is resuscitation equipment, including adrenaline, available wherever vaccinations are performed.

But something unusual happened that November morning at Penweddig School. Twelve other pupils were sent to the local casualty department within hours of receiving their BCG vaccinations. They suffered from a variety of symptoms including sweating, dizziness, nausea, breathing difficulties, shivering and blurred vision. Some of these children were probably suffering from nothing more than fainting attacks that occur quite commonly after immunisation. It is surprising, though, that a team of four doctors and three nurses, experienced at giving school children BCG, had to send ten of the children to hospital in ambulances if they thought the problem was no more serious than a faint. Ten pupils were admitted to the hospital from casualty, though seven were discharged later that day, with only three being kept in overnight.

It has been suggested that Dominic's collapse could well have triggered panic amongst the other pupils who then went on to develop symptoms themselves. That is a very plausible suggestion, but has one major flaw: most of the affected children reported feeling unwell before Dominic collapsed.[24]

Was there something wrong with the vaccine? A faulty batch perhaps (these things have happened before)? No, said Bryan Gibbons, the Welsh Minister for Health. So what was the cause of 13 out of 118 pupils being taken to hospital after receiving the BCG vaccination? We just don't know. Nonetheless, the chief executive of the local NHS trust, Allison Williams, described the students' reactions as 'normal side effects to BCG immunisation....'[25]

7
Polio
A Middle-Class Disease

Polio is unique amongst the major infectious diseases of the twentieth century in that in the early part of the century, at least in the UK, it was not considered a serious illness. It was first described in 1789, but little attention was paid to it until the 1940s when an upsurge of the illness, accompanied by heaps of publicity, resulted in outbreaks of panic to rival the epidemics of polio itself. Also, interestingly, it was a change in our habits — including increased mass vaccination — that made the disease become far more serious than it had ever been.

Polio used to be called 'infantile paralysis,' implying that it affected babies under one year old. During the 1920s and 1930s between a hundred and two hundred people (mainly children) died every year from polio in the UK. In addition, four times as many were left permanently paralysed by the disease. However, if one bears in mind that during this same period both measles and whooping cough were killing thousands of children every year, it's not difficult to understand why there was so little concern over polio.

This was to change in the hot summer of 1947 when the UK had its first large epidemic with nearly 700 deaths and over 7000 people paralysed. During the following decade, in which polio killed and maimed many thousands, the population lived in fear of what was not a new disease in itself, but one that was behaving very differently, and with far more frightening consequences, from what everyone had been used to. Paralysis from polio was relatively rare, but of those who became paralysed in some way, one in twenty died, a quarter remained moderately or severely paralysed and two thirds made a full, or nearly complete, recovery. One of the more serious effects was paralysis of the respiratory muscles used to breathe. Various breathing machines (such as the 'iron lung', which caught the public imagination) were used to keep people alive until they (hopefully) recovered the use of their muscles.

A particular reason why polio attracted special publicity was because it was affecting the wealthier and better off families more than poorer ones throughout the country. This was in contrast to the other main infectious diseases. Franklin D Roosevelt, USA President from 1933 to 1945, had also raised the profile of the disease. Ten years before his presidency, at the age of thirty-nine, he had been paralysed by polio, after which he was unable to walk.

Two factors helped turn polio from a relatively unimportant disease to one with such serious consequences. The first one, paradoxically, was increased hygiene. Everyone used to be exposed to polio, a virus that spreads from person to person in infected faeces, a journey made much easier by poor sanitation and open drains. Thus, up until the early twentieth century, most people caught polio as a baby during the first few months of their lives, when they were still protected by immunity obtained from their mothers, or as very young children. Over 99% of people were hardly ill at all, possibly suffering only a mild fever, and then going on to develop permanent immunity so that they couldn't catch the illness again. But, as cleanliness improved, children didn't come into contact with the disease until they became older, when there is a greater risk of dying from the illness and they were no longer protected by the antibodies acquired in their mother's womb.

This postponement of the age of infection applied especially to the more hygiene-conscious middle classes, who were also the first to be able to afford the new flush toilets. The proportion of adults and children over five contracting polio increased from a quarter in 1912 to two thirds by 1950. So, ironically, an increasing standard of cleanliness in society made polio a far more devastating disease than ever before: a thirty-year-old's risk of dying of polio is five times higher than that of a child below five.

The other reason for the increasing number of cases of paralysis from polio, however, is rarely mentioned. It was discovered that giving an injection (of anything) deep into the muscles of people in the very early stages of polio could actually lead to complications. It could cause paralysis to occur when a complete recovery might have been made if the injection hadn't been given (the 'injection provocation' referred to briefly in the chapter on diphtheria).[1] As the polio virus was widespread, virtually everyone came across it, usually as a baby or young child. So if many babies or young children were to be given lots more injections over a short period of time, that could trigger an epidemic of paralysed children.

Until 1940 the only routine immunisation given was for smallpox, but this did not involve a deep injection into the muscle. In 1942, however, the national immunisation campaign against diphtheria began in the UK, followed by trials of the new whooping cough vaccine in 1946. Both these vaccinations are given by deep injection into the muscle. Another new medical treatment of the 1940s, often given by injection, was penicillin, along with other new antibiotics. So, on top of cleaner living, it appears that the introduction of a national immunisation programme against diphtheria in 1942 contributed to converting polio from a usually mild illness into a national disaster.

This was later confirmed when a Medical Research Council report concluded that the risk of paralysis from polio within a month of a diphtheria or whooping cough vaccination was three times the normal rate. Between 1951 and 1953, 1 in every 37,000 diphtheria and whooping cough immunisations in the UK resulted in a case of paralysis from polio.[2] This amounted to 13% of all cases of paralytic polio in children between six months and two years of age during that period. It was no wonder that diphtheria vaccination was suspended wherever there was an outbreak of polio.

The fall

During the 1940s and 1950s there was feverish research into a vaccine against polio, which had now become such a high profile disease among the middle classes. Two types of vaccine were developed and both are still used today.

The killed, or inactivated, poliovirus vaccine ('IPV') was the first to be introduced in the UK in 1956, though not used routinely until 1958. The other type of vaccine is the oral poliovirus vaccine ('OPV') based on a live virus, which replaced IPV as the UK's preferred polio immunisation in 1962, and remained so until 2004 when we reverted to the killed vaccine.

The original trials of the killed IPV vaccine, conducted in the USA in 1954 on over 600,000 schoolchildren, were the culmination of 15 years of hard endeavour. The vaccine was, it was announced, 'safe, effective and potent' and it was, indeed, between 60% and 90% effective in preventing paralytic polio.[3] Even allowing for the fact that immunisation started slowly and was not used on a wide scale until 1959, the numbers dying or becoming paralysed from polio — though then already in decline anyway — fell impressively in the very early years after immunisation was started. In the UK it seems the killed IPV vaccine had done most of the good work before the (supposedly better) live OPV was introduced. The effectiveness of the IPV was even more notable when one bears in mind that the IPV used now is many times stronger than the ostensibly 'effective and potent' one used to kick start the immunisation campaign 50 years ago.

Furthermore, since the introduction of the live virus vaccine (OPV) in 1962, a change in the way polio is diagnosed has muddied the waters by leading to a 'drop' in the number of reported cases of polio since widespread vaccination. The vast majority of people (around 99%) who 'catch' polio don't get ill or only suffer mild flu-like symptoms, and so don't know they have encountered the polio virus. This made mild polio very difficult to diagnose unless the more severe symptoms of paralysis occurred. So a change in diagnosis of polio is likely to make an appreciable difference in the number of reports of polio.

The 'fall' in the number of cases would be similar to when, say, removing sick people from the unemployment register results in an immediate 'fall' in the unemployment figures. Before the onset of immunisation, polio was diagnosed by history-taking and examination of the patient by the doctor. Laboratory tests were rarely employed. Following the introduction of vaccination, the criteria for diagnosis became increasingly strict. The new requirement that the polio virus be detected in the stool resulted in some missed cases. The subsequent insistence that paralysis should last for a minimum of sixty days inevitably excluded most cases as few cause paralysis. The diagnosis was also tightened to exclude other conditions that were mistakenly diagnosed as polio prior to immunisation. The World Health Organisation's increasingly stringent diagnostic criteria have led to criticism that cases of polio are being missed.

*

But the really interesting questions about the live-virus OPV vaccine arise from the different way it operates. British health officials switched to the OPV in 1962, claiming that the vaccine would be more effective than the killed vaccine IPV. It was believed that the vaccine might work better because it would be excreted by vaccinated children. The living OPV virus was passed on to others, helping to immunise people who had not received the vaccine. In other words, health officials decided to release a live vaccine polio virus that would roam freely alongside the wild polio virus and keep the population's immunity up. Because the OPV virus had been weakened ('attenuated') this was considered to be safe. As soon as the oral vaccine was licensed in 1962, it replaced the IPV in the UK. Rather than being injected, it is given as drops, and initially it was administered on a sugar cube.

But whether a new and ostensibly more effective vaccine was really necessary in the first place is a seriously moot point. By 1962, the number of people being paralysed from polio had fallen from a high of over 7,000 in 1947 to a few hundred a year, with deaths falling just as spectacularly. The IPV vaccine appeared to be working extremely well in dealing with a disease that was already in rapid decline. Other countries decided not to make the switch to OPV and instead continue with the killed vaccine, protecting only those who were themselves vaccinated.

One reason why they did not make the switch is because the passage of the OPV virus throughout the community is a double-edged sword. The risk of live viruses in vaccines had surfaced only a few years before. The most notorious and serious disaster is known as 'The Cutter Incident'. The polio viruses in one batch of IPV prepared by the Cutter laboratory in California had not been adequately killed. Live viruses were inadvertently injected into 120,000 people in 1955, shortly after the onset of polio immunisation. This resulted in 260 cases of polio, nearly 200 paralysed people, and 10 deaths.[4]

Another instance was the simian-40 contamination. Polio (and other) vaccines are grown on animal cells. It is possible for the vaccines to become contaminated with an infection from the animal. The best known example of this is the contamination of both IPV and OPV with simian virus 40 (SV40) from monkey kidney cells. It's thought that between ten and thirty million Americans received a polio vaccine contaminated with the simian virus between 1955 and 1963.[5] Although both OPV and IPV were affected, contamination of a vaccine with a wild virus is more likely with a live vaccine. Despite the fact that all polio vaccines used in the UK since 1980 have been free of the problem, some vaccines used between 1962 and 1980 did contain the simian virus 40.[6] The main concern about it is that it can probably cause various cancers in humans.[7] We shall never know how many human cancers may have been caused by it, but it's a sobering reminder that vaccines can contain disease-causing impurities. Steps are taken to ensure current vaccines don't contain known viruses, but vaccines cannot be screened for viruses and other infections that we do not yet know about.

There was, in 1962, no guarantee that the live virus vaccine would not change, as it passed though gut after gut, and revert to its original 'virulent' form that could cause paralysis. And that is exactly what did, occasionally, happen. The main problem with the 'weakened' live vaccine is that it turned out it could cause polio, which can paralyse and even kill, in a similar way to the disease that it seeks to prevent.

It is now understood that there are two ways in which the 'weakened' live vaccine can cause polio. The first is associated with the people who actually received the vaccine (or those close to them). The disease occurs usually because of a mutation of the live virus. It is assumed that this type of infection stops as soon as the live vaccine is no longer used. However, vaccination experts in the USA were taken aback in 2005 when they discovered a vaccine-derived polio virus in a seven-month-old infant in rural Minnesota.[8] The live vaccine virus, presumed to be the source of the infection, has not been used in the USA since 2000, suggesting the OPV may survive undetected in communities far longer than expected.

The other way is where the infection was not caused by receiving the vaccine, but where the vaccine virus runs wild. Even before the live vaccine virus (OPV) was licensed for use, nearly half a century ago, its genetic instability was a major concern. The virus is able to mutate to a form similar to the wild virus and circulate amongst the community, causing an epidemic of polio. Between 2000 and 2015 there have around 800 cases of paralysis as a result of circulating polio vaccine.

Long-term carriers of either type have the potential to re-infect the population after the 'eradication' of wild polio. People with compromised immune systems may excrete these disease-causing viruses for many years. In 1995, for example, it was estimated that a UK resident had been spreading the virus for nineteen years. Since 2000, two additional UK residents have been discovered to be virus excreters. This is even more of a problem in countries with a high proportion of HIV positive people, who are both more likely to suffer paralysis or death after receiving OPV and more likely to be long-term virus excreters.[9]

Another problem with the live (OPV) vaccine is the association with the rare immune disorder called Guillain-Barré Syndrome (GBS) which causes paralysis of the arms or legs and, if severe, near complete paralysis. Most people make a full recovery. 'Outbreaks' of the syndrome have occurred in several countries following mass immunisation campaigns with OPV.[10,11,12] As the symptoms of GBS and polio are so similar it can be difficult for doctors to distinguish between the two. But the isolation of vaccine strain polio virus from the faeces and brain of people diagnosed with GBS provides pretty conclusive evidence that the vaccine can cause GBS.[13,14]

*

While the decision to introduce the new vaccine was defensible in 1962, if one gives the health authorities the benefit of the doubt, the same cannot be said about the decision to wait until 2004 to switch back to the killed polio vaccine (IPV).

By the 1970s the rare but deadly mutation of the OPV was well known. Norway had switched from the IPV to the OPV, as the UK had done, in 1966. However, the Norwegians switched back to the IPV twelve years later because of the risk of paralysis from the vaccine.[15]

From 1970 onwards, the OPV used in the UK was causing more cases of paralysis than the disease itself.[16] Furthermore, by the 1980s, for example, Sweden, Finland, Iceland and Holland had all eradicated polio by using only the killed vaccine IPV. Yet, despite repeated calls by doctors for the switch from OPV to IPV, health officials persisted in using the OPV insisting that it was more effective. In 1990 an article in the medical journal the *Lancet* argued that 'the case to a switch to IPV seems irresistible.'[17] In fact, an editorial in the same journal argued for the introduction of IPV into the UK immunisation schedule as long ago as 1984.[18] Nevertheless, as late as 1996, the Department of Health was officially advising doctors, 'The possibility of a very small risk of poliomyelitis induced by OPV cannot be ignored but is insufficient to warrant a change in immunisation policy.'[19]

One would like to believe that health officials stuck with their decision because of medical reasons. But there is past evidence that suggests that remaining vigilant, monitoring the risks associated with the polio vaccine and taking appropriate action to ensure the safety of the population is not the government's strongest suit. The forty-two year wait seems to be related to other things.

In 2000, the Evans / Medeva UK polio vaccine (OPV), which was made from UK calf blood between 1985 and 2000, was withdrawn because of the possibility of contamination with the variant CJD (mad cow disease).[20,21] The vaccine had continued to be made using calf blood throughout the 1990s, contravening European Union guidelines, even though variant CJD had been known about since the 1980s.[22] Thankfully, no case of vaccine-transmitted vCJD has yet been reported. Though the government described the risk from the vaccine as 'incalculably small', in a classic sleight of hand it instructed all doctors not to use any of the vaccine already in their possession.[23] 60,000 children and adults are known to have been given polio vaccine containing blood from a British donor who went on to develop vCJD.[24]

Only in January 2002 did the Joint Committee on Vaccination and Immunisation (JCVI), the body that advises the government on vaccination, decide that 'the move from OPV to IPV in primary immunisation should happen as soon as practicable.'[25] This was timed to coincide with the declaration of the WHO that Europe was free of wild polio. The UK finally switched back to the IPV in September 2004 as part of a '5-in-1' vaccine, lagging behind the vast majority of other western countries.

To this day, doctors and parents remain unaware that the mass vaccination of children between 1962 and 2004 with the cheaper OPV may not have been the great success story claimed, but instead a dangerous misjudgement, contributing no extra to the decline in polio, yet paralysing dozens of children.

8
When Is Polio not Polio?

WHO

Answer: when the WHO is trying to eradicate it.

This chapter takes a side-step from the investigation and is about the efforts of the World Health Organisation (WHO) to eradicate polio, and so some readers may want to cut to the chase and turn straight to the next chapter. I am including it here because it is a good example of how even this type of organisation has to resort to spin when protecting the star status of mass vaccination. In the interest of laudable goals, and the attempt to present vaccination as unequivocally beneficial, the twists and turns become so strained that the reality becomes hard to distinguish from fantasy.

The World Health Organisation declared Europe polio free in June 2002. The last known case of wild polio in Europe was in a two year old Turkish boy who was paralysed by the virus in 1998. The UK had, in effect, been 'polio free' for a good deal longer than this.

When reading this, however, you have to mentally adjust to the fact that this doesn't quite mean what you may think it means. 'Polio free' refers to the wild virus. People can still become paralysed from the live virus of the polio vaccine in a 'polio free' area.

There is also another adjustment worth noting. Polio is one of many causes of 'sudden floppy weakness' or AFP, acute flaccid paralysis, in medical terms. Other diseases can also cause the floppy paralysis of an arm or leg that is characteristic of AFP. When polio was widespread it was one of the most common causes of AFP. In its effort to eradicate polio, the World Health Organisation (WHO) has developed strict guidelines on diagnosing polio.[1] It doesn't want doctors diagnosing the disease unless they are absolutely sure that is what they are dealing with. It's now far more difficult to make a diagnosis of polio than it was fifty years ago. If these strict criteria aren't met, another diagnosis has to be made instead. Nowadays, the people that don't make the grade are more likely to be diagnosed as suffering from Guillain-Barré syndrome mentioned in the previous chapter, an illness causing remarkably similar symptoms to polio. Some have even suggested that Franklin D Roosevelt – the American president famous for running the USA as a polio sufferer from his wheelchair – instead had...GBS.[2]

Though GBS is not thought to be an infectious disease, 'outbreaks' of GBS have occurred in countries following mass polio immunisation campaigns.[3,4,5]

In Central and South America the number of cases of polio fell impressively from 930 a year to 6 between 1986 and 1991. But the number of AFP cases (including a large number of GBS cases), equally impressively, more than doubled from 1,000 to over 2,000 a year during the same period, more than accounting for the fall in the number of polio cases.[6] A similar trend has been seen more recently in India.[7] Could it be, as has been argued, that the 'outbreaks' of GBS that occurred after polio immunisation campaigns were side-effects of the polio vaccine, or polio proper, or live virus vaccine infections?

The Chinese were given a particularly hard time over their reclassification of 'polio' and AFP. The live virus vaccine was introduced to China in 1971, following which the numbers of polio cases started to slowly fall. But the numbers of people diagnosed with GBS increased tenfold. It was suggested, with unintended humour, they call the disease 'Chinese Paralytic Syndrome'.[8] Other doctors described a similar condition, with symptoms remarkably similar to polio, but with no polio virus detected, in other countries in Latin America and southern Asia.[9] Two Chinese doctors responded with a letter to the medical journal Lancet claiming that 'Chinese Paralytic Syndrome' was nothing new but was in fact…polio.'The epidemiological observations strongly suggest,' they continued, 'poliovirus as an agent in cases of GBS.'[10] They felt cases of polio were being misdiagnosed as both Chinese Paralytic Syndrome and GBS.

Is the WHO being over-enthusiastic in its attempt to rid the world of polio? There have been attempts to eradicate a total of seven diseases from the world: hookworm, yellow fever, yaws, malaria, smallpox, dracunculiasis and polio. The first four were total failures, the one and only famous success so far being smallpox.

The campaign to eradicate the world of polio has now become the largest international health campaign in history. Some ten million people have been involved in the eradication effort, at a cost of billions of dollars, and it may at last be reaching the end stage.

In 1988 the World Health Organisation (WHO) set a target for global eradication of polio by the end of 2000. The target date for polio eradication has since been postponed many times. At the end of 2003, the target date was the end of 2006 for the eradication of polio from the last remaining six countries in which it was still present, with a view to declaring the world 'polio-free' by the end of 2008. Towards the end of 2006, when this latest target had undeniably been missed, Bruce Aylward, of the WHO's Global Polio Initiative, promised 'We will not go into the next decade with polio', predicting eradication by 2010.[11] As I write this the most recent target for eradication is 2018.

The reality
At the end of 2003, the six countries with wild polio were Nigeria, India, Pakistan, Niger, Afghanistan and Egypt. Over 90% of cases were in Nigeria, India and Pakistan. The large numbers of cases in India and Pakistan were par-

ticularly disappointing as 90% of Indian children under five had received at least four doses of live polio vaccine (OPV), with the figure in Pakistan being 87%. Virtually all cases now diagnosed in India are in children who have received four or more doses of vaccine, with nearly half having been given ten doses.[12] Despite this, many cases of polio in India are being misdiagnosed and therefore not included in the official WHO figures.[13]

Eradication suffered a serious set-back when thirteen previously polio-free countries were re-infected.[14] By April 2006, wild polio transmission was re-established in a further eight countries. There were cases reported in a total of sixteen countries during 2005, though in the majority the virus had been imported. In 2005, there were large outbreaks in two countries (Indonesia and Yemen) that had both been polio-free for ten years.[15]

The effort to achieve eradication has been huge in many developing countries where preschool children have had to receive ten to fifteen doses of vaccine with near 100% coverage to get rid of the virus;[16] But the live OPV appears to be less effective in developing countries than in developed countries. The fight to eradicate polio is becoming increasingly frantic, with ever more children being given increasing doses of vaccine, to the extent that parents are beginning to mistrust the authorities and question the vaccine's effectiveness.[17] In 1997, 134 million Indian children were immunised on a single day, whilst Indonesia responded to polio's re-emergence there after ten years by vaccinating over five million children in a single day in 2005. Other countries have launched massive vaccination drives. Despite all these resources being poured in, outbreaks of polio have occurred in populations with 100% vaccination coverage.[18]

The total number of confirmed cases of paralysis from wild polio in the world in 2014 was 359 (plus 56 cases of paralysis from circulating polio vaccine), which appears tantalizingly close to elimination. However, only a very small number of cases result in paralysis, which means that the large majority of cases causing only diarrhoea and vomiting probably go undetected. The vast majority of cases were in Pakistan and Afghanistan.

Since 2003, numbers were steadily rising, largely because of an outbreak in Nigeria as a result of fears over the safety of the vaccine. Similar fears resurfaced in 2007 in Pakistan, where the parents of 24,000 children refused to allow their babies to be given the vaccine — there were rumours that the vaccines were an American plot to sterilise Muslim children.[19] Compulsory vaccination is now being considered. (Indeed compulsion is alive and well in Belgium where, in 2008, two sets of parents were fined 5500 (per parent) and given a suspended five-month prison sentence for refusing to have their children vaccinated.) In Namibia, at least thirty-four people developed polio in 2006, and seven died, after a ten-year absence of the disease.[20] A small victory was achieved when Egypt had its first full year of no polio cases during 2005. Also the total number of countries with polio circulating in the community (as opposed to imported cases) has been steadily falling. However, in 2008, six countries that were previously polio-free had ongoing transmission: Angola, Chad, the Democratic Republic of the Congo, Ethiopia, Niger and Sudan.[22]

However, since the turn of the century numbers have been falling. As of 2012 the big success story is that India has gone a full year without a case of wild polio, leaving Afghanistan and Pakistan and Nigeria as the only countries where wild polio remains endemic.

Another question is — what should be done after the world becomes 'polio-free' from wild polio, should that goal be reached. In 2004, the WHO warned that 'the potential risk of [mutated live-virus vaccine infection] emergence has increased dramatically in recent years.'[21]

Most countries have now switched to IPV, which cannot be transmitted to others and cause paralysis, and nearly all countries should be using the IPV by the end of 2016. However, it is more expensive and, being given by injection rather than drops, requires greater expertise to give.

This switch to the safer vaccine has become all the more urgent with outbreaks of cVDPP in 2015 causing paralysis in 8 people in Madagascar and, closer to home, 2 children in Ukraine close to the Hungarian border. Outbreaks of cVDPP were also ongoing in 2016 in Guinea, the Lao People's Democratic Republic and Myanmar.

The road to polio eradication has been very rocky, often two steps forward and one back. However, with a total of only 74 cases reported in 2015, eradication in the near future is now a real possibility.

9
Tetanus

A Country Affair

Tetanus is unique amongst all the diseases for which children are vaccinated. It is the only infection that we do not catch from other people. Like diphtheria, tetanus is caused by a powerful poison, in this case poison of the spores of the Clostridium tetani bacterium. These spores are found all over the world in contaminated soil and manure. If they infect a wound, the toxin can cause painful muscle cramps, 'lockjaw', and, if severe, spasms of the whole body which can lead to death.

No one knows what proportion of those coming into contact with the tetanus poison, in soil or manure, go down with tetanus. This is partly because about half of those who catch tetanus don't even know they've injured themselves. But of those who get ill in this country, one in five will die, even with modern treatment.

As people do not themselves transmit tetanus, it has never been a big killer in the UK. Since the beginning of the twentieth century, it has been rare for more than two hundred people a year to die in the UK from tetanus. The largest outbreak of tetanus in recent years in the UK was twenty cases in injecting drug users in 2003 and 2004, probably from contaminated batches of heroin. People nowadays no longer come into contact that much with contaminated soil and animal faeces in which the tetanus bacterium lives. For the last fifteen years fewer than ten people have died every year in this country, and no child has died from tetanus in the UK since 1975. The disease is a much bigger problem in less developed countries where tetanus of the newborn kills 180,000 children every year. This is sometimes caused by the application of animal dung to the cut umbilical cord.

At the beginning of the twentieth century, at around the same time that an 'anti-poison' was discovered for diphtheria, so one was also discovered for tetanus. It was not given as a preventive, like a vaccine, but as an antidote after the injury that put someone at risk of tetanus. As most tetanus infections are acquired from soil, fighting on the Western Front in the First World War was a high-risk environment. It was here that tetanus anti-poison was first used successfully on a large scale, and it reduced the number of cases dramatically. Unfortunately, the antidote was made from horse blood and caused frequent side-effects, the worse being fatal allergic reactions, especially after a second or third treatment.

In the same way that the tetanus anti-poison was first tried out on a large scale in the First World War, so the immunisation was first 'tested' extensively amongst servicemen in the Second World War. It seemed to work. The British and American armies had remarkably few cases of tetanus, but the disease was much more common in the Germans who had not been immunised.

This 'trial' on the army constitutes the main evidence for the effectiveness of the tetanus vaccine. Soon after the war it was recommended as part of the newly evolving childhood immunisation schedule and in 1961 was incorporated into the DTP triple vaccine along with whooping cough and diphtheria.

There have been surprisingly few proper trials to test for its effectiveness. Looking at deaths in the UK from tetanus in the twentieth century, it is clear that deaths were steadily falling throughout the century, long before the introduction of the vaccine. Some of this improvement must have been due to the use of (the somewhat hazardous) horse anti-poison, of which up to a million doses were being used every year. Nonetheless, at the time of introduction of tetanus immunisation in the mid-1950s, there were between thirty and forty deaths a year in the UK. There was no convincing drop occurring as a result of the introduction of immunisation. Deaths continued to fall as they had before, and there is currently about one death, and five to eight cases, a year in the UK. It is difficult to know how much of the fall is due to immunisation and how much to not coming into contact with the tetanus spores in the soil.

One thing that's for certain is that no immunisation is 100% effective and tetanus vaccination is no exception. There have been numerous reports of tetanus occurring in, and even occasionally killing, both adults and children who were fully immunised.[1,2] In some cases, they were known to have high antibody levels against tetanus toxin — something that is expected to offer protection.[3]

There is also some uncertainty over how many boosters are required to provide life-long immunity. Whilst the Department of Health advises that a total of five doses will provide 'satisfactory long-term protection' for most circumstances, other experts believe that this may not be enough.[4] The confusion arises because no one actually knows what length of protection five doses offer.[5] It is concerning, but perhaps not surprising when taken in the context of other vaccines, that there has been so little research on a vaccine so widely used for such a long time. A recent random sampling of adults in Ireland showed that only 7 out of 10 (70%) were immune, and that protection was less likely in older people, indicating that protection does wear off over time and that those in high risk jobs, such as those working with animals, might benefit from extra booster doses.[6]

The difference with other vaccines
Aware of the side-effects that are historically well-documented, health officials are careful with this vaccine. Tetanus immunisation often causes pain, redness and swelling at the site of the injection. The more injections any one person receives, the more common these local, but uncomfortable, side-effects

become. This is one reason why the Department of Health, quite rightly, advises against indiscriminate boosters of the vaccine. Over-vaccination has also been found to affect both the liver and kidneys.[7] Tetanus vaccination — like diphtheria vaccination — will never eradicate the organism itself because it only acts against the poison and doesn't affect the tetanus bacterium that produces it.

Children are vaccinated against the disease, regardless of whether they are likely to be exposed to the poison. But because tetanus immunisation has always been given to children in combination with other vaccines (diphtheria and whooping cough initially, then also Hib, and now polio as well), it is all but impossible to single out side-effects due entirely to the tetanus component.

Fever, drowsiness, fretfulness, vomiting, and going off feeds can all occur in young children given tetanus-containing vaccines. Neuritis, an inflammation of one or more nerves causing a partial paralysis or lack of feeling that is occasionally permanent, is a very rare complication.[8] Guillain-Barré Syndrome (GBS), the disorder of the nerves discussed in the polio chapter and causing, usually temporary, paralysis can probably be caused by the vaccine.[9] Though there are reports of arthritis, and even temporary coma occurring after a tetanus vaccine, serious side-effects caused by tetanus vaccine alone are probably very rare.[10] If this vaccine tells us anything, it is how useful it is to know what it does and also how infrequently we check whether a particular vaccine is still necessary.

10
Measles
The 'Killer' Disease

'Love is like the measles; we all have to go through it.'[1] This quote from the writer Jerome K Jerome would now land him in considerable trouble with the health authorities. Measles is one of the diseases health officials have set their sights on and will allow no heresy. In December 2006 Dr David Salisbury, the head of immunisation at the Department of Health, gave the official message on measles: 'We have consistently had evidence that parents view measles as a trivial disease. Now it may often be a trivial disease, but measles has the potential to be a very serious disease and it has the potential to kill people. And one of the priorities was to raise the parental awareness of the seriousness of measles. Now this came from the parents themselves. They said to our researchers that if we wanted their support, we had to convince them that measles was serious.'[2]

What are the facts on measles? The disease lives only on people and has very distinctive symptoms, unlike polio, for example, which is only apparent when it is quite serious. It was unknown to the famous Greek doctor Hippocrates (ca. 460 BC–ca. 370 BC), but it probably surfaced in Rome around 250 AD and is now found all over the world.

The illness is caused by the measles virus. It starts like a cold with a cough, runny nose and fever. The eyes typically become red (conjunctivitis or 'pinkeye' in the USA) and the characteristic measles rash appears around the fourth day of illness on the neck and spreads over the whole body during the next two days. By the tenth day the majority of children recover, but some develop the complications that can cause serious problems. It is very infectious and before vaccination everyone caught the disease, usually during the early years of life, with epidemics occurring every other year.

At the beginning of the twentieth century, the seriousness of the disease was at an all-time high and Dr Salisbury's official message would not have been hard to justify. The number of people dying from measles was greater than deaths from smallpox, scarlet fever and diphtheria combined. Thus, a century ago, it would have been reasonable to describe measles as a 'killer disease' — but not now.

Since then, there has been a massive decline in the total number of deaths. Between 1900 and the end of the First World War, in 1918, an average of 10,000 to 12,000 children were dying from measles every year. Over the next forty years there was a steady but steep fall in deaths so that, by the mid-1950s, the total annual number of deaths rarely exceeded 100. Reporting of measles cases (as opposed to deaths) was made compulsory in 1940, and these allow the death rate, that is the chances of dying if you catch measles, to be calculated. These figures, too, make clear that the disease has become harmless in relative terms. The death rate from measles in 1940 was one in 690. By 1960 the death rate had fallen to one in 5,000 cases.[3] These plummeting rates happened well before the introduction of vaccination. In fact, if the rate of fall of measles deaths had continued as it had done throughout the twentieth century, the numbers of children dying would have reached fewer than one death per year by 2007.

Nonetheless, since the 1960s health officials have given themselves the task to mass vaccinate against the disease in the conviction it is a serious potential killer. On what dangers does the Department of Health base its conviction that measles is so serious that it requires intervention on a massive scale with the goal of eradication?

The disease affects over 90% of children in such a way they will get through an attack of measles with nothing worse than a week of feeling rather miserable. The real danger, however, of measles is actually slightly different from other diseases. Because measles suppresses the immune system most complications are due, not to the measles virus itself, but to other organisms that 'take advantage' of the weakened child and invade some area of the body. The risks were as follows in 1963:[4]

- A fit (or convulsion) occurs in about one in 500 cases.
- A middle ear infection. This is rarely serious and can usually be successfully treated with antibiotics but can result in a permanent hearing loss. It occurs in about one in 40 cases.
- The measles virus invades the brain (encephalitis) in one in 1,000 children. This varies from being so mild that it isn't even noticed, to being so serious that it kills. It's the second most common cause of death. Around 15% of those getting encephalitis will die, though the majority will make a full recovery.
- Pneumonia or other chest infection. Pneumonia is the most common cause of death from measles. It isn't caused by the measles virus itself but by a bacterial infection that can usually be successfully treated with antibiotics. One in 26 children who develop measles go on to develop a chest infection, of which the most serious form is pneumonia. It occurs in 2-3% of children.
- SSPE (Subacute sclerosing panencephalitis) is, thankfully, very rare as it's a terrible disease in which the measles virus infects the brain. Instead of causing normal encephalitis, a slow insidious disease results in inevitable death some years later. This probably occurs in one in every 200,000 cases.
- Death. The death rate was around one in 5,000 cases in the UK.

It is important to note that the risks above were all average risks, and there are considerable differences between age and social groups, for example. Long before vaccination, it was observed that, 'measles was one disease for the rich and another for the poor.' In 1931, the death rate from measles in children aged one in the lowest social class was nearly twenty times that of children in the highest class, a distinction that still exists.[6,7]

Malnourished children from poorer families suffer from a greater proportion of deaths and complications from measles, and also have impaired antibody production, compared to healthy children.[8,9] The same applies to the chronically ill, and to those who live in overcrowded conditions; they are more likely to suffer complications and die.[10] Almost half the children who died from measles in the UK before vaccination were severely physically or mentally disabled.[11]

Treatment, such as it was, was not comprehensively available to the poor and consisted of a combination of lotions, diet and inhalations; silver nitrate would be applied to any associated conjunctivitis, whilst the most dreaded complication, pneumonia, would call for fresh air, inhalations of carbolic acid vapour, jacket poultices of linseed meal, and a little drop of brandy. Some argued that being cared for in hospital would provide a child with an 'ample supply of fresh air and suitable feeding' that was often unavailable in the 'stuffy and frequently overcrowded atmosphere of a poor home.'[12] However, others warned the high death rate of children admitted to hospital was due to the abundance of organisms that could cause a fatal pneumonia, and advised caring for children at home.

Today it is difficult to maintain measles is a killer disease. There were three deaths from measles — of which only one was in a child — reported over four years (2001-2004) by nineteen European countries.[13] Occasionally there still is a scare in the media. In 2006, for example, there was widespread media coverage of the death of a thirteen-year-old boy in England from measles. The circumstances were exceptional, though. He suffered from a chronic underlying lung condition, and was also taking immunosuppressive drugs — both of these would have increased the risks to him of measles, or many other infectious diseases.[14] A seventeen-year-old boy from West Yorkshire died from measles in 2008; he too had immune problems, having been born with a poor immune system. These were the only deaths form measles in the UK in anyone under 15 years of age from the turn of the century to 2013. The most recent outbreak of measles in the UK was in South Wales in 2013 causing over 1,200 cases of measles. There was one death in a 25-year-old man with significant underlying health problems.

An outbreak of measles in the USA in 2014 (with 644 cases) helped fuel a tightening of the criteria for vaccine exemption in a several states.

The development of the measles vaccine
The development of a vaccine to eradicate the disease did not exactly run smoothly. A live measles vaccine was first developed in the 1950s in the USA. After early trials showed unacceptable side-effects, a revised vaccine was

licensed for routine use on American children in 1963. One of the first trials of a measles vaccine in the UK was on 154 children in an area where, it was believed, an epidemic was developing. Though the vaccine used appeared to be very effective (none of those vaccinated developed measles whereas many unvaccinated children did get the disease), a fifth of the children developed severe reactions.[15]

A killed vaccine was tried next which didn't produce the serious reactions of the live vaccine, but neither did it prevent the vaccinated children from getting measles — it didn't work. So attempts were made to develop a less harmful live vaccine that would successfully prevent measles without the nasty side-effects. The only large trial comparing a measles vaccine to a placebo (nothing) was conducted in the UK between 1964 and 1969. This demonstrated an effectiveness of the live vaccine of between 84% and 95%. (Interestingly, the researchers commented on the small number of complications of natural measles that they had seen, reporting only one case of inflammation of the brain, encephalitis, in over 7,000 cases of measles, providing further evidence that measles was becoming a milder illness.)[16]

By the late 1960s, a measles vaccine was ready for the UK. But was the UK ready for the vaccine? The risk of dying from measles was only a fraction of what it had been fifty years earlier, which led to a debate in the UK throughout the 1960s on whether the vaccine should be introduced or not. A British Medical Journal editorial argued in 1963, 'measles is now a mild disease, and many parents and doctors may feel that no protection against it is required.'[17]

At that time about eighty children were still dying of measles every year. This was not many as a proportion of the whole population, but why let them die, it was argued, if vaccination could prevent most of their deaths? There were also a hundred cases of encephalitis a year, some of which resulted in permanent disability and these too could be prevented by vaccination. In addition, as many as one in fifteen children who caught measles were developing potentially serious complications such as pneumonia.

It was accepted by everyone that there was a strong case for vaccinating those at particular risk of developing measles: those, for example, with chronic diseases, or who were severely disabled, as they are far more likely to die from measles than healthy children. But the case for immunising all children was far less clear cut. 'Even before vaccine was introduced, measles appeared to be becoming a trivial disease in civilised communities,' wrote vaccine expert Professor George Dick in the leading British Medical Journal in 1980. 'There is something to be said,' he continued, 'for allowing a mild 'wild' measles virus to give a natural life-long protection to the healthy children of the community and to offer vaccine selectively to those [who are most vulnerable] or who have escaped a natural infection in the early years of childhood.'[18]

But there were concerns about the long-term implications of mass vaccination against measles. It was suggested that some sort of 'natural immunity' to measles had developed in this country, making it the mild illness it had become. If measles were eradicated with widespread vaccination, this 'natural immunity' would be replaced by vaccine immunity. It is notoriously difficult to maintain vaccine uptake for diseases that no longer exist. If vaccine uptake were to fall after measles had disappeared, the reintroduction of measles from another country might result in epidemics in both children and adults. This was not the talk of a radical anti-vaccine group, but the voice of the medical establishment:[17] don't intervene with nature unless you are sure you have to.

The proponents of aggressive vaccination, however, won and the national vaccination programme for measles began in May 1968. Two measles vaccines were initially available, but one of these was withdrawn in the following March after reports of inflammation of the brain (encephalitis) in two children after they had received the vaccine.[19]

Like live OPV polio vaccine, the vaccine consisted of live measles viruses that had been 'attenuated', or made relatively harmless when compared to the 'wild' measles virus. The measles vaccine couldn't be given with the other DTP (diphtheria, tetanus and whooping cough) and polio vaccines in the first months of life because it does not work well until the baby is twelve months old. This is because the baby is born with antibodies (cells of the immune system) to protect against measles that are supplied by the mother in the womb. These provide some protection to the newborn baby in the first months of life against wild measles, but also react against the live measles virus vaccine in the same way – preventing the baby from producing its own antibodies. In the days when all mothers caught measles and passed on natural antibodies, these provided protection against measles in babies for 6 to 12 months. The protection passed on by vaccinated mothers lasts for a much shorter time, with most babies losing immunity by 3 months of age and very few being protected beyond 6 months.[54]

Mass vaccination fell well short of what was needed to bring about eradication of the disease. The British public wasn't particularly enthusiastic and the uptake of the vaccine picked up to around 50% by 1972 where it stayed until 1980, when it slowly increased to 75% by 1987, just before the MMR vaccine was introduced. As recently as 1980 a specialist in infectious diseases predicted, 'in any event acceptance rates in Britain are never likely to reach the 80-90% that eradication seems to demand.'[20] (This is now believed to be around 95% – if eradication can be achieved at all.) The introduction and promotion of the MMR resulted in a boost in vaccine uptake.

How effective is the vaccine?

The (single) measles vaccine produces antibodies in at least 95% of children. But its actual effectiveness at preventing an attack of measles in the real world is probably 90% at most – and nearer to 70%, or even 50%, in developing countries.[16,21,22,23] That means, at best, that of every ten children vaccinated, nine will be protected against measles and one won't. But it's not that straight-forward, because the effectiveness of the vaccine depends on the age at which it is given. The vaccine is only 77% effective when given at 9-11 months but this rises to over 90% effectiveness when given over 12 months.[55] However, a study on children during a recent outbreak in Canada suggests that the vaccine is most effective when given at or after 15 months.[56] The protection is long-term. How long? Probably at least 25 years, but immunity from natural measles is always better and longer-lasting than that obtained from vaccination. So, though the vaccine appears to be reasonably effective in preventing measles, how much effect has it really had on the number of children dying from measles in this country?

The Department of Health would like us to believe that the measles vaccine is the main cause of the fall in deaths from measles. It is certainly true that deaths from measles have fallen since the introduction of immunisation. There were over 100 deaths in alternate epidemic years from 1960 that were immediately reduced, after the introduction of the single measles vaccine in 1968, to 40 deaths a year. This continued to decline until the introduction of the MMR in 1988 when the death rate was reduced to approaching zero.[24]

But it must be remembered that the death rate had been continuously falling since the First World War. It would be reasonable to assume that the introduction of antibiotics in the 1930s might have hastened the decline of measles deaths, by preventing those from pneumonia, but there's no convincing evidence for this, since the decline continued after the introduction of antibiotics much as it did before. The impact of the measles vaccine on measles deaths over the whole century was tiny, with 99% of the decline occurring before the introduction of the vaccine. The main reasons for the fall in deaths from measles were probably improved nutrition, sanitation and living standards, and possibly the development of a 'natural' immunity to the disease.

Like most vaccines, the measles vaccine works to a degree, though giving a child one, or even two, measles-containing vaccines (that is the single measles or MMR) is no guarantee that he or she won't catch the disease.

The measles vaccine consists of live measles viruses. They've been 'attenuated' to become less harmful than 'wild' measles viruses but, because they are live, and can multiply and spread in the body, they can produce most of the same complications that can occur with measles. In fact, the most common 'side-effects' of measles vaccination are symptoms identical to that of natural, or 'wild', measles infection. Measles vaccine can cause permanent brain damage and SSPE (the rare but fatal brain disease) — though almost certainly less commonly than wild measles.[25,26,27] It causes a fit, or convulsion, in one in 2,000 vaccinations.

One of the most thorough studies ever done into serious brain damage from vaccinations suggests that measles vaccination causes a 'serious neurological disorder', such as encephalitis or prolonged convulsions, in one in every 87,000 children vaccinated.[28] Between 1968 and 2005, doctors notified the Department of Health of 114 children who developed encephalitis or encephalopathy (serious brain diseases) as a result, they believed, of receiving a measles-containing vaccine.[29]

This may not sound many, but doctors probably report fewer than 10% of drug and vaccine side-effects. In fact the JCVI, the expert advisory body that advises the government, noted as long ago as 1973 that more than one case of encephalitis was being reported for every 100,000 vaccinations. Assuming a 10% reporting rate (and it's unlikely to be that high), that equates to more than one child in every 10,000 suffering encephalitis as a result of the measles vaccine.[30] One study from Germany found the risk of any sort of brain damage to be as common as one in 17,650 vaccinations, though nearly all made a good recovery and the risk is still fewer than that from the disease.[31]

Measles vaccine can also cause the rare auto-immune bleeding disorder ITP (Idiopathic Thrombocytopenic Purpura) once in every half a million vaccinations. Though ITP is potentially serious, most children make a full recovery within six months. Children with severe immune disorders (which are very rare) have died following measles vaccination because the measles vaccine contains live viruses which their damaged immune systems were unable to eliminate.[32] It's not always possible to detect these children in advance.

Most children who catch measles get a rash. Some children, unusually, get an 'atypical measles,' which may involve an unusual rash, or no rash at all, often with a higher likelihood of complications. Children who appear to have suffered measles without getting any rash are particularly prone in later life to disorders of the immune system such as arthritis, skin problems or cancer. Atypical measles occurred more commonly following use of the killed measles vaccine, which is no longer in use; however it can also occur after the live vaccine used today.

Finally, the measles virus has been implicated in some children's autism. This is particularly so for a sub-group of children who suffer from regressive autism, and bowel disease. The measles virus has been found in the gut, blood and even brain of these children. In most cases the measles virus is believed to have come from the MMR vaccine but, in a small number, could have come from the single measles vaccine.

Vaccination has changed the profile of the groups at risk, too. Before vaccination, nearly all children caught measles before 10 years of age, with babies protected during the first months of life by maternal antibodies. The expected effect of large-scale vaccination against measles was to increase the average age at which children caught it. This was predictable, because it's an inevitable consequence of vaccinating against a childhood illness. Before vaccination, virtually all children acquired natural life-long immunity from the illness. But once you start vaccinating children, they stop getting the disease at the normal young age that they used to; instead, measles is caught by older children and adults who were either never vaccinated, or whose immunity obtained from vaccination has worn off. The protection given by natural infection is life-long whereas that from vaccination is far shorter. And the problem with more teenagers and adults getting measles is that the disease is more likely to cause serious complications in these age groups. The other group at greater risk than before vaccination are the under one-year-olds. Their mothers are now more likely to be vaccinated and not to have had measles; these babies no longer receive the same protection from their mothers' wombs and now are more susceptible to measles. The risk of getting the rare, but deadly, slow encephalitis (SSPE) is sixteen times higher in children under one year of age.[33] The risk of death, though still small, is higher in babies under one year and adults.

Is mass vaccination against measles necessary today?

This is answered by the question whether there is any point in following the 1960s dream of eradicating the disease. The term 'herd immunity' describes the percentage of the population that needs to be vaccinated (or is naturally immune to a disease) to prevent it spreading through the community and so, potentially, eradicating it. The herd immunity is different for different diseases and depends on how easily a disease is spread from one person to another. The herd immunity required to eliminate measles was originally thought to be around 80-90%, but is now believed to be 95%.

We're told that if we can get 95% of the population vaccinated against measles then it will disappear. Unfortunately experience does not bear this out. There have been several outbreaks of measles in schools and colleges where over 99% of the children had been vaccinated, many twice, or even three times.[34,35,36] A report of one outbreak stated, 'We conclude that outbreaks of measles can occur in secondary schools, even when more than 99% of the students have been vaccinated and more than 95% are immune.'[37] The vaccination rate in one school outbreak was as high as 99.9%.[34]

Back in 1982, there was anticipation that 'measles could be the next human disease [after smallpox] to become extinct.'[38] The World Health Organisation (WHO) more recently recommended that measles be eliminated from Europe by 2007, a target that was extended to 2010 and then 2015. It hasn't happened. However, some European countries, such as Iceland and Finland, appear to have already succeeded in getting rid of measles from their countries. The Americas were officially declared 'measles-free' by the WHO in September 2016. But the global elimination of measles is turning out to be a tough challenge. 'Eradication of measles has been much more difficult than originally anticipated' wrote a group of vaccination experts in 1998.[39] The WHO has more recently modified its aim of eradication. Bjørn Melgaard, head of vaccines at the WHO, admitted in 2001 'we may not be able to eradicate measles, and it may not even be worth it to try.'[40] There is evidence that the measles virus can circulate in an apparently immune population.[41] It's now questionable whether giving every child two measles vaccines during childhood — an impossible task in itself — would lead to eradication of the disease.

If children don't get vaccinated, then of course there will be outbreaks of measles. It doesn't take a medical degree to figure that one out. However, outbreaks can occur despite an extremely high level of vaccination coverage (over 95%).

But there are many things, other than vaccination, that will help children get through measles without becoming seriously ill. A healthy immune system is dependent on numerous factors in our lifestyles. Eating well, living in a healthy, unpolluted environment and being free of chronic diseases and health problems all help promote a healthy immune system. Not living in overcrowded conditions helps prevent serious complications from measles, and a well-ventilated house helps prevent others in the house catching the disease. Giving vitamin A to children with measles is proven to have a huge effect on reducing deaths and serious complications in developing countries where the illness is still a 'killer disease': it may also help reduce the severity of the disease in developed countries.

Finally, there's disturbing evidence that the measles virus may be beginning to become resistant to the measles vaccine.[42] Outbreaks of an extremely dangerous form of measles, caused by a mutant measles virus, have caused dozens of deaths in India.[43] Some measles viruses are changing their genetic sequences — possibly galvanised by vaccination; we may be creating a more dangerous, mutant strain of measles because of the worldwide vaccination campaign.[44]

Could measles be good for you?

There is a belief among some parents that catching measles could actually be good for their child. Although this sounds suspiciously like an old wives' tale, research suggests that there may be some truth in it.

For example, in 1998 there was an outbreak of measles in a largely unvaccinated anthroposophical community (followers of the spiritual philosophy of Rudolph Steiner) in Gloucestershire.[45] Nearly all the 126 cases were relatively mild, though one child was admitted to hospital. Only three parents felt their child's illness had changed their negative opinion on vaccination. Interestingly, many parents felt their child had strengthened and matured, both physically and mentally, as a result of the measles infection.[46]

In fact, the belief of followers of Rudolph Steiner's anthroposophical teachings, that catching measles 'strengthened' their children, is receiving increasing support from scientific research. Children from a Rudolph Steiner school in Germany who had suffered measles were less likely to have allergic eczema than other children.[47] In another group of children, doctors noticed a clear improvement in their eczema after they had suffered an attack of measles.[48] Recent research suggests that catching measles protects the child from getting asthma and other allergic diseases later in life.[49 53] It's also known that children in West Africa who suffered, and survived, an attack of measles were less likely to die over the next four years than children who didn't catch measles.[50] However, this is a controversial subject and other research refutes this.

Do health officials still believe themselves?

The Department of Health has appeared confused as to when an outbreak may, or may not, occur. Ever since MMR levels started slipping below 90% in the late 1990s we have been repeatedly warned of imminent measles epidemics. However, at the same time as other doctors were warning of imminent measles outbreaks, in January 2002 the government's Chief Medical Officer, Sir Liam Donaldson, was reported as saying: 'There is no epidemic of measles and there is no concern that there will be.'⁵¹ (In the following month, there was an outbreak of measles in London with 90 confirmed cases, some of whom had received the MMR vaccine).

At the same time that Sir Liam was reassuring the country, there was concern in North Cheshire that MMR rates were dropping to a dangerous level. The health authority ordered doctors to give a 'single message' to encourage uptake of the MMR vaccine. The title of the health authority's campaign?

'Killer disease ready to strike.'⁵²

11
Whooping Cough

A Campaign of Terror

Whooping cough is the one infectious disease that remains a real threat to this day, but it also reveals most about how health officials spin results. It is also the one I grappled with myself as a parent when my son required vaccination, and I was particularly interested in investigating this vaccine for this book. At the time, after initial misgivings, I was persuaded by expert opinion to have my son vaccinated. Would I have done so if I had completed the research for this book?

What is the disease like?
Whooping cough is an infectious disease that has three characteristic phases. The initial stage consists of a cough, runny nose and temperature — just like a bad cold (the 'catarrhal' stage). This is typically followed, after a week, by uncontrollable spasms of coughing which, when severe, are separated only by the 'whoop' as the child forcefully breathes in between coughing bouts (the 'paroxysmal' stage). The final 'resolution' stage heralds an improvement in the child's condition and the road to recovery, though this can take some time, which is why the disease is also known as the 'hundred-day cough'.

It is, therefore, a very apt name for the disease that used to be a frequent killer. In the nineteenth century, many children died from the disease. Along with smallpox, measles and scarlet fever, it was one of the most common causes of death in the first 10 years of life. At the start of the twentieth century, 10,000 children a year were dying from whooping cough but the death rate fell sharply during the first half of the century.

During this period, there was no effective treatment for whooping cough. Apart from fresh air and adequate nourishment, the only treatments offered by doctors in the first half of the twentieth century would have included belladonna (deadly nightshade) and barbiturates to calm the child during the uncontrollable spasms of coughing. The advent of antibiotics in the 1940s brought hope, but these were disappointingly ineffective in treating the disease. Antibiotics did, however, help treat pneumonia, the complication that was by far the most common cause of death.

Nowadays, most cases are relatively mild with fewer than half developing the characteristic 'whoop'. As most children with whooping cough only have what appears to be a bad cold followed by a cough, it's very easy to miss now.

Serious complications can still occur though.[1]

The whooping cough vaccine has had a long and chequered history like some others discussed so far. Though the vaccine had been in use as early as the 1920s, the first trials in the UK started in 1942. During the 1940s, some areas of the country introduced vaccination if their medical officer recommended it. Healthcare was far less centralised then. The introduction of a vaccine in some parts of the country, but not others, would never be considered now. But it made sense even if it probably wasn't a conscious decision. The effectiveness and side-effects could be tested in the 'real world' over time. We can still learn something from the more cautious pace and greater rigour of sixty years ago.

The early trials in the 1940s were disappointing, showing no benefit to children from vaccination. During the late 1940s, the Medical Research Council organised an excellent trial with four different whooping cough vaccines. All vaccines tested worked, with an average effectiveness over the first twenty-seven months of 78%. But the vaccines weren't all equally effective. It varied from vaccine to vaccine, from 61% to 89% — a large difference.[2]

Following the results, a standard vaccine was prepared from one of the more effective vaccines in the trial. By the late 1950s the whooping cough vaccine was in widespread use in the UK, and in 1961 it was launched nationally in a triple vaccine along with diphtheria and tetanus (DTP).[3]

*

Lethal side-effects

Doctors were alerted to the potential dangers of the vaccine as long ago as 1933, when two babies died immediately after receiving the whooping cough vaccination.[4] Over the next 20 years there were numerous reports of brain damage following immunisation, resulting in convulsions, permanent physical or mental disability or even death.[5,6,7,8,9] It led to widespread acceptance amongst all doctors that the vaccine could occasionally cause brain damage. What doctors couldn't agree on was how common, or rare, this was. Estimates of the frequency of brain damage occurring after whooping cough immunisation varied from one in a million to an alarming one in ten thousand.[10]

Though the whooping cough vaccine was introduced into the national immunisation programme in 1961, doctors also disagreed publicly on the necessity or value of immunisation. Those who supported vaccination believed that the partial use of the vaccine had caused the fall in deaths from whooping cough during the 1950s. Others disagreed, arguing the fall in death rate was mainly due to better social conditions. They also felt that whooping cough was becoming a milder illness, killing very few children compared to the early decades of the century. Moreover, they felt the potentially serious side-effects of the vaccine meant it shouldn't be used on a widespread basis.

Nevertheless, by the late 1960s over three quarters of all babies were being immunised against whooping cough. A first small scare flared up when two batches of apparently 'toxic' whooping cough-containing vaccine were given to babies in the UK and Ireland between 1968 and 1970. The vaccine was reported to be between eight and fourteen times more potent than the standard dose.

Another 14 batches, containing thousands of vaccine doses, were not put through toxicity tests. The vaccine, 'Trivax', was made by the British company Wellcome. The concerns of parents and some experts were brushed aside at the time and it was only decades later that the truth was made public. Wellcome is now part of multinational GSK, which does not accept that the batches were harmful.

As if that were not enough, it also emerged that ostensibly some babies in Ireland might have been given Wellcome's veterinary vaccine by mistake. GSK has said this is most unlikely. The batch numbers of Trivax and Tribovax, intended for cattle, were remarkably similar and the company has suggested that the batch numbers may have been incorrectly recorded.[11,12,13]

The 1970s whooping cough scare

The real whooping cough crisis, the one I recall as a parent, started several years later. It began with the findings of a distinguished doctor relating to a small group of children. Dr John Wilson was a consultant paediatric neurologist at Great Ormond Street Hospital. He saw children, with conditions such as severe epilepsy or brain damage, who came to Great Ormond Street for specialist assessment and treatment. He became aware that many parents were telling him a similar story. Their child had been immunised with the whooping cough vaccine and within a few days − most often only a few hours − started to fit uncontrollably, often screaming or becoming unconscious. Over the following months the fits would become more frequent and the child would become mentally or physically disabled. In 1973, Dr Wilson stood up at the annual meeting of the British Paediatric Association and described, to the medical audience, thirty-six of the children he had seen at Great Ormond Street. The majority of these children were left mentally retarded and with persistent fits. The cause of the brain damage in these children was, he felt, the whooping cough vaccine. He recommended caution in giving this vaccine.

His speech and subsequent published paper triggered a vaccine scare, the like of which was not to be seen again until the MMR furore of more recent years.[14] The widespread media coverage resulted in a sharp drop in take-up of the whooping cough vaccine. Whereas around 78% of children were having the vaccine in the early 1970s, this dropped to a low of 31% in 1978.

The government acted promptly to make the components of the triple DTP vaccine available separately. Parents who didn't want to give their children the whooping cough (the P, for pertussis-'violent cough', of the DTP) component were still able to immunise them against diphtheria and tetanus. Concern wasn't confined to parents; a survey of family doctors in 1974 showed that over half had seen convulsions and other serious side-effects of the whooping cough vaccine, and they were divided on whether to continue vaccinating or not. A third of family doctors no longer gave children the whooping cough vaccine, a third continued giving it and a third followed parents' wishes.[15]

There was widespread misinformation on both sides. The frenzy of media publicity was unprecedented, and has an uncanny resemblance to later events surrounding the MMR. Television documentaries and newspaper reports dramatised tragic stories of brain-damaged children who were, their parents claimed, injured by the vaccine. Even the sober *Sunday Times* ran a story with the headline 'Boy's brain damaged in vaccine experiment.'

The Department of Health responded to this adverse publicity to the whooping cough vaccine with its own propaganda campaign of exaggeration that a senior doctor at the time called a 'campaign of terror'. It resulted in the pro-vaccine headlines: 'Killer Disease Strikes Again,' and 'Epidemic Claims New Victim'. Dr Herbert Barrie was a consultant paediatrician at London's Charing Cross Hospital during the period. He describes the extraordinary next move of the health officials. 'A pre-recorded phone-in service was installed...to 'inform' parents about the vaccine. Anybody calling this number was greeted with a blood-curdling series of spasms of coughing, followed by a diatribe on the imminent dangers of brain damage, lung damage and demise. The message ended, like a bad commercial, with a high-pitched hysterical exaltation, 'If your child has not been vaccinated, do not delay. There is an epidemic. Get your child vaccinated now!' This was followed by another paroxysm and what sounded like a last gasp.'

The message being put out by the government was epitomised by a poster stating, 'Whooping Cough is a Killer'. As Dr Barrie pointed out 'With 13 deaths and 65,772 survivors this is overstating the case.' This children's doctor felt that priorities were misplaced 'when we have an annual total of 1,500 cot deaths, 2,000 child deaths from accidents and 2,500 avoidable perinatal deaths.'[16]

Though its tactics over later years were a little more subtle (to parents at least), the government's attempt to strike fear in their hearts has disturbing similarities to more recent efforts to boost the uptake of the MMR vaccine by scaring parents as much as possible.

The epidemics

The scare created an unplanned experiment. Never before had immunisation, once it was in place, dropped off to such a spectacularly low level where fewer than one in three children was vaccinated. By sheer chance the whooping cough debacle offered for the first time a unique opportunity to assess the real value of a vaccine. If vaccination made a real difference, deaths would be expected to go up as vaccination plummeted. If it did not have an effect, or only a modest one, the general trend would continue.

It looked at first as if the worst was happening. Following the 'brain damage' scare and drop-off in vaccination rates, there were reports of several large outbreaks of whooping cough. Such reports are based on the number of notifications of whooping cough. Having fallen dramatically during the 1960s, they rose again during the late 1970s and early 1980s as the immunisation rate fell following the scare.

These notifications are voluntary reports of cases of whooping cough made by family doctors and hospitals to the Department of Health. They are notoriously unreliable, however. Under-reporting is common, as the majority of reports are often made by a small number of dedicated doctors. The accuracy of such reporting also relies on the correct diagnosis being made by the doctor.

Whooping cough is quite difficult to diagnose, as there are many other causes of a bad cough. Doctors are more likely to have diagnosed whooping cough during the widely publicised epidemics of the late 1970s and early 1980s.[17] As the Department of Health repeatedly notified family doctors that epidemics of whooping cough were imminent, these warnings became self-fulfilling prophecies: doctors suspected that children with a prolonged cough must have (mild) whooping cough.[18] Also, doctors were more likely to diagnose a prolonged cough as whooping cough in an unvaccinated child compared to a vaccinated child. Their assumption that the vaccine worked led to evidence, based on reported cases, that it did work.[19]

The first two reports of epidemics that occurred following the scare were expected as part of a roughly four-yearly cycle of whooping-cough epidemics. Nonetheless, it certainly appears from the notification figures that they were the largest epidemics for thirty years. But could this have been due to over-reporting by family doctors, wrongly assuming most coughs in their surgery were whooping cough? An editorial in the *British Medical Journal* admits in 2002, 'surveillance is so incomplete that enhanced awareness... can result in apparent epidemics'.[20]

A conclusive way of measuring what happened after the drop in vaccination is not that difficult to find. If the epidemics really were three times the size of the previous two epidemics in the early 1970s, as the notifications suggested, then we should expect to see three times as many deaths. The severity of the disease is unlikely to change much over a few years. Even today, it is true that whooping cough can kill. The numbers of people dying of whooping cough are more accurate than notifications. Even though the cause of death on a death certificate can be wrong, it's more likely to be correct than a busy consulting-room diagnosis.

The figures are startling. The total number of children dying from whooping cough in the two epidemic years with low immunisation rates (well under one in two uptake) is identical to the number of children who died in the 1974/5 epidemic when over three quarters of children had been immunised. What is more, the number of deaths is far fewer than in the 1970 epidemic when, again, four in five children were immunised. This shows convincingly that the percentage of children immunised has little bearing on the numbers of children dying from whooping cough.

The reported massive epidemics of whooping cough beg another question. If many more children were apparently catching whooping cough, why weren't larger numbers dying from it?

Pro-vaccination doctors, whilst admitting that 'death rates from whooping cough have fallen unexpectedly', have tried to explain the figures away by suggesting the disease suddenly shifted to higher social classes (who were less likely to die), that treatment had improved (but over ten years it hadn't really) and that more milder cases had been notified.[21] Everyone agrees about the last reason, though it does mean of course that in fact there were no massive epidemics.

Furthermore, during the 1978 epidemic, a period of high notification, only one in twenty unvaccinated children were reported to have caught whooping cough, the remainder apparently escaping the disease. Even Professor Elizabeth Miller, the government immunisation specialist at the Health Protection Agency, conceded in 1980 that not only were more cases of whooping cough notified in the 1978 outbreak but, even allowing for this, the death rate was lower than in previous epidemics.[22] In other words, even at the time, health officials were admitting that whooping cough was becoming less of a killer disease despite the drop in vaccination.

During the ten years of low immunisation uptake (1978-1987), a total of sixty-two children died of whooping cough. But this is an improvement on a hundred-and-one children who died during the previous ten years — a time of high immunisation uptake.

The facts put in stark contrast the government's claims at the time of a 'Killer Disease' that would claim victims among the unvaccinated as a result of the inevitable epidemics that would follow. The total number of deaths was lower. The death rate (the proportion of children catching whooping cough who died) was actually the lowest ever recorded. In fact, nearly as many fully vaccinated children were catching whooping cough as unvaccinated children.

The official view

Though these are the official figures, this is not, however, the official view. Despite the government's prompt measures during the scare, their propaganda machine stuck to the mantra of a 'Killer Disease'. It is not wrong as such — whooping cough can still be a dangerous disease — but it placed spin on the seriousness of the disease by ignoring the continuing decline of its severity. Had there not been a scare, the same figures would no doubt have been used as proof of the success of the vaccine.

So it comes as somewhat of a surprise that in 2001 Dr David Salisbury, the government health official then in charge of immunisation, went on record to say 'Parents thought they were choosing the safer option by not having the whooping cough vaccine, but in fact they were putting their children at risk. There were at least 200,000 extra cases of whooping cough recorded and 100 deaths from the infection in the 1970s and 1980s. That situation resonates very loudly with where we are today with MMR.'[23] It is a statement that is very economical with the truth.

Salisbury went on to say that it took five or six years to discover that the original suggested link (by consultant Dr John Wilson) between whooping cough and brain damage was false.

It is certainly one take on the whooping cough scare. But there is a problem with it. The government is unlikely to have paid out large sums in compensation to brain-damaged children under the vaccine compensation programme (introduced in 1979 as a direct result of concern over the side-effects of the whooping cough vaccine) if the vaccine had not been the cause. What does medical research say about the 'false link'?

As early as the 1950s and 1960s doctors were reporting that a small number of children appeared to have a severe reaction to the whooping cough vaccine that could result in brain damage. The Department of Health noted in 1953 that the risk of brain damage from the vaccine may be 'of an equal risk' to that of brain damage from the disease itself.[24] Even a doctor from Eli Lilly, the drug company that manufactured a whooping cough vaccine, admitted in 1963, 'It is obvious that severe neurological reactions have occurred in children after immunisation with pertussis vaccines.'[25]

Once the scare of the 1970s had brought this issue to the attention of the whole nation, the government felt that this problem had to be addressed at last. Numerous committees and sub-committees were set up, with some senior doctors calling for the whooping cough vaccine to be abandoned.[26] One committee concluded that brain damage had probably occurred after one in every 155,000 whooping cough vaccinations. In effect, this meant that, with children receiving three vaccinations each, nearly one in every 50,000 children had been brain damaged following a full course of vaccination.[27]

This caused genuine concern and the government then set up The National Childhood Encephalopathy Study (NCES), which was, and still is, the largest and most detailed study ever performed on the relationship between whooping cough vaccine and brain damage. It looked at children admitted to hospital over three years between 1976 and 1979. The study concluded that the vaccine caused brain damage in one in 110,000 immunisations and that the damage was permanent in one in 310,000 immunisations.[28] This was confirmed in a follow-up study published thirteen years later.[29]

The results of an American study using the same criteria as the NCES suggested a similar risk for brain damage, though the doctor in charge of monitoring drug and vaccine safety at the Department of Health had even greater concerns. He estimated that serious reactions were occurring in one in thirty thousand vaccinations — ten times more than the British study.[30,31] Estimates of serious reactions, usually resulting in permanent brain damage, have been as high as one in seventeen thousand.[32] The USA Institute of Medicine concluded in 1991, and again in 2000, that the vaccine could cause brain damage.[33]

After forty years, the medical evidence demonstrating that the vaccine can cause brain damage is strong, but doctors are still arguing the point. What is certainly wrong, however, is the conclusion that within six years of the 1970s scare it was clear that the link between brain damage and the whooping cough vaccine was false.

Other side-effects

It was not the only point on which health officials were wrong. The vaccine often causes a high fever, and can cause persistent, uncontrollable screaming, abnormal drowsiness and restlessness as well as redness, swelling and pain at the site of vaccination. These symptoms occur more commonly after whooping cough vaccination than most other vaccines. More worryingly, the baby sometimes 'collapses' and becomes unresponsive and impossible to arouse. I have seen a baby go floppy and death-like after whooping-cough vaccination, and it is very scary, both for the parent and the doctor. Convulsions, sometimes prolonged, can occur, as can severe neurological reactions, including brain damage. In addition, the vaccine can cause babies to stop breathing (apnoea), at least temporarily,[34,35] and this is believed to be a cause of cot deaths. (There is an unresolved controversy over the possible link with vaccination.)

These side-effects have manifested themselves more in Britain because of the type of vaccine used in the UK for over half a century. The whole-cell whooping cough vaccine is made from the whole of the bacterium, which was killed and injected whole. There had been concern over the side-effects of this type of vaccine for as long as it existed, and scientists had been working on a safer vaccine for decades: over half the babies immunised suffered a side-effect of some sort. During the 1960s and 1970s, Merck and other vaccine manufacturers developed vaccines that contained only the bits of the bug thought to be necessary to produce immunity. These 'acellular' vaccines are therefore far less 'dirty'. They were both safer and thought to be more effective than their whole cell counterparts.

It is alleged that pharmaceutical companies decided against marketing, at least for more than a short period of time, their new, improved (but more expensive) vaccines on economic grounds. As countries continued to use the more dangerous vaccines, denying children the safer option for decades, they found no takers. They then stopped making all whooping cough vaccines for a while. Why? They could be legally liable for marketing inferior vaccines when they had a safer and more effective product that they declined to sell.[25]

However, in Japan in 1975, following the deaths of two babies within a few hours of receiving the whole-cell whooping cough vaccine, the Japanese temporarily suspended the vaccine and then reintroduced it only for children over two years while research on a safer vaccine was completed. Furthermore, in Sweden, the 'whole cell' vaccine was withdrawn in 1979 because of safety concerns (and worries that it wasn't working). Japan was the first country then to switch to the new 'acellular' vaccine in 1981. Other countries followed, including the USA in 1996, and by 2000 the majority of western European countries had introduced the safer vaccine for their baby immunisation schedules.

The UK belatedly followed suit in 2004. The Department of Health not only stubbornly persisted in using the 'whole cell' vaccine, it insisted the vaccine was more effective than the acellular vaccine. The whole-cell vaccine was not replaced by another one. Instead the safer acellular vaccine was introduced as a part of the new 5-in-1 vaccine.

At the launch of the '5-in-1' vaccine in 2004 Dr David Salisbury, the doctor in charge of vaccination at the Department of Health, kept the pressure on parents, saying, 'If you delay and you do not protect your baby against, particularly, whooping cough, at a young age, then you are putting your baby at very high risk.'[36]

Apart from death, the government cites the risk of brain damage as one of the reasons to vaccinate against whooping cough. How common (or rare) this is has been hotly debated, but, as no case of encephalitis (infection of the brain) — whether or not resulting in brain damage — was seen in either of the two epidemics following the 1970s vaccine scare, it would appear that the risk of brain damage must be much less than the government's estimate of 1 in a 1,000.[37]

Dr Herbert Barrie, a consultant in paediatrics working during the 1970s, said, 'I can honestly say I have never knowingly seen brain damage caused by this disease — in contrast with a few cases of vaccine damage — and have encountered only two deaths, both preventable, in 25 years.'[16] He described the chances of surviving an attack of whooping cough as, 'excellent and, indeed, overwhelmingly superior to crossing the road.'[38]

How effective is the vaccine since the scare?
As long ago as 1966, when deaths were still relatively high, Sir Graham Wilson, the senior doctor responsible for the control of infectious diseases in England and Wales, said 'Whooping cough has now such a low death rate that the advisability of continuing vaccination against this disease must be seriously questioned, particularly when there is reason to believe that...vaccination has played little part in bringing about its fall.'[39] At the same time as the start of the scare, Professor George Dick, a senior UK doctor and immunisation expert wrote in 1974, 'I am not entirely convinced that the community benefit of whooping-cough vaccination outweighs the damage which it may be doing.'[40]

The effectiveness of the vaccine has been calculated as being anywhere between 37% and 92%.[41] In reality, it's probably near the bottom end of that estimate. To take an example, an epidemic of whooping cough hit the Shetland Isles in 1974. The same proportion of immunised children caught the infection as unimmunised children, suggesting the vaccine offered no protection at all.[42]

In another example, in the 1970s the immunisation rates in three similar countries, France, Britain and West Germany, varied between 95% and 10%. However, the death rate from whooping cough remained the same in all three countries, again suggesting the vaccine made no difference.[43] Between 1981 and 1983, when no whooping cough vaccinations were given in Sweden, there were only three deaths, and two of these were in severely disabled children.[44] More recently, there was an outbreak of whooping cough in a Florida kindergarten in 2013. Of the 33 children, aged between one and six years, who contracted whooping cough, 28 had received at least three doses, and 23 at least four doses, of vaccine. The vaccine effectiveness was calculated as 45%. What is of particular concern is that the average length of time between the last dose of vaccine received by a child and the onset of symptoms was fewer than two years; seven children had been vaccinated during the previous year.[64]

Has the return to a high vaccination rate after the 1970s scare made a difference to the occurrence of whooping cough in Britain?

It is certainly not disappearing, and has actually become more common over recent years than most people realise. A study in a General Practice in Birmingham showed that up to a quarter of adults, and half of all children, with a prolonged cough had whooping cough.[45] Research in London showed half of twenty-five to thirty-five year olds with a persistent cough had whooping cough. Despite a high vaccine uptake of around 94%, the disease is both common and widespread. Other countries are experiencing similar problems, where outbreaks of whooping cough have even occurred amongst children who have been fully vaccinated.[47,48]

In the 1990s it had, furthermore, become apparent that, whatever protection the vaccine did offer, it didn't last long. It seemed to be between four and fourteen years for the UK whole-cell vaccine in use at that time, though usually not more than five years.[43,49] The newer acellular vaccine is no better: only one child in ten will still have protection against whooping cough 8-9 years after the primary course. Health officials, therefore, decided that another dose of the vaccine was needed. 5 November, 2001, marked the introduction of a booster dose of whooping cough vaccine into the immunisation schedule.[62] This was added to the tetanus, diphtheria, polio, and second MMR, already given at four years of age. The new, safer 'acellular' vaccine was used.

The addition of the booster is doing little, if anything, to reduce the number of cases of whooping cough in the country. Why? Though it provides good protection in the short term, this only lasts for a few years[50]. In the four years (2001-5) following the introduction of the booster, over a third of all school age children in Oxfordshire with a persistent cough had evidence of whooping cough, one study concluded. 'Our research suggests', the authors wrote in 2006, 'that in the United Kingdom pertussis is...endemic [widespread] amongst younger school age children'.[51] Even more recent research carried out in the Thames Valley found that 1 in 5 children aged between 5 and 15 years with a cough lasting between two and eight weeks had evidence of recent whooping cough infection. Most of these children were fully immunised with four doses of whooping cough vaccine including the pre-school booster.[53] The USA added a sixth booster dose for adolescents in 2006 but the protection afforded by this only lasts two to three years.[54] The vaccine offers, at best, short-term protection. The currently used vaccines will never eradicate the disease.

Vaccinate pregnant women
Despite fifty years of high vaccination coverage in many western countries, it is now accepted that 'pertussis cannot be controlled by the current immunisation programs.'[52] Worryingly, cases were increasing in newborn babies in whom the disease is most severe.[46] An increase in reported cases in 2011 and 2012, partly — if not solely — due to improved lab tests and increased awareness (increased awareness, remember, resulted in the so-called epidemics in the 1970s and 1980s), resulted in the startling recommendation that all pregnant women should receive the whooping cough vaccine between 20 and 32 weeks of pregnancy. The reasoning behind this cavalier suggestion was that 4-5 babies were dying from whooping cough every year on the England and Wales. Most were under 10 weeks of age and nearly all under 16 weeks of age. As most were too young to have received any vaccine it was hoped that the

vaccine would stimulate the pregnant mothers to make protective antibodies which would be passed on to the baby in the womb and provide protection during the early weeks of life. So far so good. However, the DoH had to use what was available, which was a 4-in-1 vaccine which also protects against tetanus, diphtheria and polio. Not only had this vaccine never been tested for safety or effectiveness in pregnant women, but the assumption that the mother would pass on adequate quantities of protective antibodies to her baby was just that – an assumption. Once again the government undertook a mass vaccine experiment, this time on pregnant women.

The policy appears to be a double edged sword. Giving the vaccine to pregnant women, ideally between 27 and 30 weeks of pregnancy, provides the new born babies with good levels of antibodies which do appear to give babies good protection, at least for the first 8 weeks of life.[55, 56] However, it reduces their response to the whooping cough vaccines given at two, three and four months. Thus vaccinating pregnant women may protect babies against whooping cough in the first few weeks of life at the expense of reduced protection over subsequent months.[63] Interestingly some, but far fewer, babies born to unvaccinated mothers are also born with immunity to whooping cough.[57] Vaccinated mothers also pass on some antibody protection to their babies through breast milk.[58] The most effective time to have the vaccine appears to be between 27 and 30 weeks of pregnancy.[59] Limited research has now been done into the safety of giving pregnant women the four-in-one vaccine containing whooping cough. One study found a 19% increase in the risk of chorioamnionitis, an infection of the placenta and fluid surrounding the baby in the womb.[60] The infection causes a fever in the mother and pain and tenderness over the womb. Chorioamnionitis results in an increase in caesarian sections, abscesses and postpartum haemorrhage. If the baby is affected, then brain damage, death or long-term developmental problems can all occur. Chorioamnionitis affects 1 to 4% of all births and so a 10% increase would be important. Another study detected a 20% increase risk of intrauterine growth retardation / low birth weight, but this finding was not (quite) statistically significant.[61] A couple of other studies have been more reassuring.

Whooping cough can still be distressing and unpleasant, lasting for several weeks. The greatest distress is often suffered not by the children, but by parents experiencing weeks of sleepless nights looking after their child with prolonged coughing fits. The most common complication, affecting around 1% of children, is pneumonia and this is normally readily treatable with antibiotics. The risk of a child dying from whooping cough is probably around 1 in 30,000 cases.

The question is whether vaccination makes a difference that is worth the risks it introduces. It is a personal decision that every parent should make for themselves. On balance, I would not have had my son vaccinated with the old whole cell vaccine that was on offer at the time; however, the new vaccine is much safer and one that I would consider giving to prevent the undoubted distress the illness can cause.

12
Rubella

Good Sense

The rubella vaccine was introduced on the tail end of the 1960s' spirit of optimism and before the whooping cough scare of the 1970s. Rubella is itself a mild infection that is normally of little consequence. The one exception is the damage it can do to the unborn baby. It was first recognised as an illness in its own right, rather than being confused with scarlet fever or measles, in the early nineteenth century. At this stage the disease was still nameless. The Germans were the first to label the illness, calling it Rötheln. Henry Veale, a Royal Artillery surgeon, serving in India in the mid-nineteenth century, took offence to this name, which he described as 'harsh and foreign to our ears....'[1] He proposed rubella, meaning 'little red.' Rubella was, for years, thought of as being like a mild case of measles, and so was also called 'three day measles' or German measles.

Rubella causes a pink-red rash, mild fever and, typically, swollen glands (lymph nodes) at the back of the neck. The disease is harmless and serious complications are almost unknown. Up to half of all people who catch German measles do not even get ill at all.

The infection itself is harmless in anyone who is not pregnant. It is also harmless in a pregnant woman provided she is immune to rubella. The infection commonly causes temporarily painful joints in adults. It rarely causes a mild inflammation of the brain (encephalitis) in about one in six thousand infections, though recovery is normally complete. A rare bleeding disorder called ITP (Idiopathic Thrombocytopenia Purpura) very occasionally follows an attack of German measles.

Little attention was paid to the disease by the medical profession until Norman Gregg, an Australian ophthalmologist, noticed an unusually large number of babies being born in 1941 with cataracts, and other birth defects, shortly after a particularly large and widespread epidemic of rubella. From this time, it was recognised that children born to mothers who had contracted German measles in the first three to four months of pregnancy were at risk of a variety of congenital abnormalities.

The most common disability is deafness, often partial, but sometimes severe. The eyes are often affected, most often with cataracts (a clouding of the lens that can cause blindness), but also damage to the retina at the back of the eye, and abnormally small eyes. The heart is the next most frequently affected organ, typically with congenital heart defects such as a 'hole in the heart'. Over half of all affected babies suffer only from deafness, with the remainder suffering a combination of deformities, including mental retardation. The affected baby is said to suffer from 'congenital rubella syndrome' (CRS).

It is surprisingly difficult to calculate the exact risk of a baby being affected following an episode of German measles in the mother. Rubella can be such a mild and non-specific illness that it is often not easy to diagnose. Though blood tests are now available to confirm a suspected case of rubella in the mother, only a few women are known to be affected every year, again making the calculation of risks problematic. In the first eight weeks of pregnancy there is a roughly two in three chance that the baby will be born with one or more of the abnormalities of CRS; this risk falls to around one in two between the ninth and twelfth week, and a one in seven chance in the following four weeks. After the sixteenth week of pregnancy there is virtually no risk to the baby.[2,3]

Overall, it is probable that around one in four of all babies whose mothers catch German measles in the first four months of pregnancy will be born disabled. A very few affected babies, probably around one in every hundred, will be stillborn and a few may also miscarry.[4]

Before the introduction of immunisation most people caught rubella as children, which then gave them lifelong immunity. This meant that most pregnant women were protected. If they did come across the infection, which was likely because it was common, they would be able to resist it naturally, and so prevent their baby from becoming infected.

But some babies were still being born deaf and with heart defects. No record was kept of affected babies so we don't know the size of the problem. There were absolutely no figures on rubella itself as it was considered a trivial disease that everyone got, and for which there was no need to keep any national records.

When immunisation against German measles was introduced into the UK in 1970, there was no attempt to eradicate the disease. It was actually thought that it would be better to keep the infection circulating in the community, as natural infection provided women with lifelong immunity. There was no doubt that the best protection a woman could get to prevent her baby catching rubella when she was pregnant, was to have caught the illness as a child.

But some women were becoming pregnant without having had the illness, and their babies needed protecting. For this reason vaccination was introduced in 1970, but only for girls between eleven and fourteen years of age. Most children would have had the infection by then, so the new vaccination would not make rubella any less common in the community. But it would provide protection for those girls who, for one reason or another, had not yet caught the disease. The vaccine was given at around twelve years of age for a good reason: it would give protection at just the time girls needed it — before their fertile years when they were likely to have children. The vaccine is a live vaccine (like measles and mumps), made from a virus that has been altered ('attenuated') to make it relatively harmless.

The UK only started to keep records of babies born damaged with CRS in

1971, following the introduction of the vaccine, and so it is difficult to assess how effective the vaccine initially was. There is no doubt that, since the introduction of immunisation, the numbers of babies born damaged from German measles, though fluctuating, have fallen. What we don't know is whether or not the numbers had also been falling before immunisation. It has been estimated that between 200 and 300 babies a year were born with CRS before the onset of vaccination. But this seems unlikely, as it is improbable that the number of babies affected would plummet by 80% immediately after the introduction of vaccination for twelve-year-old girls, most of whom would not have got pregnant for some years. What did happen is that the number of cases of CRS steadily fell as the vaccinated girls started to become mothers.

The cyclical pattern of rubella, with epidemics occurring every few years, meant that the number of babies affected varied from a high of sixty-eight in 1979 — as a result of a particularly large epidemic in 1978 — to lows of ten. Nevertheless, the overall trend remained downwards. In the years that the single rubella vaccine was given to twelve-year-old girls, on average around thirty babies a year were born in the UK with signs of damage from congenital rubella syndrome (CRS).

Routine screening of all pregnant women was also started during the 1970s. Any woman found to be susceptible (that is, not immune to, or protected against, rubella) was offered vaccination after delivering her baby. In contrast, any woman found to have rubella antibodies in her blood was considered to be protected against rubella. An indirect measure of the effectiveness of the vaccination policy, therefore, is the proportion of women of child-bearing age who are immune to rubella, as measured by this blood test. Throughout the 1970s and 1980s, when the single vaccine was in use, increasing numbers of pregnant women, and women of child-bearing age passed the screening. In other words, the number of women susceptible to German measles was falling throughout the time that schoolgirls were getting the single vaccine. The immunisation appeared to be working. Routine screening of pregnant women for rubella antibodies was stopped in England in 2016.

The number of babies born with CRS was falling, the number of pregnant women remaining unprotected against rubella was also falling, and the uptake of rubella vaccine amongst schoolgirls was slowly increasing.

The effect of the selective immunisation can also be measured against other data. Though the most important problem associated with German measles is children born with congenital rubella syndrome (CRS), there is one other undesirable outcome that should not be overlooked. That is, women who have their pregnancies terminated because of the possibility that their baby may be damaged by rubella. Abortion had been legalised in 1967, and the suffering involved with this is not included in the numbers of CRS.

The figures for abortions due to suspected CRS show an encouraging downward trend from a high of over a thousand in 1971 to fewer than a hundred by the late 1980s, despite a blip following the 1978 rubella epidemic. However, the rubella vaccine cannot take all the credit for this. As twelve-year-old girls were being vaccinated from 1970, most would not have become pregnant for at least six or seven years. Therefore the rapid decline in abortions between 1970 and 1977 cannot be attributed to the vaccination programme. One likely contributory factor was the declining birth rate which fell by nearly 30% from 1970 to 1977.

It should be noted that not all terminations are carried out because of the risk of infection; some are also done because a pregnant woman was given a rubella vaccination. As a proportion of total abortions, terminations because of vaccination were becoming more important and in one year (1989) equalled the number due to infection. All these terminations were undertaken as a precaution; it is not known how many of them were actually necessary. No baby is known to have been born damaged because the mother was vaccinated in early pregnancy, but tests suggest that the baby can be 'infected' by the live vaccine virus, and so damage is a theoretical possibility.

Good sense

The question arose whether more should be done to lower the number of CRS cases further. One option was to continue with the current policy of vaccinating all girls at around twelve years of age, at least until no more improvement was seen. Another suggestion was also to screen teenage girls (with a blood test) for immunity, offer all unprotected girls vaccination, and then re-test them to make sure that the vaccine had worked. In one area of Scotland, girls were already having an immunity blood test and only those who were not protected were then given the vaccine. This appeared to be successful with 'high' levels of immunity being achieved. The supporters of this plan argued that girls should still be given the opportunity to acquire natural immunity (by catching rubella) as this was preferable.

In 1986, the powerful Joint Committee on Vaccination and Immunisation (JCVI) felt that 'there was insufficient evidence to justify a change' in rubella vaccination policy.[5] However, pro-vaccination doctors, of whom there were many at the Department of Health, felt that the policy of selectively vaccinating only girls at twelve was not effective enough in preventing the problem. They argued that, on average, thirty babies a year were still being born damaged with CRS and that 2-3% of adult women (97-98% of whom now had immunity, largely naturally acquired) were still not protected against rubella.

The position of the JCVI made good sense. Unless a vaccine is both very effective for a long time and has a high uptake, immunising children increases the average age at which one gets the disease. Why? The immunity against the natural disease is replaced by the antibodies induced by the vaccine. But as the antibodies lose their effectiveness over time, the natural disease can strike again later. This is something that happened in Greece after the introduction of the MMR vaccine on an optional basis in 1975, when the vaccine uptake was fewer than one in two people. This was sufficient to shift upwards the age people were likely to contract German measles, but not enough to eradicate it. The twenty five cases of CRS that resulted from an outbreak of German measles in 1993 was the largest number recorded in that country since 1950.

But this good sense was not to last.

13
MMR/Mumps
Who Wanted the MMR?

In 1988, no new immunisation had been introduced for almost twenty years, while deaths from infectious diseases were continuing to fall to unprecedented low numbers. There did not seem to be an overriding need for any change at first sight. Nor had any major new vaccine discoveries been made that required changing the national schedule. After the 1987 election, the Thatcher government was keen on tax cuts and an increase in the immunisation budget did not seem a likely priority. Nor do I, as a GP at the time, recall any major medical problem that needed urgent action. Nonetheless, in that year a new type of vaccine was launched by the government, the MMR. It is the only vaccine that has ever been routinely used that contains three live viruses, a unique idea. It aimed to protect the population against measles, mumps and rubella (German measles). We were told by the government that the vaccine would save lives and prevent babies from being born disabled. It seemed a goal no one could disagree with, and the high profile introduction was uneventful.

However, it was an unusual move by the government that was not quite as uneventful as all that. Underlying the seemingly smooth launch was a dramatic change in the way health officials were now using vaccines. Without any debates in parliament, or wide consultation in the medical profession, the focus was now no longer on combating the major diseases alone. The focus had all of a sudden widened and now included minor diseases. Given the whooping cough scare some ten years earlier, it was a very high risk strategy that health officials were pursuing — and it is not easy to comprehend why — but the government clearly must have thought it worthwhile. Because there were no debates, not much can be said about the motivation for this sea change. It is not clear who had been promoting the change, who had wanted it, or in whose interest it was. A major change in thinking just happened as a fait accompli, the health officials' preferred way of operating with regards to vaccines.

Mumps
The 1988 MMR, with one of its three components, all of a sudden introduced a new vaccination for all children against an infectious disease — mumps. The reason why is not clear. Like rubella, mumps is an extremely mild disease and before immunisation nearly everyone caught mumps, typically when between five and ten years old. It rarely causes anything more than a harmless illness.

One third of those who catch it do not even get ill at all, and one attack of mumps gives immunity for the rest of one's life. It is also a well-known disease.[1] First described over 2000 years ago by the Greek physician Hippocrates, it most commonly causes an inflammation, or swelling, of the glands[2] in front of and underneath the ears on either side of the face.

Though generally mild, there can be certain complications. The UK government cited this as its main argument for introducing the mumps vaccine: mumps was the biggest cause of viral meningitis in children. This sounds scary and it is, strictly speaking, true. But it is also misleading. Mumps meningitis is not like the serious (bacterial) meningitis that can kill within twenty four hours. It is nearly always harmless; the most that children are likely to suffer is a mild headache and a stiff neck. Nearly all children make a complete recovery.[3]

Other complications of mumps are that about 1 in 3,000 children suffer from inflammation of the brain (encephalitis). Most will make a full recovery, but permanent hearing loss may occur in about 1 in 30,000 cases of mumps, though in children it is even rarer.[3,4] It will usually affect one ear, and the risk for children is probably around 1 in 100,000. Then there is swelling of the testicles (orchitis), rarely a problem before puberty. Finally, it may cause an inflammation of the pancreas gland behind the stomach which can cause abdominal pain, but this usually settles in a few days.

As a sign of the medical consensus of the gravity of the disease, doctors had not been required to notify cases of the mumps and there are no figures. The only evidence is that during much of the twentieth century, ten or twenty deaths a year were recorded as being caused by mumps. But it is quite likely that most of these deaths were due to some other cause.[5,6] The results of a large study on two and a half thousand people admitted to hospital over twelve years between 1958 and 1969 in England and Wales puts the complications of mumps into perspective. There were no deaths, and the only long-term problem was deafness in one child.[3] As the vast majority of people with mumps are not admitted to hospital, the survey would have looked at only the most serious cases of the disease. A survey in Scotland of all cases of mumps covering eight years found that every patient made a complete recovery.[4]

Official medical opinion before 1988 was also quite clear that vaccination was not a necessity. In 1967 an editorial in the *British Medical Journal* (*BMJ*) concluded: 'there is no obvious need immediately for mass immunisation with a view to eradication of the disease.'[7] In 1974 a UK survey on the complications of mumps stated: 'It seems clear from the results of this survey that there is little need for general vaccination against mumps', a view endorsed by others.[3] In 1978, Professor George Dick, an adviser to the government on immunisation and Joint Committee on Vaccination and Immunisation (JCVI) member, wrote, 'there is little good reason for introducing mumps vaccine as a routine procedure, for the disease is usually mild, complications such as pancreatitis [inflammation of the pancreas] and orchitis [swelling of the testicles] are rare, and the prognosis of the common complications, namely meningitis and meningo-encephalitis, is good.'[8] The JCVI itself conceded in 1974 that 'there was no need to introduce routine vaccination against mumps.'[9]

Was the mumps vaccine new, then, in 1988? Not really. The single mumps vaccine had been available in the UK since 1971. But it generated little interest before its introduction in the combined MMR vaccine. The problem with the mumps vaccine is the same as with the rubella vaccine (and all child vaccines). Mass immunisation replaces the immunity gained by the natural infection and pushes the age of infection up as medically-induced immunity does not last a lifetime. For this type of strategy to be effective, the induced immunisation needs to eradicate the disease, as in the case of smallpox. Failing this, all that is done is that a dependency on the vaccine is created to keep the disease under control.

A problem in the case of mumps, however, is that it is more serious in later life, especially for men and adolescent boys. All complications of mumps are more serious at a higher age, but two in particular stand out: permanent hearing loss and the painful swelling of usually one, but occasionally both, testicles (orchitis). Though the 1958-1969 mumps survey in England and Wales showed deafness in one child only, it recorded deafness in four adults as a result of mumps.[3] Around one in four males who contract mumps after puberty will suffer orchitis. This can be very painful, but it is extremely rare for it to cause infertility, if it can at all, partly because it usually only affects one testicle (government doctors agree that 'there is no firm evidence that orchitis causes sterility.[10]). Nonetheless, mumps orchitis may increase the risk of testicular cancer.[11]

Mass vaccination of mumps meant taking the risk that the disease would become less trivial by pushing up the age of the sufferer. Recognition of this risk is one of the reasons why vaccination was not introduced earlier on.

The sensible thing would have been selective vaccination, as in the case of rubella, which was initially only offered to adolescent girls and mothers after giving birth. Teenage boys who had not had mumps could have been vaccinated in order to prevent an attack in adulthood and its attendant risk of complications. But this is not what officials chose to do, even though it was foreseeable what was going to happen. In 1980, a *BMJ* editorial reiterated the journal's earlier reservations against immunisation and warned that widespread vaccination might have an overall negative effect and cautioned, 'to attempt [mumps] prevention on a mass scale might well increase its incidence in adults with all the troubles and risks that implies.[12]

Although the reason for the introduction of the mumps immunisation is somewhat of a mystery, it is inconceivable that health authorities in 1988 wanted to cultivate a more harmful disease, or make the population dependent on a vaccine. The only remaining motivation, it seems, was that they had returned to the 1960s optimism of eradicating disease and had set their sights on the (somewhat trivial) mumps.

A vaccine is believed to work primarily by tricking the body into thinking that it has come across the real illness, so that it produces 'antibodies' against the disease, which should prevent future attacks. Though no vaccine has this effect in 100% of the population, the effectiveness of the mumps vaccine at preventing mumps was originally considered to be very high: around nineteen out of twenty people would produce the antibodies.

Experience has shown that this trust in the vaccine was grossly misplaced. Outbreaks of mumps have even occurred in populations where 98% of children have been vaccinated. [13] In one outbreak a greater proportion of vaccinated children caught mumps than unvaccinated children, the opposite of what should have happened.[14]

Natural immunity lasts a lifetime, but how long does the MMR vaccine remain effective? When the MMR first came out, we were assured that only one shot was necessary to confer life-long immunity. Studies in the UK measuring the level of antibodies, however, have shown that one in five children were not protected against mumps four years after vaccination with the MMR.[15,16]

In other words, the MMR, instead of eradicating mumps, is now pushing up the age when people contract it. It is turning the disease from a trivial one into a more serious one than before, for boys and men in particular.

The aftermath

Is this prediction borne out by the facts? The figures available for mumps cases are 'notifications' (when a doctor clinically suspects mumps) and laboratory reports (lab confirmations) since 1988. Mumps became a 'notifiable disease', meaning that doctors are required to report cases to the Department of Health, in 1988, when the MMR was introduced. Even so, it is certain that doctors did not report all, or even most, cases. After all, a third of cases do not produce any symptoms, and so cannot be diagnosed.

The official figures suggest a sharp fall since 1988 in cases after introduction of the vaccine. In the first year, 1988, not all children would have been vaccinated and they would continue to get the disease naturally. Their number would drop in the next year as twice as many children were immunised. Most of them would no longer get the mumps because the antibodies they produced would prevent them from contracting the disease.

Eight years on the situation was no longer looking so rosy. The discovery that the mumps vaccine was less effective than at first thought was one of the reasons for the introduction of the second MMR in 1996. At that time, UK government doctors estimated that the effectiveness of the vaccine was around 70%, much lower than the original 95%. With the optimism we have come to expect from immunisation officials, it was predicted that a second dose 'should eventually eliminate mumps.'[17]

Having added the second MMR vaccine to the immunisation budget, it was expected that mumps would continue to decline and, as was predicted, disappear. Indeed, from 1996, the decline in reported cases continued, but only just, helped by the 'catch-up' element of the 1996 second MMR campaign.

Then, from the end of 2000, the number of cases of mumps started rising again. Walsall was the first area to report a large rise in the number of mumps cases, mainly in teenagers. Of 200 people getting mumps in Walsall in the year 2000, over two thirds had received the MMR vaccine — and nearly a fifth had been given two doses.[18] The rest of the country followed. The over-fifteen-year-olds were predominantly affected, though cases were rising in all age groups. In fact, since 2002, there has been a huge increase in the total number of notifications of mumps.

Some have tried to insist the mumps component is effective, and explain away the increase in the numbers of older teenagers and young adults getting mumps, saying they were too young to have got natural (life-long) immunity, but too old to have received the MMR vaccine, or at least to have received two doses. It is hard to share this optimism about a product that, on its launch, was said to be far more effective than it proved to be in the real world.

Sadly, the propaganda machine swung into action. The subsequent self-inflicted rise in cases around the country resulted in media headlines like 'Britain put on Mumps alert' and "Vaccinate' plea as mumps cases soar.'

The pro-vaccination propaganda then really got underway, with a public health consultant warning that 'The danger is that mumps is one of the most common causes of viral meningitis'. In his enthusiasm to promote uptake of the vaccine, he probably forgot to mention the harmless nature of mumps meningitis, but it sounded really frightening. In August 2001, a tabloid ran a story under the headline 'Jab fears lead to mumps outbreak.' In the report, a Department of Health spokesman warned, 'Mumps is a very serious disease.'[19]

In May 2004, the silly season started early at the Department of Health when a message was sent to all GPs in the country warning us that a single student had been 'infectious with mumps' whilst attending a student games in Spain, which over two thousand students from all over the UK had attended. Doctors were advised to consider 'opportunistic vaccination of all at-risk students at the forty-one universities affected,' and were reminded that 'no opportunity to immunise should be missed.'[20]

British doctors could be forgiven for thinking that an outbreak of the plague was imminent. By the summer of 2004, cases of mumps were reported as having reached 'the highest level since records began.'[21] On returning to colleges in the autumn, students were being offered MMR jabs in a bid to stem the threat of a mumps epidemic in universities. Ironically, in 2005, this was turning into panic at the universities as a massive rise in mumps in sixteen to twenty-five-year-olds was reported. Universities were holding huge vaccination clinics with queues of hundreds of students stretching outside medical centres. Some Universities are now asking all new students to ensure that they have received the MMR vaccine before starting their courses.

It is not only in Britain where the mumps vaccination is having an unwanted effect. When mumps broke out at a summer camp in New York State in 2005, all twelve campers who caught mumps, aged between ten and fifteen years, had been vaccinated with two doses of the MMR vaccine.[22]

Side-effects

In 1998, it was clear there would be a cost of achieving eradication. The mumps vaccine consists of the live virus that has been attenuated – that is, made harmless. However, occasionally it infects and harms in the same way as the wild virus. As the illness itself is so rarely serious, this is not often a problem. A little fewer than 1% of children will get the classic swelling of the salivary glands typical of mumps. Swelling of the testicles occasionally also follows mumps vaccination.

Perhaps most importantly, live viruses can interfere with each other. Controversially, given with the measles vaccine (as in the MMR), or within a few weeks of a single measles vaccine, there may be an increased risk of side-effects such as autism and bowel disease. This will be discussed in greater detail later on. The emergence of mutant strains of mumps virus that the vaccine does not protect against may be another consequence of immunisation.[23] The implications of this are currently unknown.

Health officials in Britain have stubbornly refused to offer the single vaccines as an alternative to the MMR. This not only denies parents choice, but is probably also denying them a more effective vaccine. The effectiveness of the mumps vaccine to prevent mumps in the real world has been calculated at rates from as low as 46% up to 97% with an average of around 75%.[24] Two studies looking at outbreaks of mumps found that, whereas a little over 3 out of 5 children vaccinated with the mumps vaccine bundled into the MMR were protected, more than 4 out of 5 children who had received the single mumps vaccine were protected.[14,25] The single mumps vaccine appears to be considerably more effective than the MMR at preventing mumps.

The disappointing effectiveness of the MMR was confirmed by research from London, which showed that the mumps component of the MMR vaccine is only 65% effective after one dose, rising to 88% after two doses, suggesting that even two doses of MMR will never eradicate mumps but will, instead, simply push the illness into older children and adults.[25] Even staunch, pro-vaccine doctors are conceding that there is a problem: 'perhaps the protection against mumps is not as good as we had thought,' said one immunisation co-ordinator, whilst the immunisation spokesman for the Royal College of GPs admitted that the effectiveness of the mumps component of the MMR 'may be much lower than we have thought in the past.'[26] Over recent years, there have been numerous outbreaks in students and young adults, the majority of whom had received two doses of the MMR vaccine. To take one typical example, in an outbreak of mumps in Belgium in 2013, of the 4061 people contracting mumps, nearly all (99%) had received at least one dose, and over two thirds (69%) had received two doses of the MMR vaccine.[27] A study into 114 cases of mumps in France during 2013 showed that nearly three quarters (82) had received two MMR vaccines. Further analysis found that protection against mumps, even after two doses of MMR vaccine, only lasts, on average, for ten years.[30]

There can be little doubt that the original aim of introducing the mumps component of the MMR has been an unmitigated failure. Even scientists at the UK Health Protection Agency (HPA) have reluctantly conceded, 'In the absence of natural boosting, therefore, future mumps epidemics may be unavoidable in vaccinated populations living in crowded, semi-enclosed settings such as colleges.'[28] The average age of infection has risen over the past two decades, making the disease less trivial than it used to be, and the population is now dependent on two vaccinations rather than none. The vaccine appears to be doing more harm than good.

14
MMR/Measles
A Bold Plan

Given the sea change that the MMR heralded — a brand new type of vaccine with the purpose of disease eradication — one would expect health officials to have worked diligently on the introduction of this first new vaccine in a generation. In particular, that they would have ensured the vaccine had been tested for safety and effectiveness, like any other type of medication. As this vaccine would be given to every healthy child in vast numbers, such safety studies should of course follow enough children for long enough to uncover side-effects that are not particularly common, say affecting one in a thousand children. It took, after all, fifteen years of research to introduce the whooping cough vaccine.

For the MMR this means that at least ten thousand children should have been 'actively' followed up for a minimum of twelve months. The word 'actively' is important. It means that the researchers are keeping track of the children and looking for possible problems. 'Passive' follow up relies on family doctors, or hospital doctors, to report side-effects they believe may be caused by the vaccine. Such 'passive surveillance', though useful in helping to pick up rare side-effects after the introduction of a vaccine, is obviously inadequate to demonstrate that a new vaccine is safe.

Not one of the safety trials on the MMR 'actively' followed up the vaccinated children for more than six weeks, and most for no longer than three weeks.[1,2] This is all right for detecting immediate side-effects such as fever or fits, but it is useless for picking up possible long-term consequences of vaccination such as autism and chronic bowel disease. In fact, diarrhoea and vomiting and other symptoms such as ear infections, allergy and abdominal pain did occur remarkably frequently in children receiving MMR, but the doctors conducting the trials considered these to be unimportant and unrelated to the MMR.

It seems there is only one conclusion possible, and that is that the safety studies performed before and around the time of the introduction of the MMR were woefully inadequate. They followed up too few children for too short a time and could not hope to pick up any more than the most obvious side-effects. The potentially more serious side-effects that were picked up were too easily dismissed as being 'unrelated' or of no significance, instead of being taken up as leads for further investigation.

This is not just one view, it is a view shared by health officials. Dr Peter Fletcher was a senior doctor at the Department of Health responsible for the licensing (approving for use) of drugs and vaccines. He has written that 'caution should have ruled the day', and that 'the granting of a product licence [for the MMR vaccines] was premature.'[3] It is also the view of a senior doctor who worked at the Department of Health at the time and said: 'a vaccine didn't get the same scrutiny as a drug would have got.' The expertise of the JCVI, he told me, was 'looking at large-scale epidemiological studies. It was not drug safety or toxicity.' Because they look at efficacy 'vaccines bypass quite a lot of the scrutiny that the CSM [the Committee on Safety of Medicines] would give it.'

An influential European study by the independent and respected Cochrane Collaboration concluded in 2003 that 'the design and reporting of safety outcomes in MMR vaccine studies, both pre- and post-marketing, are largely inadequate.'[4] A more recent review from the same organisation is hardly any more reassuring. The authors mention a specific concern that safety studies followed up children for no more than three weeks, except for one study that lasted six weeks. Remarkably the paper concluded, 'The safety record of MMR is probably best attested by its almost universal use.'[5] In plain English, the best evidence of safety of the MMR is not good medical research, but simply the fact that it has been given to so many children, who were, in effect, being used as guinea pigs. The discerning authors of this review were clearly unimpressed by the flurry of published research over the subsequent decade purporting to demonstrate the safety of the vaccine. In the most recent Cochrane review, published in 2012, they came to the identical conclusion: 'the design and reporting of safety outcomes in MMR vaccine studies, both pre- and post-marketing, are largely inadequate', rebuffing the government's confident reassurances at a stroke.

A generation on, curiously, we are still waiting for that large, systematic study following at least ten thousand children for an adequate length of time.

The Urabe scandal

There were, initially, three different MMR vaccines that were used for nationwide immunisation. The first to be licensed – though not the first to be used – was MMR-II. It was made by Merck, which obtained its license from the Department of Health in 1987 ('MMR-I' had been licensed way back in 1972 but was never used in the UK.) The MMR-II contains the Jeryl Lynn strain of mumps vaccine, and is still used today. The other two MMR vaccines contained the 'Urabe' strain of mumps virus and were called Pluserix, made by Smith Kline & French (SKF), and Immravax, made by Merieux UK. Pluserix was licensed in June 1988 and Immravax in September 1989.

The different strains of mumps vaccine used in the different MMR vaccines turned out to be rather important.

A senior doctor working at that time in the Department of Health, in an interview with me, revealed that the Department of Health was reluctant to use the MMR-II, the first vaccine it had licensed, because of its high price. It therefore asked a competing vaccine manufacturer, SKF, for a cheaper MMR vaccine.

However, SKF's MMR vaccine contained the Urabe mumps vaccine strain. Though all mumps vaccines can occasionally cause viral meningitis – the mumps complication of choice for the Department of Health, when scaring parents – it seemed to be occurring more often in children who had been given the Urabe strain than in those given the Jeryl Lynn strain used in the MMR II.

There had been serious concerns in Canada over the safety of the Urabe mumps component of their MMR (called Trivirix) before the UK licensed Pluserix and Immravax, both of which were similar to Trivirix. The Canadian authorities had, in fact, removed Trivirix from the market in February 1988, and subsequently revoked its license in 1990.[6,7]

There was also concern in Japan, where the proportion of children getting meningitis after Urabe-containing MMR varied from one in six-and-a-half thousand to as many as one in three hundred and thirty children. By October 1989, the Japanese Ministry of Health, too, was urging caution in the use of MMR and later withdrew it.[8,9] In Australia the Urabe vaccine was (secretly) withdrawn in May 1991.[10]

The Department of Health had been aware of increased reactions to Urabe-containing mumps vaccines before they were either licensed or introduced in the UK, but kept this information to itself.[11,12]

SKF were naturally concerned about these safety issues and were, understandably, reluctant to obtain a UK license for their Urabe-containing MMR. But the UK government was intent on obtaining the cheap MMR. The senior doctor at the Department of Health stated to me that the UK government was asked by a pharmaceutical company to offer them indemnity against possible legal action taken against them as a result of the introduction of their MMR vaccine. The UK government, in its enthusiasm to get a cheap MMR onto the market quickly, agreed to this request. The senior doctor told me, 'They wanted an MMR that was cheap...some very funny licensing decisions were made between 1984 and 1989 and MMR was one of them.' A second source has since suggested the existence of a 'legal waiver' given by the Department of Health.

The Department of Health denies providing indemnity for any manufacturer of the MMR vaccine, though it concedes that indemnity was granted to SKF against any loss outside of its control as a result of storage or distribution failures by Farillon, the national vaccine distributor. JCVI minutes from May 1993 refer to an unnamed MMR manufacturer that 'continued to sell the Urabe strain vaccine without liability.'[13]

In November 1988, just after the launch of the Urabe MMR, a fourteen-month-old girl was admitted to Charing Cross Hospital intensive care unit in West London. She had a high fever and continuous fits that could only be controlled by heavy sedation and being paralysed with drugs. She was so ill that she required life support for four days. She recovered slowly and, when she was discharged four weeks later, she was still behaving oddly and had visual problems. When seen four months after discharge, the doctors described her as being 'well'.

She had suffered from severe encephalitis (swelling of the brain), which was considerably more severe than the cases of meningitis that were being caused by the Urabe-containing MMR vaccines. The doctors felt the cause of her illness was the MMR vaccination, again probably the Urabe mumps component, that she had received just less than four weeks before her admission. The doctors were sufficiently concerned to make further enquiries and discovered that other cases of encephalitis had occurred after the MMR vaccine. They published a report in the *British Medical Journal* (*BMJ*), suggesting MMR could be causing encephalitis in as many as one in 100,000 vaccinations (roughly six cases a year given that the vaccine was given to around 600,000 children).[14] The authorities weren't impressed.

Professor A Campbell, the chairman of the JCVI committee that had recommended the introduction of the MMR vaccine (reversing its earlier policy statement) argued in the *BMJ* there was 'no proof' that the mumps component of the MMR had caused the girl's encephalitis and that 'it would be a pity if current initiatives to improve the protection of British children from measles, mumps and rubella were to be affected adversely by the publication of such a speculative case report.' In any case, the little girl had 'recovered completely.'[15]

A week later another letter appeared in the *BMJ*, this time from two government-funded doctors who wrote, 'Publication of cases where a link has not been established may cause unnecessary harm by damaging professional and public confidence in a vaccine whose benefits clearly outweigh its risks.'[16]

After a few weeks a doctor from Merck, the manufacturers of MMR-II (the one not containing the Urabe mumps), wrote to the *BMJ* to point out that these cases were caused by the Urabe mumps and not by Merck's vaccine.[17]

During 1989, there were reports, too, from other doctors of cases of meningitis occurring after the MMR.[18,19] Doctors in Nottingham estimated that it affected one in three thousand eight hundred children. These were children ill enough to be admitted to hospital. There may have been more cases that did not require hospitalisation. All children did appear to make a full recovery.[20] By 1990, the Scottish Health Department was concerned by the high rate of adverse reactions occurring in Scotland, possibly because of its above average use of Urabe-containing MMR vaccines (the other type was also in use).

The Department of Health continued to feel there was 'insufficient evidence of a problem', but three health districts disagreed and, in 1990, took matters into their own hands by abandoning the Urabe-containing MMR vaccines in favour of Merck's MMR-II, which was by then available on the market throughout the UK.[21] By September 1990, the subcommittee at the Department of Health responsible for monitoring adverse reactions to vaccines was aware of an increasing number of reports of viral meningitis and encephalitis occurring in recipients of Urabe-containing MMR vaccines. The committee members agreed that SKB's Pluserix was causing more reactions than Merck's MMR-II. However, they also felt that Pluserix was more effective. They were still pursuing, at that time, the revisionist dream of eliminating mumps, which they felt was a 'realistic prospect in the near future.' They declined to issue any warnings about the Urabe-containing vaccines.[22]

Further research done on behalf of the government by Dr Elizabeth Miller (who also did the trial on the safety of the MMR before its launch) during 1990 and 1991 confirmed an increased risk of 'aseptic' meningitis from the Urabe vaccine. But it took a leak to the national press on 14 September 1992 finally to force the Department of Health to hastily announce the withdrawal of the two Urabe-containing brands of MMR, Pluserix and Immravax.

The manufacturers' licenses weren't cancelled — as they had been in Canada in 1990 — as it was felt that this would have caused a world-wide vaccine crisis.[12] In a letter dated 14 September, Dr Kenneth Calman, the Chief Medical Officer at the Department of Health, informed doctors, in typical government doublespeak, of the 'new arrangements' for the MMR vaccine.[23] One insider told me how, after the withdrawal of both Pluserix and Immravax, a senior Department of Health official had to fly across the Atlantic on Concorde 'cap in hand' to the bosses at Merck, the company the Department of Health had initially snubbed because of their high price, to request they divert extra supplies of their MMR-II to the UK to avoid running out of the vaccine. A new MMR from SKB, Priorix, this time containing the Jeryl Lynn strain of mumps, was licensed, in December 1997, and introduced in 1998.

Following the leaks in 1992, a medical spokesman for one of the manufacturers of the Urabe-containing MMR vaccines dismissed the cases of vaccine meningitis as 'only a bad headache and they all recovered.'[24] This is correct, mumps meningitis, as opposed to bacterial meningitis, is mild — which is exactly why there was no reason for mass immunisation against this disease in the first place.

However, numerous children were admitted to hospital with vomiting and fever after the MMR, making it an important side-effect in its own right.[20]

The rush for a licence

Why was the government so successful in both getting the MMR vaccine licensed and in starting its use for a three-pronged attack to eradicate two mild diseases along with measles?

The approval, licensing and control of all drugs and vaccines introduced into the UK is the responsibility of the medicines division of the

Department of Health. During the late 1980s, it was in a shambles. A senior member of the division described it as a 'pig's ear'. There was so much concern about the running of this important department that an official inquiry was launched. The subsequent report described the department as 'showing signs of overload' and making 'frequent errors'. There was 'slipshod working... poor morale... and... ample opportunities for errors to creep in.' This, in civil-service-speak, was damning criticism.[25]

There was also Dr David Salisbury, then (and up until 2013) head of immunisation at the Department of Health. He was widely seen as one of the driving forces behind the introduction of the MMR into the UK. A highly efficient civil servant, he ably coordinated the path of the MMR through the official implementation process.

There were further political considerations that made the MMR highly attractive to the government. There had been hope that the European Bank would be located in London, but this had been lost to Frankfurt. The European Medicines Agency was up for grabs and the UK government wanted it for London. A senior doctor in the Department of Health described how there was 'pressure to rush through the licensing process [of the MMR] not only from the drug companies, but also from the government, to try to get the European Drug Medicine Agency based in London,' where it was subsequently located.

Not all the members of the Joint Committee on Vaccination and Immunisation (JCVI), the body that advises the government, were in agreement that the introduction of the MMR vaccine was necessary.[26]

The launch
The morning of 3 October 1988 was warm and sunny as, presumably, was the mood of Edwina Currie, the Tory Health Minister. At a high profile launch of the MMR vaccine at the Queen Elizabeth Conference Centre in London, she promised 'lifelong protection with a single jab.'[27] She was to be proven wrong on both counts: the protection obtained is not lifelong for any of the three diseases, and within eight years a second MMR vaccine was to be introduced into the UK vaccination schedule. The aim was elimination of all three diseases.

There was much huffing and puffing at the MMR launch with Sir Donald Acheson, the chief medical officer, warning that compulsory vaccination might have to be considered if the new MMR campaign failed to reach its target of 90% of all children (this target has since been revised upwards to 95%).[28]

At the same time, Edwina Currie, in the 'get-on-your-bike' language of the time, was ordering doctors to 'pull their socks up' to achieve these vaccination targets.[29] The launch was accompanied by an advertising campaign and leaflets advising parents to vaccinate their children 'against brain damage, blindness and deafness' because 'Measles, mumps and rubella are much more a cause for concern than people used to think'.

It was a curious rabbit out of the hat. Even if the seriousness of all three illnesses had been far more serious fifty years ago and this had gone unrecognised, the three diseases had certainly become so much less relevant by 1988 that it really didn't matter what people used to think.

At the time of the launch of the MMR in 1988, the government was preoccupied with the crisis surrounding BSE ('Mad Cow Disease'). In an effort to control public panic, agriculture minister John Gummer was to make a show of eating a hamburger with his daughter.

This preoccupation may also have contributed to the sloppy introduction of the MMR.

Mad cow disease

The concern that BSE could be transmitted in childhood vaccines first arose in 1988, before the launch of MMR.

The problem was that most vaccines were made using the blood from cows, many of which were potentially BSE infected cows from the UK. The Department of Health was concerned that letting slip a mere hint of a problem to the public would replicate the whooping cough vaccine scare of the 1970s and undermine the whole vaccination programme.

After years of reassuring the public that there was no risk to humans from BSE in cattle, the government finally realised that it had a 'serious problem' on its hands. The Chief Medical Officer (CMO), the principal government adviser and head of all medical staff at the time, Sir Donald Acheson, was so concerned about the possibility of vaccine contamination that, in an unusual step, he intervened personally to 'stir up more activity' in the Department of Health as a matter of urgency.

He warned the Secretary of State in 1989 that 'At the present time, we cannot give any complete guarantee of safety for human medicines that use bovine [cow] materials, in manufacture, such as most vaccines.'

One of the vaccines made using UK cows' blood was the MMR vaccine Pluserix. However, the Department of Health's view was that the benefits of continuing to use potentially contaminated vaccines far outweighed the 'remote' risk to children of being infected with BSE from the vaccines.

Not all the experts agreed. Dr Hilary Pickles, a government doctor, had 'serious concern about the safety of bovine-based vaccines'. After all, the risk of becoming infected with BSE was greater from contaminated injections than from contaminated food. The government's response was to issue 'guidelines' (advice) to drug companies; in March 1989, they were requested to use non-infected cows' products in vaccine manufacture 'wherever possible'.

In practice this meant that potentially contaminated vaccines, including MMR, continued to be used for an unknown period whilst alternative supplies were obtained.

The Department of Health, obsessed with public perception, was concerned that 'certain elements of the press did not get the wrong impression about the safety of vaccines', and continued to reaffirm their safety.

The BSE Enquiry of 2000 criticised the Department of Health for not being sufficiently open with the public about the risks of BSE from vaccines and other medicinal sources. It damningly added, 'we believe that a policy of giving the public full information about risk is... the correct one.'

The official report offered further advice:'We believe that vaccine scares, like food scares, are likely to be fostered by a belief, on the part of the public, that the full picture is not being disclosed.'[30]

Did the government and Department of Health take to heart this warning?

The virtual epidemic

In 1994 the Department of Health announced there was likely to be a large epidemic of measles in the UK in 1995. This is despite the fact that the previous year, 1993, had seen the lowest numbers of reported cases of measles ever, and uptake of the MMR vaccine was running at over 90%. The government forecast an outbreak of between 100,000 and 200,000, and the deaths of no fewer than fifty children. It was, we were told, 'definitely' going to happen unless there was a vaccination campaign.[31]

The arguments are complex and convoluted and rely on 'mathematical modelling' to predict the outbreak. The forecast relied on a recent outbreak of measles in Scotland, a rising number of measles notifications in England and Wales during 1994 and blood tests showing that nearly 9% of children were susceptible to measles. It seems quite possible, however, that there was no such degree of certainty.

Over six million children were vaccinated with MR (measles and rubella) vaccine in the first ever mass vaccination campaign conducted in an industrialised country.

It was, in effect, an experiment. Over a quarter of all children had already received two measles vaccines (a single measles vaccine and the MMR introduced six years previously).[32]

The Department of Health pressed on. Under its own guidelines there must be 'informed consent' for any medical intervention, including vaccination. Many of the children being vaccinated (up to sixteen years of age) were mature enough to make their own decision on whether to have the vaccine. Yet they were rarely informed. One consultant paediatrician wrote that there was an 'apparent disregard of children's rights' during the MR vaccination campaign.[33]

The MR vaccine shouldn't have been given to any child who was unwell, who had impaired immunity or who had an allergy to any of the ingredients of the vaccine. But when children were being lined up to receive vaccines at thirty-second intervals it is difficult to see how there was time to ensure that all these safeguards involving contraindications were met.

The Department of Health's own guidelines state that the MMR vaccine shouldn't be given to pregnant women, but, during this campaign, doctors were advised not to try and find out whether any of the older girls up to sixteen years of age were pregnant. The department advised doctors that enquiring about girls' menstrual histories 'is likely to cause considerable difficulties and will not be helpful.'[34]

The government's obsession to vaccinate millions of children caused disruption in schools. Developmental checks and routine vaccinations were all delayed. Schools ran out of soft mats to cater for children who fainted or were distressed by the vaccination.

The Department of Health promoted the MR vaccine with a multi-media campaign involving the press, radio and some particularly hard-hitting television advertisements. The parent information sheets stated, 'Measles can be much more serious than most people think. School-age children who get it are likely to be very ill. Measles can cause pneumonia, blindness, deafness and even brain damage. Measles can also be fatal.' The literature goes on to reassure parents about the vaccine, 'Side-effects are uncommon. They are usually very mild and disappear quickly,'[32] though the reality is that a high fever is common, as is a painful arthritis (inflammation of the joints), especially in older girls.

After the campaign, it was acknowledged that the TV advert 'had been a little frightening' and that children and their parents had not been warned enough about possible side-effects.[35] However, the spin had its desired effect: the proportion of parents that felt that measles was serious rose from 15% before the campaign to 40%. It was hard to see, though, who had benefited.

Why no mumps?

A puzzling feature of the MR campaign is why rubella (German measles) was included but not mumps. The reason the Department of Health gave for including rubella was 'to hasten the elimination of the congenital rubella syndrome [CRS]'.[36] But there was only one baby born with CRS in 1993 and only four or five were being born a year on average, and the JCVI knew that 98-99% of women were immune to rubella.

A more plausible explanation for using measles and rubella, but not mumps, was the withdrawal of two Urabe mumps MMR vaccines in 1992. It left two companies, Smith Kline and Merieux, with a lot of surplus measles and rubella vaccines that they were unable to use.

A paper written later by government doctors admitted, 'a mumps component was not included... because there was no suitable mumps component available at the time.'[37] Was it mere coincidence, then, that the only two companies approached by the Department of Health to provide the MR (measles and rubella) vaccine were SKF — by then Smith Kline Beecham — and Merieux? Apparently so, according to the Department of Health.[38]

Nonetheless, some have questioned the government's need to spend £20 million on a campaign of dubious justification. 'If the predicted epidemic was to be prevented, prompt action was required,' argued public health doctors in defence of the campaign.[39] Under pressure, they conceded that, 'it is impossible to prove that an epidemic of measles would have occurred.'[40]

It is impossible to give over six million doses of vaccine without side-effects. The Department of Health received 1202 reports of a total of 2735 suspected 'adverse reactions' to the MR vaccine (roughly 1 in 2000). Five hundred and thirty were serious and included encephalitis, convulsions and Guillain-Barré syndrome. However, 'side-effects', it was asserted, 'are outweighed by improved disease control.'[41]

The number of babies born disabled with CRS from German measles was little affected by the MR vaccination campaign. As for the predicted fifty deaths from measles, the last time that had happened in the UK was nearly twenty years earlier, in 1968, when The Beatles topped the charts with 'Hey Jude'.

The second MMR
Hot on the heels of organising the MR campaign, the Department of Health announced the addition of a second MMR vaccine to the childhood vaccination schedule. It was introduced in October 1996 and was given to four-year-old children along with their 'pre-school booster'.

As was now becoming the norm, it was introduced along with a 'catch-up' programme to vaccinate those children who had recently had the pre-school booster but had not had two measles-containing vaccines (most likely MMR and MR). The reasons given for the introduction of a second MMR were not unlike those of the ad hoc MR, namely to 'prevent the possibility of future epidemics and to build on the success of the MR campaign.'[42]

As for safety studies, if there had been disturbingly little done before the introduction of the initial MMR vaccine, there were none on the safety of a two-dose schedule.

In any case, the introduction of a new booster contradicted the claims of Edwina Currie eight years previously that a 'single jab' would provide 'lifelong protection.' The Department of Health offered no explanation.

Ripples of unrest − the start of the legal cases
Richard Barr, a solicitor based in Norfolk, had previous experience in obtaining compensation for victims of drug side-effects. In 1990 he was approached by a woman whose son had become ill with meningitis shortly after receiving the MMR. She was concerned that it could be linked to the vaccine and wanted his help.

Over the next few years he was contacted by several hundred families, who all had children whom they believed had been damaged by the MMR vaccine.

Initially the solicitor thought that, even if most of the cases were caused by the vaccine, they were probably very rare side-effects. He started to become concerned as the numbers continued to rise and a clear pattern started to emerge. Most of the children had been developing normally until they received the vaccine. They then started 'regressing' or losing skills they previously had: they stopped talking, lost their potty-training skills, and no longer played and socialised as they had done. This was often accompanied by bowel problems. Some were diagnosed with autism. In 1994 Richard Barr joined forces with solicitor Paul Balen and managed to obtain legal aid funding for over a hundred children.

By 1996 Barr was becoming so concerned that he wrote to the Committee on Safety of Medicines (CSM), the body responsible for vaccine safety at the Department of Health. By then he had three hundred and sixty cases on his books, including children with autism, epilepsy, bowel problems and behavioural disorders. A few children had died.

He acknowledged in his letter that it was possible the vaccine had nothing to do with the disorders suffered by the children, but he urged that the numbers and similarities of the children he was seeing warranted further action. 'If our observations do no more than raise the possibility of a link between the vaccines and the injuries that I have described,' he wrote, 'then it is incumbent on you and your colleagues to take steps to carry out a thorough investigation.'[43]

Professor Rawlins, Chairman of the government Committee on Safety of Medicines (CSM) had already dismissed Richard Barr's concerns as 'unconvincing'.[44] He declined to meet the solicitors.

Professor Rawlins also turned down repeated invitations to view the medical records of the children.

The government on the offensive
The JCVI, having been aware of the alleged link between MMR and autism for some time, felt that 'This was likely to be a long running issue.'[45]

When doctors suspect side-effects have occurred as a result of any drug or vaccine, they are meant to report these on 'yellow cards' which are sent to the Department of Health, though only a small minority, probably 10% at most, get reported.

The JCVI knew of the 'big increase in yellow card reports after MMR vaccine.'[46] These all came from doctors, not parents, and many referred to autism. The 'big increase' occurred before the furore that would erupt in the national media, caused by a paper published in the Lancet, co-written by twelve authors including the then unknown Dr Andrew Wakefield.

15
MMR/Rubella

A Further Mystery

As already discussed, in 1986 the powerful Joint Committee on Vaccination and Immunisation (JCVI) felt that 'there was insufficient evidence to justify a change' in rubella vaccination policy. Nonetheless, just as had mysteriously occurred in the case of mumps, two years on and this long-held view had been moved aside to make way for the MMR vaccine. All of a sudden, health officials decided that the new medical aim was to eradicate mild diseases such as rubella (and mumps). The new objective was not merely to prevent cases of CRS, as had been done with increasing success, but to eliminate the disease. Every baby was to be vaccinated in the second year of life, no longer just twelve-year-old girls and non-immune mothers after having given birth.

The risk of this strategy, as with mumps, was that it could actually increase the complications – specifically the number of children born with CRS. The manufacturers of the vaccine had warned in the late 1970s that, for mass vaccination of pre-school children to work, the vaccine had to be more effective than the natural disease at producing immunity – something the rubella vaccine clearly isn't.[1] It otherwise risks pushing up the age at which most people get infected into the very group we are trying to protect – child-bearing women.

In the UK it had been predicted that the uptake of the rubella vaccine (and therefore the newly introduced MMR) had to be at least 84% to prevent making things worse.[2] The rubella vaccine is generally considered to be one of the more effective vaccines, working in around 95% of immunisations – the same figure that was originally, incorrectly, put on the mumps vaccine, but with more evidence because of its widespread use since 1971. As a safety measure, the vaccine given to twelve-year-old girls was, for a while, continued. There was optimism, at this stage, that rubella – and therefore CRS – could be eliminated from the UK by 2000.

Six years after the introduction of the MMR, in 1994, the Department of Health was concerned that women may have been at increased risk of catching rubella. The number of children born disabled (with CRS) due to rubella was by then in single figures, with only one case reported in 1993, so one might be forgiven for thinking that there wasn't really any need for an extension to the rubella vaccination programme. From the routine test given to women, it was also clear that nearly all pregnant women had antibodies against the disease and were immune. The Department of Health reasoned, however, that there were still young men getting rubella who could then pass it on to pregnant women, and it presumably still wanted to eradicate the disease.

At a cost of £20 million, a national campaign was started in which all children aged between five and sixteen years were offered a combined measles and rubella vaccine. It may have seemed an overreaction, but 7 million schoolchildren were vaccinated in order to prevent two or three cases of CRS a year. It turned out that the susceptibility (that is those remaining unprotected) to rubella of fifteen to nineteen-year-old boys, one of the main target groups, fell by only 4% — from 16% before the campaign, to 12% shortly after, a disappointing return considering the size and cost of the campaign.[3]

In the next year, 1995, the vaccination of twelve-year-old girls was stopped, to be replaced in October 1996 by the addition of a second dose of MMR vaccine to the childhood immunisation schedule at the age of three to five years. This meant that all children were now having two rubella vaccinations before five, but none afterwards unless, in the case of women, they were found to be susceptible when tested during pregnancy. This new policy relied on the vaccine having a long-lasting effect — at least 40 years, to cover women until their mid-40s.

Unfortunately, for many women, protection does not last this long — or anywhere near it. The routine blood tests on pregnant women suggest that not only may the vaccine not be as effective as 95%, but there is also a falling-off of immunity after vaccination. Of particular relevance to the UK is a study from Finland that showed that one third of girls given the MMR twice, at one year and six years of age (very similar to the current UK schedule) had lost all the protection they may have had by fifteen years of age.[4]

Other studies have since confirmed this loss of protection by the late teenage years in a substantial proportion of women despite having received two MMR vaccines. This is particularly worrying as this is just the age at which it is so important that they are protected, namely before they have children. However, only 9% of those girls who received a second rubella vaccine at the later age of twelve years were unprotected at fifteen. This suggests that the UK policy of abandoning the vaccination for girls at twelve years of age, in favour of vaccinating four-year-old boys and girls, may have been a mistake.

Between 2005 and 2015 there were 23 known cases of pregnant women contracting rubella, though the figure is likely to be higher because of the mild nature of the illness. Most of these are believed to have been acquired abroad. The 23 cases resulted in seven babies being born with CRS or with evidence of infection, two babies died in the womb and four women had terminations. Ten babies were born unaffected. These low figures suggest that the current policy is working with regard to CRS.

After the introduction of the MMR vaccine for children in 1988, the single rubella vaccine remained available on the NHS to protect women who were not immune to rubella. In late 2003 the Chief Medical Officer announced, however, that the single vaccine would no longer be available and that women should be given the MMR vaccine as a 'suitable alternative'. He alleged that the NHS was 'unable to secure supplies of licensed rubella vaccine.'[5] It seems extraordinary that a purchaser as large as the NHS could not, if it really wanted to, obtain a supply of the single rubella vaccine. The single rubella vaccine continued to be available privately until 2015 when the last remaining manufacturer, the Serum Institute of India, ceased production, concentrating instead on the MMR vaccine.

Did the rubella component of MMR achieve its goal?

In twenty years, a generation later, there has been a reduction in the number of children born damaged by rubella (with CRS) from an average of thirty a year, when the single vaccine was given to girls at age twelve, to only one or two a year after all children, boys and girls, were being given two doses of MMR. The next years will be crucial. Women first vaccinated as children in 1988 are now in their late twenties and have started to give birth to the next generation. Given that childbirth happens later and later in life, the effects of the rubella component of the MMR vaccination will be put to the test. Thankfully there is so far no sign of an increase in CRS.

During the three years 2001-3, there were only forty-seven cases of CRS reported in all of Europe, including Turkey and a large part of the former Soviet Union.[6] Nonetheless, the target of eliminating CRS has been abandoned in Europe and rubella remains widespread. Some countries, including France and Germany, do not even attempt to count the number of rubella cases.[7]

The number of babies born with CRS in the UK is now very small. Against this should be set the fact that no medicine, vaccines included, is ever harmless. The introduction of the second MMR vaccine means that four times as many vaccinations are now being given compared to when the single vaccine was in use (all boys and girls twice, compared to just girls once).

If one discounts all doubts and assumes that all the reduction in CRS cases is due to rubella vaccination, then each year an additional million MMR vaccinations are given to achieve this result.

Whether this is really a worthwhile trade-off depends on the risks of giving the MMR vaccine.

There was no debate in 1988, or in 1996 when the second MMR was introduced, on this trade-off.

However, the side-effects of the rubella vaccine are fairly well known since the vaccine was selectively introduced in 1971. The rubella vaccine contains a modified form of the live rubella virus and so can cause any of the symptoms of rubella. Painful or inflamed joints (arthritis) are a common side-effect, more common in adult women than in children; though symptoms generally settle within a few days, they can occasionally persist for over a year.[8] It has been suggested that rubella immunisation may be a cause of chronic fatigue syndrome, or ME, though other infections and vaccinations have also been implicated.[9]

Breast-feeding mothers who have been vaccinated transmit the rubella vaccine virus to their babies in the breast milk.[10] Whilst there is no known danger to the baby, that is not a guarantee of safety. The vaccine virus can spread to close contacts, but this is probably very rare. The rubella virus appears in the throat of some children after the MMR vaccine; though there is no evidence of this being passed to anyone else, one vaccine expert has advised caution in giving the MMR to any child in whose household someone is in the early stages of pregnancy.[11]

As with all vaccinations there will always be some people who just don't 'take' the vaccine. One unfortunate baby boy was born with CRS whose mother had been properly vaccinated against rubella three times.[12]

Live viruses can interfere with each other, and it is unknown as yet how the live rubella vaccine interacts with the other two live vaccines of mumps and measles.

16
MMR Scare

Dr Andrew Wakefield

The MMR was in many ways the catalyst for my investigation into vaccines. The furore surrounding it to this day has made one thing clear. While the danger of infectious diseases has declined dramatically over the past fifty years, paradoxically the danger of questioning, even gently, the perceived truth about vaccines has risen dramatically. It seems that any discussion, even a medical one, is considered heretical. The case of Andrew Wakefield, who inadvertently started the furore, speaks volumes. Had I thought his story remotely possible when I was first alerted to the MMR by a newspaper in 2001?

At the time, I would have said no.

A rising star

In the early 1990s, Dr Andrew Wakefield was a rising star at The Royal Free Hospital in north London. He was working there as a gastroenterologist (gut specialist) and was particularly interested in inflammatory bowel disease in children. Crohn's disease, an inflammation of the bowel, was unheard of in children before measles vaccination, and Dr Wakefield had found the measles virus in the gut of some of these children.[1] What appeared to trigger bowel disease in these children was an 'unusual exposure' to the measles virus. Crohn's disease was more common in children born during or just after a measles epidemic.[2] Also, of four mothers who contracted measles while pregnant, three had children who went on to develop Crohn's disease of the bowel, a 'coincidence' that is all but impossible to have happened by chance.[3]

Andrew Wakefield first contacted Dr David Salisbury, the most senior doctor in charge of vaccination at the Department of Health, in 1992. His concern was not the MMR at that stage, but rather that children who had been vaccinated against measles were three times more likely to develop bowel disease.[4] A year later, he became aware of the imminent MR campaign, in which the measles and rubella vaccine was to be given to over six million children.

He again contacted Salisbury to share his concern that this campaign was likely to provide the children with the very 'unusual measles exposure' from which some would go on to develop bowel disease. Sir Kenneth Calman, then the government's Chief Medical Officer and head of all medical staff in England, wrote back to reassure Wakefield that other countries had two-dose measles vaccination policies (though no western country had ever undertaken a campaign on the scale the UK was about to embark on with six million doses), and that 'because so many young lives are at imminent risk we felt it right to go ahead with the measles campaign as planned.'[5] Sir Kenneth did finally meet with Wakefield for twenty minutes in January 1995, but nothing came out of this meeting and Wakefield's impression was that the Department of Health saw him as a 'pain in the neck', and that they were not really interested in his concerns.

Until the mid-1990s Andrew Wakefield hadn't been concerned with the MMR vaccine, and he knew little about autism. However, as part of his work as a specialist treating children with bowel disease at the Royal Free Hospital, he saw something that started to puzzle him.

Parents who were bringing their children to see him were telling a remarkably similar story. The children had been developing entirely normally, both physically and mentally, until they received the MMR vaccine. They then regressed, stopped talking, became clumsy and irritable and would stare with glazed eyes instead of interacting normally. Intriguingly, to Wakefield, the children also suffered from bloating, abdominal pain, diarrhoea and weight loss; they became extremely thirsty and developed cravings for certain foods. The children were often 'allergic', with asthma or eczema, and got frequent colds and ear infections, often requiring multiple courses of antibiotics. Some had already been diagnosed as autistic and many more were later to be given that label.

Dr Wakefield and the other Royal Free doctors were initially sceptical of the parents' belief that the MMR vaccine was the cause of their children's problems. But when they examined the children's guts, they were all found to be inflamed in a similar, but unusual, pattern quite unlike any bowel disease they were used to seeing. What's more, they found measles virus in the gut of some of these children.

It didn't 'prove' anything, but it certainly raised questions that needed to be investigated with further research. Andrew Wakefield wondered whether the MMR vaccine could represent another form of 'unusual measles exposure' that, as he had already found, could cause bowel disease. After all, these children certainly had bowel disease and giving a live measles virus together with two other live viruses in an injection is not a 'normal' exposure to measles.

A meeting with the minister

As Dr Wakefield saw more and more children with the same story he became increasingly worried. Some families of the children he saw were investigating legal action with the help of solicitor Richard Barr, who contacted Dr Wakefield to ask him if he could help by providing clinical evidence that might support their cases. By 1997 Richard Barr had on his books twelve hundred children whose parents felt had been damaged by MMR.

Wakefield, Barr and others felt that there might be something in this and felt obliged to alert the government to their concerns. They, along with some concerned parents, had a meeting with Tessa Jowell, a member of the shadow health team when the Labour Party was in opposition. After that meeting, Ms Jowell wrote to one of the parents: 'I was deeply disturbed by the evidence presented in the course of our discussion and hope very much that after the election we may be in a position to provide greater safety and certainty about these vaccinations'.[6]

After Labour was elected to government, Wakefield had another meeting with Tessa Jowell, then Labour's health minister, and Dr Kenneth Calman. Professor Walker-Smith, a colleague of Dr Wakefield's at the Royal Free Hospital, and Jackie Fletcher, who knew of another five hundred possibly affected children through her organisation JABS, were also at the meeting, as were other officers of the Department of Health. Tessa Jowell and Dr Calman were told of the (now many) children who had been developing normally before receiving the MMR jab, following which they had regressed, lost skills such as speech, developed bowel problems, appetite changes, disturbed sleep patterns and increased thirst.

Andrew Wakefield wanted to alert the government to his worries in order to prevent a vaccine scare that he felt might happen if his fears were correct. Tessa Jowell appeared concerned. At Dr Wakefield's request it was agreed the government would convene a meeting of experts to look at the issue, but nothing was to happen until after the publication of a medical paper that was to spark the biggest vaccine scare for a generation.

MMR & autism – the 1998 Lancet paper

The Royal Free team felt that they were on to something new. As mentioned, the children had a unique bowel problem that was not the same as other known inflammatory bowel diseases.

The majority were found to be suffering from what the researchers described as 'ileal-lymphoid-nodular hyperplasia' (ILNH), a meaningless term to most people, but it accurately described their finding. It is like swollen lymph glands in the neck when, for example, someone has a sore throat. But in this case the swollen glands are in the gut. The finding was important because this pattern of disease could easily be causing the pain and diarrhoea or constipation from which these autistic children were suffering. Up until now these symptoms had usually been dismissed as something that autistic children just had, possibly because of a poor diet.

The finding of ILNH, along with inflammation of the gut, in autistic children (which the researchers later labelled 'autistic enterocolitis') represented a new disease, not previously described.

As is normal practice when doctors make a new discovery, the team of thirteen doctors wrote a paper describing the children. The paper, published in the *Lancet* on 28 February 1998, was entitled 'Ileal-lymphoid-nodular hyperplasia, non-specific colitis, and pervasive developmental disorder in children.'[7] It is not the sort of title expected to trigger a stampede of media excitement. The paper was a report of twelve children who had all lost skills, including language, had diarrhoea and abdominal pain, and who all had the unusual changes in their guts described in the title of paper.

Though Andrew Wakefield and his colleagues were not yet convinced the MMR vaccine had actually caused the problem, and wrote as much in the paper, they noted, 'In eight children, the onset of behavioural problems had been linked, either by parents or by the child's physician, with measles, mumps, and rubella vaccination.' Most of the children had by this stage been diagnosed with autism. Though a Danish mother had first suggested that the MMR vaccine had caused autism in one of her children back in 1993, they were the first doctors to publicly suggest a link.

The press conference

Even this tentative suggestion of a link might have passed by unnoticed had the Royal Free Hospital not, rather unusually, arranged a 'press briefing' to announce the findings of the paper. Questions from the press on what parents should do about the MMR vaccine had been anticipated. Most of the doctors felt the benefits of the vaccine far outweighed any possible risks that may occur. However, Dr Wakefield told Arie Zuckerman, the Dean of the Royal Free Hospital's medical school who was chairing the press conference, that, if asked about the vaccination issue, he would urge caution and recommend the three components of the vaccine be given separately.

When, as expected, a journalist asked this very question, Professor Zuckerman directed the question not to any one of the other doctors who would have encouraged parents to continue giving their children the MMR, but to Dr Wakefield who notoriously advised that children should continue to be vaccinated, but with the three vaccines given singly and separated by a year. 'There is sufficient concern in my own mind,' he told the journalists, 'for a case to be made for vaccines to be given individually at not less than one year intervals.' He went on, 'For the vast majority of children, the MMR vaccine is fine, but I believe there are sufficient anxieties for a case to be made to administer the three vaccines separately.'[8]

It was this challenge to the established view that was to signal the beginning of his downfall.

Dr Wakefield wasn't the only member of the research team who, at that time, felt single vaccines were preferable to the MMR. His colleague, Professor Roy Pounder told the BBC, 'In hindsight, it may be a better solution to give the vaccinations separately. When the vaccinations were given individually, there was no problem.'[9] Professor Pounder had written to Sir Kenneth Calman six weeks earlier to warn him that, 'it seems likely that at least some members of our team will recommend that there is a switch from MMR to monovalent [single] vaccination,' advising that he increased the NHS stocks of the single measles vaccine. Two other senior co-authors of the paper, though publicly supporting government policy on the MMR, confided in Andrew Wakefield their real feelings: 'In private our view is that the government should institute urgently a comparative study of MMR and monovalent vaccines.' Both doctors have since publicly supported the MMR vaccine.

'Child Vaccine Linked to Autism' ran the headlines on the following day. The Department of Health acted quickly to try to reassure worried parents, stating, 'Our advice remains to have your child immunised. Measles, mumps and rubella can kill and cause serious illnesses.'[10]

Two weeks later an editorial in the *British Medical Journal* (*BMJ*) defended the vaccine, comparing the scare to that of the whooping cough vaccine in the 1970s, 'which resulted in much suffering and many deaths from pertussis [whooping cough] both in Britain and internationally.' The editorial went on to dismiss the whooping cough scare as unfounded. 'Unproved theories are no basis for dropping a vaccine of global safety and effectiveness,' argued the *BMJ*, 'The pertussis experience must not be repeated with the MMR vaccine.'[11] The World Health Organisation (WHO) weighed in with a fax from its Geneva HQ to Tessa Jowell, expressing alarm at suggestions that MMR could be causing autism. WHO was, its Assistant Director-General wrote, 'offering you and your colleagues support in remaining firm in supporting the continued use of this highly effective vaccine which has such an outstanding safety record.'[12]

Shaken by the media storm, the government's Chief Medical Officer, Sir Kenneth Calman, belatedly convened an 'expert scientific seminar' to look at the possible link between MMR and Crohn's disease and MMR and autism.

Ken Aitken, a clinical psychologist and autism specialist, was one of the thirty-seven experts present at the one-day meeting. He remembers the general feeling of the meeting as 'one of concern.' This was reflected in the minutes, which concluded, 'Further research, probably on an international basis in order to include a sufficiently large number of patients, would be needed to settle the question of any possible association between autism and MMR vaccination.'[13] The seminar had made him worried that there was a problem that needed to be addressed.

Aitken was, therefore, surprised to read a Department of Health press release issued on the following day entitled, 'MMR vaccine is not linked to Crohn's disease or autism — conclusion of an expert scientific seminar,' in which Sir Kenneth Calman, who had been present throughout the seminar, was quoted as saying, 'I have concluded there is no link between measles, measles vaccine or MMR immunisation and either Crohn's Disease or autism.'[14] Could both men have attended the same meeting?

Sir Kenneth followed this release with a letter to all doctors, in which he wrote that although he didn't know what caused Crohn's Disease or autism, it certainly wasn't the MMR vaccine. He dismissed the *Lancet* paper as demonstrating 'normal variants in a highly selected sample, with no reason to believe that MMR vaccine played a part in their condition.' He dismissed the option of separate vaccines writing, 'I cannot endorse an opinion that jeopardises child health.'[15]

Also present at the 'expert scientific seminar' was one of Andrew Wakefield's co-researchers. This scientist was so concerned at the way that the government's Chief Medical Officer (CMO) had misrepresented the outcome in 'an almost 'tabloid' fashion,' that he wrote to Sir Kenneth himself. He stated to Sir Kenneth the opinion that his language conveyed 'neither the substance nor the tone of the meeting'. The letter Sir Kenneth had sent to every doctor in the country was, the researcher felt, loaded in a 'pejorative and damaging way.'

In his letter to Sir Kenneth, the researcher was especially critical of Sir Kenneth's dismissal of the gut abnormalities as 'normal variants.' The Royal Free team, he pointed out to the most senior doctor in the land, had examined the guts of more children than any other unit in Europe and had an international reputation. They wouldn't have dreamed of publishing a paper to describe a clinical condition unless it had been both unusual and important. The CMO's turn of phrase, was, he commented, 'unnecessary, insulting, and liable in time to be viewed as propaganda rather than the measured response required in these circumstances.'

Even within the Department of Health there were doubts. At that time it was far less certain about the safety of the MMR than it admitted in public. There were concerns about the lack of robust safety trials; a significant minority of senior medical advisors felt that the department's support for the MMR was rash, and that single vaccines should be made available, at least until further research was done. Despite this, it was finally decided to fully back the vaccine and not allow the option of single vaccines — with cost being a factor in the decision.

What happened next?

Consultant colleagues at the Royal Free Hospital were initially very supportive of Dr Andrew Wakefield's work, which was felt to be extremely important. A presentation of the first seven cases of children with bowel disease and autism following MMR vaccination had been made in 1996, not by Dr Wakefield, but his colleague Dr John Walker-Smith. However, those at the top of the medical school hierarchy (Dr Wakefield was officially employed by the Royal Free Medical School), were becoming increasingly concerned about the 'unwelcome publicity' that the research looking at the MMR would attract. The majority of medical research in UK universities is funded by drug companies. By coincidence the Royal Free set up its vaccine research unit in 1993 funded by Smith Kline Beecham (now GlaxoSmithKline), one of the manufacturers of the MMR who were, at that time, embroiled in the legal action by families of children allegedly damaged by the MMR vaccine.[16]

The Medical School Dean, Professor Arie Zuckerman, was particularly concerned about the damage to the school's 'reputation' that this controversial research might cause. Despite the concern felt by some, the board of the medical school unanimously approved Dr Wakefield's promotion in the middle of 1997.

However, once Dr Wakefield had stood up and suggested single vaccines might be a safer option than MMR, his relationship with the medical school deteriorated. The Royal Free quickly dissociated itself from his comments referring to the MMR. The Dean exerted increasing pressure on Dr Wakefield and his colleagues not to talk publicly about their research — imposing, in effect, a gagging order.

Wakefield doesn't know who was tapping his home phone line, as it could have been one of several organisations: he was a thorn in the side of the government, was unpopular with the powerful multinational drug companies and he had lost favour at The Royal Free Hospital, where continuing with his unpopular and controversial research might have jeopardised future research funding to the hospital.

Once a rising star in research on gut disease at the hospital, by late 1999 Wakefield was told in clear terms that his work on the MMR vaccine was no longer going to be supported. During the next two years the relationship between him and the Royal Free became increasingly strained and hostile. In early December 2001 the inevitable happened and Dr Wakefield and The Royal Free Hospital parted company 'by mutual consent' – at least that was the official line. The reality was that he was forced out. The Royal Free hospital's explanation was that his research 'was no longer in line with the department of medicine's research strategy'.[17]

By now his work was pilloried by the government and senior doctors. Every paper he published (and there were lots) was vociferously criticised. Dr Elizabeth Miller is reported to have described him as 'naïve', saying his research methods contained 'basic errors.'[18]

Dr Wakefield's departure affected the care of some of the children with bowel problems. Parents were forced to seek treatment elsewhere. 'Our children were effectively pushed out of the Royal Free', one mother told me. 'We were told that the funding had stopped for our children who, we were told, were putting other children at risk.'

Spurred on by John Reid, then health secretary, the General Medical Council (GMC) announced it was investigating Dr Wakefield's conduct,[19] something Dr Wakefield welcomed as he believed, wrongly it turned out, it would clear his name from any wrongdoing. 'I've lost everything,' he told me, referring to his job, security, income and, to some extent, his family because he moved to the USA where he was, at least for a while, able to continue his research.

Reconciliation of the two sides appears improbable. An article in *The Times* referred to Dr Wakefield as 'the Abu Hamza of the medical profession', and chastised his 'followers' as 'hysterical middle-class parents who, in the name of love, risk dragging Britain back to an era of high child mortality'.[20]

The legal cases

By 2003, over sixteen hundred families had been granted legal aid to seek compensation from the manufacturers of MMR – GSK, Merck and Aventis Pasteur. More and more evidence was accumulating to implicate the vaccine in the children's disabilities, and a date for the start of a preliminary court case had been set for April 2004.

Then something unprecedented happened: after years of funding (some of the children had been receiving funding for nearly ten years), with mounting evidence against the MMR, the support of twenty-nine experts and with a trial date only months away, the Legal Services Commission withdrew funding in September 2003. The commission wouldn't even pay the legal team to inform the parents of their decision.

The Legal Services Commission (LSC) decided 'the litigation is very likely to fail' even though Merck's leading barrister had acknowledged in court the strength of the parents' evidence.[21] The LSC argued that £15 million had already been spent and that a full trial would cost another £10 million that couldn't be justified. The pharmaceutical companies are believed to have spent £80 million on the case by this point.

Various appeals against this decision all failed. The cases never went to court as the cost to the families (who would also have to pay the drug companies' costs) would have been prohibitive. Solicitors acting for Merck, one of the MMR manufacturers, sent letters to parents in May 2004, promising not to seek legal costs from the parents if they, in turn, promised by the end of the month, never to sue Merck in the UK or anywhere else in the world. Merck, by sending parents an intimidating letter, urging parents to give their 'offer the most serious consideration', appeared to be trying to take advantage of the parents' vulnerability and fears of bankruptcy if they continued.[22] However, the trial judge in the case ruled this was out of order and declared the letters invalid, saying the parents should be given far longer to consider their position.

The High Court appeal on funding was heard by Mr Justice Davis, the younger brother of Sir Crispin Davis. Sir Crispin was then on the board of directors of GSK where he remained until 2013. He was also Chief Executive of Reed Elsevier, owner of the *Lancet* which had recently expressed its 'regret' at having published the notorious paper, from 1999 to 2009. A spokesperson for the judge said that 'The possibility of any conflict of interest arising from his brother's position was not raised with him and did not occur to him. If he was wrong, any possible remedy must be sought from the court of appeal.' The appeal against the decision to withdraw funding was declined, though funding would later be reinstated for certain families. The legal cases floundered. Goliath had beaten David, at least in the legal arena where the parents were left on their own, and the public at large remained no clearer on the issue.

The LSC took an even more surprising partial U-turn in December 2004 when it reinstated legal aid to a minority of families who are claiming that their children suffered from an array of diseases, including epilepsy, arthritis and encephalitis, from the vaccine, but not autism, though even this was withdrawn in 2006. One of the parents claimed she was told by the LSC that the decision to stop legal aid came from the government;[23] it may have found a public trial, in which dealings between it and the drug companies would have come out into the open, rather uncomfortable.

17
MMR Research

The Science

The MMR furore started in February 1998 when Dr Wakefield suggested at a press conference that, in his view, it might be safer to use single vaccines than the MMR vaccine. In advance, he had informed his colleague, Professor Zuckerman, who led the Royal Free press conference that, if asked, that would be his response.

Contrary to public perception, the 1998 *Lancet* article did not argue that autism was caused by the MMR; it merely sought to notify colleagues of a gut disease not previously known, ILNH, an inflammation of the lymph glands in the gut, in twelve children.[1] The twelve authors also noted that the children with INLH had impaired learning skills, and that in eight cases parents, or the child's doctor, had made a link to the MMR.

Wakefield did not say that autism and the MMR were linked. It is an important distinction to make. His was not a plea to warn people off immunisation against the three diseases. Nor did he question the medical necessity of the government's goals of immunising the British population with three vaccines. The sole issue he raised concerned the bundling of three live vaccines into one. This bundling may have been attractive to the government for practical, political and financial reasons, but not because the MMR would offer the child more protection than its separate constituent parts from a medical point of view. In his opinion as a doctor, separate vaccination was the safer option.

In other words, Wakefield was not anti-vaccination, and did not state anything outrageous that his peers would have thought lacked any medical foundation. If that were so, Professor Zuckerman would no doubt have handed the question to someone else.

Nor was Wakefield's view based solely on having seen a modest number of children at the Royal Free Hospital. As a scientist, he was concerned about the cursory safety trials of the MMR. He was also concerned by the fact that people who had caught measles and mumps within a year were six times more likely to develop inflammatory bowel disease.[2] Though in an attenuated form, the MMR exposes all British children to both these viruses at the same time. In addition, research shows that exposure to measles, mumps or rubella in the womb or in early infancy may, albeit rarely, trigger autism.[3]

Another factor on his mind was the well-documented rise in autism. A survey in 1964 suggested that there were around three thousand autistic children in England and Wales. Over five decades later, there are over forty times that number — well over one hundred thousand. In Scotland, the figures are more precise: 3,484 schoolchildren were registered as autistic in 2005, compared to only 820 in 1998. Other countries have also reported huge increases.

But his single suggestion was enough to bring him on a collision course with the government and health officials. Like the colour black of the first ever Ford motor car, one was free to be in favour of any type of immunisation against rubella, mumps and measles — as long as it was called MMR.

There can be little doubt that Wakefield's point was legitimate, then, and that it remains a legitimate one after considering scientific studies in favour and against.

Mass immunisation against rubella, mumps and measles was introduced by health officials for two reasons. One was the eradication of these diseases (so far a failure), and the other was to prevent deaths and disabled children. In 1987, the year before the introduction of the MMR, the combined number of deaths caused by all three illnesses was 7 children and 4 adults and the number of disabled children was 29 from CRS plus a few disabled from measles. In 2014 (the last year for which complete figures are available) the total number of deaths caused by the three illnesses was 1 — in an adult aged in their late 70s — with, probably, extremely few disabilities. Discounting the historical decline of the three diseases, it points in a certain direction.

Whether this is a good result, however, also depends on any downside of mass vaccination — over a million doses of the MMR every year are given to British children. We know fairly well what the effects of single vaccination against three diseases are if given on their own, but, in the absence of proper studies, we still don't fully understand what happens when you bundle three live viruses together.

Every year the number of children estimated to develop autistic spectrum disorder (ASD), the broader classification of autism, is about twelve thousand (based on the latest research findings that around 1 in 60 children have ASD).[4] If one in eight hundred MMR vaccinations triggered an autistic disorder, this would result in around twelve hundred children a year in the UK being made autistic by the bundling of the vaccines. This is probably the worst case scenario. In medical terms this would still be described as an 'uncommon' side-effect of the MMR, but it would actually account for 10% of all autistic children in Britain in a year.

When this supposition was queried by me in an interview, Professor Elizabeth Miller, an epidemiologist and currently Head of the Immunisation Department at government-funded Public Health England (previously the Health Protection Agency), conceded that there is no one epidemiological study disproving that the MMR could be causing up to 10% of autism cases.[5] This is because such a small proportion cannot be picked by epidemiological studies. And it is exactly the reason why further research like Dr Andrew Wakefield's is required.

The aftermath

A few weeks after the paper and press conference, the Department of Health announced a national campaign to persuade parents that the MMR is safe. 'We are not making the running on this issue,' said Dr David Salisbury, head of immunisation at the Department of Health.[6] Later in the year, two-and-a-half million leaflets entitled 'MMR — The Facts' were sent to family doctors' surgeries.[7]

The leaflet repeated the usual spin:

Leaflet: 'Measles...kills and disables both adults and children'
Fact: this is strictly true, but omits to mention the dramatic decline in complications. The chances of death or disability are extremely small.

Leaflet: 'Mumps was the leading cause of meningitis in children under the age of fifteen years before the introduction of the MMR vaccine'
Fact: Mumps meningitis is not the lethal bacterial kind, but is relatively harmless.

But then, the Department of Health also added:

Leaflet: 'There is no evidence of any link between MMR and autism or Crohn's disease'
Fact: A factually incorrect statement, little short of deceit. There clearly was evidence — whether the evidence was strong enough was the issue.

As happened in the whooping cough 'scare' of the 1970s, the Department of Health then reached for its four-pronged strategy:
(1) side-effects of the vaccine are played down,
(2) risks of the illnesses are exaggerated,
(3) benefits of the vaccine are exaggerated, and
(4) leading critics are discredited.

The promised meeting of experts

Sir Kenneth Calman did finally arrange the 'scientific meeting' that had been promised at his meeting with Dr Andrew Wakefield in 1995. The 'Working Party on MMR Vaccine' first met on 27 February 1998. Dr Andrew Wakefield was not invited.

The eight experts (two of whom sit on JCVI) met four times between February 1998 and March 1999. The 'working party' based their report on questionnaires filled in by parents of children believed to have been damaged by the MMR vaccine. This was a fruitless exercise because it relied on incomplete information from parents, only ninety-five children were included (despite five hundred and thirty-one replies) and children were automatically excluded if their problems started more than six weeks after receiving the vaccine.

The working party concluded: 'It was impossible to prove or refute the suggested associations between MMR vaccine and autism / PDD or inflammatory bowel disease.'[8] This conclusion was inevitable considering the limited information they had.

The government used this report to reassure parents that the MMR was safe.

Ever since, there has been a vocal debate over whether the MMR vaccine does, or doesn't, cause autism in some children. There have been lots of medical articles published, which both sides in the dispute claim support their argument. There are too many papers to discuss each one in detail here. However, examining a couple of the most talked about papers from each side will help throw light on the debate.

The North London study[9]

The first study to be published after the one identifying ILNH was also published in the *Lancet*. This paper, published in June 1999, was called 'Autism and measles, mumps and rubella vaccine: no evidence for a causal association.' The lead author was Professor Brent Taylor, a 'community paediatrician' from the Royal Free Hospital, the same hospital where Dr Wakefield was working. Another author of the paper was Dr Elizabeth Miller, a government epidemiologist and subsequently head of immunisation at the HPA (Health Protection Agency), later brought under the wing of Public Health England as part of cost savings. This study was 'epidemiological', which means that it looked not at individual children but at groups, or populations, of children. They looked at all children (around five hundred) with autism in an area of North London who had been born since 1979. The researchers wanted to see whether autism had increased since the introduction of the MMR in 1988.

The authors looked at the numbers of children with autism for each year of birth. So if a six-year-old boy was diagnosed with autism in 1989, he would be plotted under 1983, his year of birth. What the study showed is a dramatic increase in numbers of children diagnosed with autism, either 'classical' autism or a group of similar diagnoses that fall into the 'autistic spectrum disorder' (ASD) category, here described as 'atypical' autism. Professor Taylor has argued that the rise in autism was not a real increase, but was probably the result of increased recognition, a greater willingness on the part of educationalists and families to accept the diagnostic label and better recording systems.[10]

The authors argued that there was 'a steady increase in cases by year of birth with no sudden 'step-up' or change in the trend line after the introduction of MMR vaccination.' In other words, if MMR were causing an increase in number of children with autism after its introduction, there should have been an even greater increase after 1988. As they could see no such increase, therefore, they concluded, the introduction of the MMR did not increase the incidence of autism.

Leaving aside the fact that a 10% increase would not show up in these figures, there are a few other problems with this study. The authors were assuming that before 1988 no children received the vaccine, while after that year all (or at least most) children did receive it. When the MMR was introduced in 1988, there was actually a 'catch-up' campaign to vaccinate children up to five years of age. Thus children born as early as 1983 would have received the vaccine. I should know: my son was born in 1983 and was given the MMR, long before I had any concerns. The first group of children to receive the vaccine routinely between one and two years of age would have been born in 1987. It is exactly around this date that numbers of children diagnosed with autism started to take off, as this study showed.

Only children with autism diagnosed before their fifth birthday were included in the study. But, as any parent of a child with autism will confirm, it often takes years from the beginning of concerns for autism to be diagnosed, and many children are not diagnosed until after five years of age.

The study discovered that parents of autistic children were most likely to become concerned five to six months after receiving the MMR vaccine but dismissed this as probably being caused by parents' difficulty in remembering when they first started having worries.

The most serious flaw, however, has to do with its scientific value. Despite requests from several doctors (including myself) to see the 'raw data' of the study, which were not in the published paper, Professor Taylor has declined to share this information. Until this information is available, it is not possible to draw a sensible conclusion from the article.

A year after publication of the paper, Richard Horton, the editor of the *Lancet*, had become concerned. After being made aware of the comments of epidemiologist Professor Walter Spitzer, whom he felt was a 'reliable advisor,' he sent a letter to Professor Brent Taylor. 'It was therefore with some anxiety,' he wrote, 'that I read his comments that your study was 'un-interpretable due to its inferior scientific quality'.'

Professor Taylor wrote back, explaining that not only did Professor Spitzer have a 'vested interest,' but that also, 'he is obviously out of his depth with the specialised statistical methods necessary to examine possible adverse effects from vaccinations,' an extraordinary criticism for a non-epidemiologist to make of a professor of epidemiology. Professor Taylor asked Richard Horton to 'stay firm,' and reassured him about the quality of his study. Another vaccine expert and epidemiologist told me that — despite Professor Brent Taylor's undoubted expertise in community paediatrics — 'the only thing [this study] proved was that Brent Taylor can't write a paper.'[11]

The North London study was published on the same day as the Department of Health's 'Working Party' report discussed earlier. The two together enabled the Department of Health's Deputy Chief Medical Officer, Dr Jeremy Metters, to conclude: 'The fact is MMR vaccination does not cause autism or Crohn's disease.'[12]

The Danish study[13]

I have selected this study because it's regarded as one of the strongest pieces of evidence that MMR doesn't cause autism. The study looked at all children born in Denmark between 1991 and 1998, sought all children diagnosed with autism or 'autistic spectrum disorder' (ASD), and then calculated whether more children with autism or ASD had received the MMR vaccine compared to normal children. The MMR vaccine was introduced in Denmark a year earlier than in Britain, in 1987. Over half a million children were followed up, so the study appears large and straightforward.

As in many epidemiological, or population, studies, a lot of adjustments of the figures are made. Before these adjustments, children who were vaccinated were 45% more likely to get autism. After adjustment for various factors such as age, birth-weight and mother's education, the authors calculated that vaccinated children were actually less likely to develop autism than those who were not vaccinated. (The conclusion that they were less likely to develop autism was not 'statistically significant' or, in other words, could easily have happened by chance.)

The study concluded, 'This study provides strong evidence against the hypothesis that MMR vaccination causes autism.' The senior doctor in the study, Dr Kreesten Madsen, told journalists: 'In the scientific community this should put this debate to rest.'

This study has, nonetheless, been criticised on a number of counts.

First, the researchers picked up a rate of autism of one in seven hundred and nine children, which is much lower than the UK rate at the time of one in one hundred and sixty-seven. Either they missed a lot of children with autism or autism is a lot more common in the UK.

The lower rate in this study has been explained by the fact that some children weren't even two years old when the data was collected. At that age it's very unlikely, even if they were autistic, that a diagnosis of autism would have been made, especially as autism can only be diagnosed in Denmark by specialists in child psychiatry. This would delay the diagnosis further. The average age of diagnosis of autism in Denmark is four to five years of age. The average age of the children looked at in the study was four, so it would seem that half of the autistic children wouldn't have been diagnosed. The authors confused their study by using 'person years' instead of actual numbers of children with autism, making the study difficult to interpret.

A different study has found an eight-fold increase in autism in Denmark since the introduction of the MMR, which actually supports the hypothesis that MMR causes autism.[14]

After hearing these, and other, criticisms, the lead researcher, Dr Kreesten Madsen, backtracked somewhat: 'We can say that MMR vaccination is not one of the common causes of autism. But we cannot prove anything.' Like Professor Miller, he seems to allow for the possibility that a 10% increase in autism followed the introduction of the MMR.

Other published evidence in defence of the MMR

Other research consists nearly entirely of epidemiological studies like the 'North London' and 'Danish' studies. One looked at the rise in autism during the late 1980s and early 1990s in the UK and, because the uptake of the MMR was fairly constant during this time, concluded that MMR couldn't be the cause of the rise in autism.[15] Some experts have argued that there hasn't been a real rise in autism and, in particular, no increase in the proportion of autistic children with 'regression' (though few autistic experts would agree with this). Several papers relied on looking at family doctors' computerised records for information on children with a diagnosis of autism. This is unreliable as a source of information for this sort of diagnosis, which can take so long to be confirmed.

The most that one can conclude from all these studies is that MMR is not the only or even, at least on its own, the major cause of autism.

But then nobody ever suggested that it was. A 10% increase will affect 300 children a year. The problem is that none of these epidemiological studies has addressed the main hypothesis or concern, which is that the MMR vaccine causes, or triggers, autism in a small subgroup of susceptible children, not in a small random selection of the whole childhood population.

The Dublin paper[16]

The Royal Free's 1998 paper describing twelve children was, rightly, criticised as being far too small to jump to any conclusions about the safety of the MMR vaccine.

The 'Dublin Paper' describes a study from Professor John O'Leary's laboratory in Dublin, where scientists looked for the measles virus in the gut of ninety-one children whom Dr Andrew Wakefield and his team had diagnosed with bowel inflammation and 'ileal lymphonodular hyperplasia' (ILNH) — the new disease he and his team had discovered. One would not expect to find the measles virus in the gut.

The children were also suffering from developmental problems, such as autism. For comparison ('controls'), they looked at the gut of seventy children with no developmental problems, but many of whom had some sort of bowel problem, such as appendicitis or other inflammation. Seventy-five of the ninety-one children with ILNH and autism (or other developmental problem) had measles virus in their gut, whereas only five of the seventy comparison children had measles found in their gut. That's 82% compared to 7% — a vast difference that had odds of one to ten thousand against happening by chance.

This paper was criticised on several fronts:

- The presence of measles virus in the gut of these children does not mean it caused the problem; it could be a 'consequence' of the disease rather than a 'cause'. This is indeed the million dollar question.
- The measles virus may have nothing to do with the MMR; it could just as well have come from the 'wild' measles virus, which would actually strengthen the argument to vaccinate with the MMR. This criticism was answered when the Dublin team presented the results of later work which showed that, of 12 samples further analysed, all the measles viruses were found to be vaccine strain.[17] That means that the measles virus hadn't come from a wild ('natural') measles infection, but from a measles vaccine, either the MMR or a single measles vaccine. As the vast majority of children had only received the MMR (though a couple had received a single measles vaccine) this confirmed an 'association' with the MMR vaccine. This doesn't answer the question of whether it is a 'cause' or a 'consequence'

- Though the research was done in Dublin, the gut specimens came from Dr Wakefield at The Royal Free Hospital, and, so the argument goes, anything he is involved in can't be trusted. The issue about the gut specimens was addressed by a presentation at the Fifth International Meeting for Autism Research in Montreal, Canada, in June 2006 by a group of American doctors, independent of Dr Wakefield. They had also been examining the bowels of children with autism and bowel disease and have confirmed Professor John O'Leary's findings of measles virus in a large proportion of these children's guts.[18]

The double whammy[19]

In a further study, Dr Wakefield studied two groups of twenty-three children each — forty-six children in total. All developed bowel problems, along with developmental regression (mainly autism), after receiving a 'measles-containing vaccine' (MCV), which was nearly always the MMR or MR. The two groups were similar in all respects apart from one: one group had received only one MCV, whereas the other had received two MCVs. Dr Wakefield's thinking was that if the children's disorder had nothing to do with the vaccine, then both groups should follow a similar pattern at the time that half of them received a second vaccine. If, on the other hand, the vaccine were causing the problem, those who were given a second dose of the vaccine would be expected to fare worse than those who weren't.

The children given a second MCV developed a recurrence, or aggravation, of symptoms including diarrhoea, blood in the stool, and faecal incontinence, whereas not one of the children who had received only the one vaccine was affected in this way. There is a one in ten thousand possibility of this difference occurring by chance.

When samples of gut from all these children were examined, acute inflammation was seen in 61% of those who had received two MCVs, but only 13% of those who had been given only one MCV. In other words acute inflammation was between four and five times more likely to be seen in the children who had received two vaccines. Many of these physical problems were accompanied by behavioural regression. The onset of symptoms after one MMR vaccine could be a coincidence, but for similar symptoms to recur in the same child after a second MMR (or MR) vaccine a few years later is most unlikely to be down to chance.

An American Institute of Medicine (IOM) report on MMR and autism from 2001 concluded that MMR was unlikely to cause autism 'at the population level' but acknowledged that 'MMR vaccine could contribute to ASD [autism] in a small number of children.' The report went on to say, 'Well-documented reports of similar outcomes in response to an initial exposure to a vaccine, and a repeat exposure to the same vaccine, referred to as 're-challenge', would constitute strong evidence of an association.'[20] In other words evidence of a double whammy effect would be powerful evidence implicating the MMR vaccine, at least in those particular children.

Other published evidence against the MMR

This consists mainly of clinical research on the affected children. Three children with regressive autism have had the measles virus found in the cerebrospinal fluid (CSF) surrounding the brain.[21,22] Other groups of researchers (that is doctors not working with Dr Andrew Wakefield) have described how some autistic children have 'leaky guts' and have confirmed Dr Wakefield's original finding of bowel inflammation and ILNH in autistic children.[23,24,25] A researcher from Utah in the USA, Dr Vijendra Singh, has found unusual antibodies to both MMR, and to parts of the brain, in autistic children, that he did not find in normal children[26] Dr Singh has also found higher measles antibody levels in autistic children compared with normal children.[27] His research suggests autism in some children may be an auto-immune disease as a result of an abnormal immune reaction to the measles component of the MMR vaccine. Dr Wakefield, working with some Japanese researchers, has also found the measles virus in the blood of autistic children, though, to confuse matters, another group of researchers has failed to confirm this.

Dr Andrew Wakefield

Many allegations have been made against Dr Wakefield, who has also been the victim of a string of extraordinary and disturbing accusations made by a freelance journalist, Brian Deer.

One that appears to have stuck is that, at the time the 1998 *Lancet* paper was published, Dr Wakefield was already receiving substantial payments from the Legal Aid Board to investigate children in order to help the parents — should the research go their way — with their legal claim for damages against the vaccine manufacturers. More importantly, it is alleged he had not told his colleagues of this 'conflict of interest.' — 'Revealed: MMR research scandal' was the headline on the front page of the *Sunday Times* introducing an article written by Mr Deer, who claimed to have 'uncovered a medical scandal at the heart of the worldwide scare over MMR.'[28] Though all twelve children in Wakefield's original *Lancet* paper had been referred to the Royal Free because of their bowel problems, some were involved in an entirely separate study that was funded by the Legal Aid Board. During his investigation, Brian Deer was advised by a company called Medico Legal Investigations (MLI), according to MLI's newsletter of March 2004. The Association of the British Pharmaceutical Industry (ABPI) is the trade association representing the major British drug and vaccine (including MMR) manufacturers. Not only does MLI claim to have 'the full weight of the ABPI' behind it, but, of the five company employees listed on its website, three have links to ABPI. The Chairman of MLI is a Vice President of ABPI, one of MLI's directors is the Medical Director of ABPI, and another Director and Medical Advisor is a past Chairman of ABPI.[37]

In actual fact, Dr Wakefield had written to his colleague, Professor Walker-Smith, a full year before the publication of the *Lancet* paper to explain his need to get involved with the legal cases in order to do what he could for these severely disabled children whom, he felt, had been neglected by both the medical profession and society. Some of his colleagues were uncomfortable that the medical school would receive funding for studies that could demonstrate problems with a widely endorsed vaccine. At one stage, Dr Wakefield requested that the legal aid funding be returned to the solicitors as it was becoming such a thorny issue. Ultimately, it remained with the Royal Free, and the research went ahead. He also wrote, in a letter to the *Lancet* three months after his paper was published, that he was receiving funding to study some of these children on behalf of the Legal Aid Board.[29] Should he have declared a 'conflict of interest' with the publication of the paper? He believes not, as he saw no conflict. Not everyone agrees.

Others involved as 'expert witnesses' for the drug companies in the legal action also failed to declare this when publishing articles declaring MMR to be safe. Professor Elizabeth Miller, from the government's Health Protection Agency, wrote several papers in which she failed to declare this potential conflict of interest. Despite being an expert witness for three vaccine manufacturers, from one of which she was also receiving work-related funding, she was not widely condemned in the manner that Dr Wakefield was.[30]

Brian Deer also made a documentary for Channel 4 which appears to have been a crusade against Andrew Wakefield.[31] He claimed that Wakefield was developing a commercial rival to the measles vaccine, that he was involved in selling dubious remedies for the treatment of autism, and was generally a disreputable character.

Since 1988, Dr Andrew Wakefield is often portrayed, by those who are attempting to discredit him, as a 'maverick', a lone figure with no support from any other credible scientists. He may not object to being called a maverick, defined as 'an independent-minded person', because he certainly is that. However, the implication that he is the only scientist claiming the existence of 'autistic enterocolitis'[i], or to suggest there may be a link between MMR and autism, simply does not stand up to examination. Neither does the repeated claim that Dr Wakefield's 1998 paper is the only published study on the subject. Inflammation in the gut of autistic children, and other children with behavioural disorders, and the unusual finding of bowel inflammation along with ileal-lymphoid-nodular hyperplasia (ILNH), has been reported by other clinicians independently in Europe, North and South America.[32] Dr Wakefield, working with other doctors, has demonstrated ILNH in well over one hundred autistic children.[33] Dr Arthur Krigsman, Professor of Pediatric Gastroenterology at New York University School of Medicine examined 143 children with ASD and chronic bowel problems; nearly three quarters had evidence of ILNH.[37] There are also other published, peer-reviewed scientific papers supporting a probable link between the MMR and autism.[34,35] However, there is pressure on researchers not to publish uncomfortable findings.

A doctor who held a high position at the Department of Health told me, 'There are a lot of people who are afraid to publish work that will displease the Department of Health and Big Pharma.'[36]

As more time passes I fear that we may never find out the truth about the MMR.

18
MMR, Conclusion

'Russian Roulette'

As a doctor with a surgery in London, the safety issues relating to vaccines had a direct relevance to my practice. I came to the conclusion, not long after the controversial 1998 *Lancet* paper was published, that I would serve the health of the babies in my practice better if I were to offer single vaccines rather than the combined MMR.

After hearing health officials' strong, though to my mind unfounded, attack on the use of the single vaccines, I expected a rough ride. However, I felt able to defend my position with a sound rational argument. When MMR was introduced in 1988, the single vaccines remained available as an acceptable (if not recommended) alternative for those parents who didn't want to give their child the MMR vaccine. In 1996, the official 'Green Book' on immunisation, provided to all doctors, also said, 'single antigen measles, mumps and rubella vaccines are available.'[1] Though I would have liked to have given all children the single vaccines, I was concerned that this would be seen by the Department of Health as one step too far and so, as a compromise, I offered all parents the choice, continuing to offer the MMR alongside the single vaccines.

What happened next, however, was astonishing. After the introduction of the MMR, in 1988, coverage had risen rapidly and remained at or above 90% until the mid-1990s. But this figure was now dropping fast as a result of the doubts cast over its safety. One option for the government would have been a campaign to offer the single vaccines to those who were concerned so that the high immunisation rates against the three diseases could be maintained.

Yet, despite unprecedented demand — from both parents and doctors — for the single vaccines to be made available following the publication of the *Lancet* paper in February 1998, the single measles was withdrawn before the end of the year.[2] As the single mumps had never been in widespread use, that left the single rubella vaccine as the one exception which continued to be available for women who were unprotected. However, even this was withdrawn in late 2003, forcing women who, quite rightly, want to be protected against rubella, to have the MMR, containing vaccines for two diseases against which they do not need protecting.

The screw was tightened in another way, too. GPs aren't paid a salary;

their income depends on the services they offer. One part of their pay comes from achieving targets for childhood vaccinations. A large practice that successfully vaccinates over 90% of its children can receive many thousands of pounds a year in this way as a bonus. As this is a target-based payment, the decision by parents whether or not to vaccinate a single child can make a substantial difference.

Reports emerged in 2001 of families being 'struck off' by their doctors for refusing to have their children vaccinated with the MMR jab. In an attempt to persuade wavering parents, some doctors told them their children would die if they didn't have the jab. One couple claimed they were accused of being 'child abusers'.[3] Another doctor, Dr Eric Holliday, justified removing a family in order to prevent a loss of income of over £3,000 a year to his Swindon practice. Though he was not abusive to the family, and offered to continue treating them 'for free', he was still on shaky legal and ethical ground.[4] There was strong support for Dr Holliday from other doctors who claimed they'd been doing the same thing for years, that is treating children who don't have the MMR for free as 'private patients.' Doctors blamed the government's 'heinous' target payment rule.[5,6]

Nonetheless, the practice of removing 'refusenik' children from family-doctors' lists continued. In 2005, Dr Michael Duggan, a doctor in Stevenage, Hertfordshire, caused a local storm when he wrote to eight families threatening to remove them from his list because their refusal to accept MMR was, as he put it, 'adversely affecting my pay.' Following intervention by the local medical authorities the families weren't removed, though three subsequently left the practice.[7]

The real motivation behind the government's intransigence was revealed in JCVI minutes from as early as 1998: 'it was felt that supporting the use of single vaccines would undermine the whole argument on the safety of MMR.'[8] It has been suggested by one insider that the real reason was that single vaccines were 'withdrawn for purely financial reasons,'[9] a view supported by a government publication, which, arguing against the use of single vaccines, warned against the 'allocation of health service resources on the basis of subjective opinion.'[10] Another motivation may have been the indemnity allegedly given by the government to the vaccine manufacturers.

Whatever the reason, the results of the government's policy have proved to be disastrous for achieving its 1998 MMR goals. The uptake of vaccination with MMR steadily fell to a nadir of 80% in 2003.

Hysteria

One contributing factor for this failure was the hectoring tone medical officials started using to coax parents into giving their babies the MMR. Within two years of the 1998 *Lancet* article, a senior doctor from the British Medical Association was reported as saying that it was a form of child abuse to give babies three injections when one was effective.[11] The Chief Medical Officer (CMO) of the National Health Service, Professor Liam Donaldson, picked up the theme in a letter to all doctors in March 2001. He instructed doctors not to give single vaccines because there is (in bold) a 'clear risk of harm from such a practice.'[12]

Throughout Britain, local officials added their perspective to the government's MMR hysteria. In the same month as the letter from the CMO, Dr Judith Moreton, Oxford's Immunisation co-ordinator, questioned the 'ethics' of offering the single vaccines.[13]

The Glasgow Health Board compared parents who chose the single vaccines for their child with people who drink and drive. 'It is for this reason that we do not allow people to choose to drink and drive, because their choice is a selfish and reckless one which will eventually inflict pain and suffering on others.' The leaflet had been toned down from its original version, which stated, 'An unimmunised child is the infectious equivalent of a drunk driver.' The leaflet was co-authored by Dr Mike Watson, medical director of Aventis Pasteur, manufacturer of the MMR vaccine.[14]

In 2001, Dr Martin Schweiger, public health consultant in Leeds wrote, 'If parents do not ensure their children are protected then there will be a real price to pay later.' The price he was referring to was a rise in the number of cases of mumps. 'In older children mumps can lead to inflammation of the brain or pancreas. There is no cure and all we can do is make sufferers as comfortable as possible. There can be no stronger warning.' It sounded as if he were talking about some terminal illness.[15]

At the same time, the Department of Health launched the second advertising campaign in three years in an attempt to reassure worried parents. 'Measles... can still kill' it reminded us. Mumps 'was the biggest cause of viral meningitis in children,' failing to mention the benign nature of the disease.[16] As a cornerstone, the campaign included a television advertisement: a little baby lies alone and unprotected on a cliff edge while a lion prowls menacingly nearby. The voice-over tells viewers, 'as a loving parent you wouldn't put your child in unnecessary danger'.

In the USA the government's hard-sell went even further. Children in Washington DC who hadn't been vaccinated were barred from attending school, while their parents faced a fine or a short jail sentence.[17]

Then there were the repeated warnings of measles outbreaks. 'Measles epidemic this winter,' and 'Warning over 'real threat' of measles deaths' were typical headlines. 'We are going to start to see dead babies,' cautioned Dr George Kassianos, the immunisation spokesman for the Royal College of General Practitioners. Dr Bernard Schlecht, the consultant in charge of infectious disease control in north Cheshire, had similar forebodings: 'There is a very real chance of children catching this killer disease this winter if they are not protected with the MMR vaccine', he warned in January 2002. He then started hitting well below the belt when he added, 'Those who lived through the devastating outbreak of measles in Warrington in 1930 will never forget it,' forgetting to add that measles in the early twentieth century was a far more serious disease than it is now.[18]

In fact, what is surprising is that, despite intense publicity, the number of cases of reported measles has fallen along with the decline in uptake of the MMR. There were far more cases reported in the five years before 1998, when the scare started, than in the five years after. Since 1994, there have been well under 10,000 notifications of measles a year. Despite the steady fall in MMR uptake, there has, remarkably, been no rise in measles cases.

Then, in 2002, the CMO Professor Donaldson, made the official tone to the public yet more shrill than the one in his letter to doctors. 'We would,' he cautioned, 'literally be playing Russian roulette with our children's health.'[19] He even threatened to resign rather than allow the single vaccines to be available nationally.[20] These were the same single vaccines – the 'Russian roulette' – that had been freely available on the NHS for ten years. The *Independent* reported from Dr David Salisbury – head of the immunisation department during the entire period – what appears to have been a case of amnesia: 'The health service has never given parents the choice to do harm before';[21] the harm being the single vaccines that had been available during practically all of his watch.

The outcome
The government's tactics to deal with the 1998 *Lancet* article were not dissimilar to its strategy towards the whooping cough scare some quarter of a century previously. Again, it had an effect. Research in 2004 found that a large majority of parents felt that measles, mumps and rubella were severe illnesses.[22]

Unfortunately, the fear did not influence the dropping vaccination rate against the three diseases. The fall continued through two national advertising campaigns, including television adverts. The government's key objective, maintaining a high level of immunity in the population, was a complete failure.

The uptake of the first MMR by two years of age fell to a national low of under 80% in 2004, following which it increased steadily to a high of nearly 93% in 2014, falling again slightly in 2015, though the uptake in London remains well below this. The national average remains below the WHO target of 'at least 95%' coverage.

Had single vaccinations been offered to concerned parents, it could have been the safety net the government was looking for. Their availability would have helped prevent the very outbreaks that health officials were predicting. Yet, the government's intransigence made this all but impossible. The single measles vaccine was offered by some twenty-odd providers over the country. Over 1 in 20 (5.2%) of UK children born between 2000 and 2002 received one or more single vaccines by their third birthday. This number includes as many as 1 in 12 (8%) London children, but only 1 in 62 (1.6%) of children from Northern Ireland. [24]

Many doctors certainly felt parents should be able to choose single vaccines for their children, if they wished. A survey in 2001 found that over 43% of family doctors thought separate vaccines should be available on the national health.[25] Even doctors who supported MMR argued that it was preferable for children to have the single vaccines rather than no vaccines.

This argument wasn't shared by the Department of Health, which paid for a full-page advertisement in a doctors' magazine, headed 'MMR — why single vaccines are bad medicine.'[26]

The government does not accept that its horror tactics are to blame for the appalling results.

It has, instead, pointed its finger at the media, accusing it of being irresponsible in its reporting of MMR concerns. It believes the media has been unbalanced, favouring the scare story over the sound science — conveniently forgetting how the government itself had miraculously transformed the three diseases into its own scare stories.

The reality is that most of the media reports on TV, radio and in the national press were well balanced and explained the government's arguments as well as those of people with concerns. Whilst some editorials were critical of the government's apparent refusal to allow the single vaccines on the NHS, others were just as vehemently in support of the government's stance.

In the summer of 2006, the media was accused of posing 'a clear and present danger' to children's health through its 'biased' reporting of the alleged link between MMR and autism. 'End the anti-MMR campaign now,' ordered a doctor from the British Medical Association. 'Your irresponsible reporting is damaging public health.'[27]

The science

The Chief Medical Officer, Professor Donaldson, said in 2001 there was a 'clear risk of harm' from single vaccinations. The government seems to have explained this harm in four ways, more social than medical.

a) There will be a period in between vaccinations when the child will be unprotected against one or more of the illnesses whilst waiting to have the next vaccine. This risk applies far more, of course, to children who do not receive either the MMR or the single vaccines. In the case of unvaccinated children, the danger the government has identified stretches to their whole life instead of a short period.

b) Giving single vaccines necessitates more injections.

c) Parents may not bring children back to have all the vaccines.

d) The vaccines are not licensed in the UK.

What does science actually say about single vaccines compared to their bundling in the MMR? The effectiveness of the vaccines used on their own is well established, but there is practically no research on the effectiveness of the MMR after all this time (as described in the earlier chapters). An influential review damningly concluded, 'We could not identify studies assessing the effectiveness of MMR that fulfilled our inclusion criteria;'[28] in other words, the studies were judged to be of too poor a quality to be meaningful. It could be that another reason why the government's aim of eliminating the three diseases is failing dramatically is because it refused to offer the single vaccinations.

The effectiveness of the mumps vaccine to prevent mumps in the real world has been calculated at rates from as low as 46% up to 97% with an average of around 75%.[29] But these studies include both the single mumps vaccine and the MMR. Two studies comparing the effectiveness of the single vaccine with the MMR found the MMR was less effective in preventing mumps.[30,31] It's difficult to calculate exact figures but, averaging all studies, they look like this:

Vaccine	Effectiveness in preventing mumps
Single mumps vaccine	83%
MMR triple vaccine	62%

This calculation is supported by research in 2005 from London, which shows that the mumps component of the MMR vaccine is only 65% effective after one dose, rising to 88% after two doses.

It suggests that even two doses of MMR will never eradicate mumps but will, instead, simply push the illness into older children and adults, the age group where the disease causes more harm.[29] Even staunch pro-vaccine doctors are conceding that there's a problem. 'Perhaps the protection against mumps is not as good as we had thought,' conceded Dr David Elliman, a consultant in child health at Great Ormond Street Children's Hospital and a supporter of MMR. Dr George Kassianos, the immunisation spokesman for the Royal College of General Practitioners, admitted the effectiveness of the mumps component of the MMR 'may be much lower than we have thought in the past.'[32] Unfortunately, the single mumps vaccine is no longer manufactured and so the only vaccine now available to protect against mumps is the relatively ineffective MMR. We know how ineffective it is because of the numerous reports of outbreaks of mumps in teenagers and young adults nearly all of whom have received one — if not two — MMR shots.

Quite separately from the autism and bowel inflammation issue first discussed by the writers of the 1998 *Lancet* paper, the MMR has acknowledged side-effects. Sixteen recipients of the MMR have been awarded damages by the government-run Vaccine Damage Payments Unit after being severely mentally or physically disabled by the vaccine. The government thus accepts that the vaccine, like all other vaccines, does cause severe harm to some children.

Reported side-effects of the MMR
In 1988, a case of severe encephalitis following MMR vaccination four weeks earlier had been reported by doctors from the Charing Cross Road Hospital in London. The fourteen-month-old girl recovered, but Daniel, whose case was reported by doctors in 1999, was not so fortunate.[33]

A healthy child, he wasn't prone to infections and was growing and developing well. Shortly after his first birthday he was given the MMR vaccine. All remained well until Daniel was twenty months when he became irritable with a high temperature and started to vomit. He was taken to hospital where a diagnosis of encephalitis was made. Despite treatment, he went in and out of consciousness and developed convulsions. He was treated in intensive care and was put on a life support machine. Tragically, Daniel continued to deteriorate, becoming more deeply unconscious and having increasingly uncontrollable convulsions.

During his eighth week in hospital, Daniel died. In a desperate attempt to find out what was causing Daniel's illness, and so possibly find a cure, the doctors performed a brain biopsy by cutting a hole in his skull and taking a small sample of brain for testing. Much to their surprise, the doctors found that measles virus had invaded the brain, a highly unusual place; what's more, it was vaccine strain measles virus. The only place this virus could have come from was the MMR vaccine Daniel had received ten months previously. Further tests also revealed that Daniel's immune system was impaired, but no one could possibly have known that at the time of his vaccination, as he had always been so healthy.[33]

Daniel's story clearly shows that the MMR vaccine can cause fatal encephalitis in an apparently healthy child. What is remarkable is that Daniel didn't become ill until nine months after being given the vaccine, at a time when few would think his illness could be due to the vaccine. It was only because he was so intensively investigated that the doctors discovered the role the vaccine played. How many cases like his have gone undetected and therefore unreported?

ITP is a rare auto-immune bleeding disorder. It can be serious, even fatal, though most children make a full recovery within six months. The MMR vaccine causes a first attack of ITP in one in 25,000 vaccinations. This is serious enough to warrant hospital admission in one in 32,000 children given the MMR. Members of the pro-vaccine JCVI had a run-in with the more safety-orientated Committee on Safety of Medicines (CSM)[34] on the importance of this side-effect. The CSM had recommended all children who had ITP after their first dose of MMR shouldn't receive a second dose of the vaccine, a view endorsed by other specialists.[35,36] The JCVI disagreed and felt they should receive the second vaccine and asked the CSM to reconsider its position.[37] This the CSM did, and came up with the compromise proposal that all children who had ITP after their first MMR should have a blood test, and only be given the second MMR if still unprotected against one or more of the three diseases. The JCVI would still not be swayed and dispatched two of their committee to attend the next CSM meeting at which ITP was to be discussed.[23] The JCVI appeared to have won their case when 'the Department had agreed the JCVI recommendation on this', so that children who suffered ITP as a result of the MMR vaccine would be given a second dose of the vaccine.[38] It's surprising that the expert body responsible for advising on the safety of drugs and vaccines should have its safety recommendations challenged by the JCVI. However, the CSM reiterated its earlier advice for antibody testing before the second dose, which remains the current Department of Health recommendation.

Like some other vaccines, MMR also stimulates the immune system in an allergic-like direction. So it should be of no surprise to learn the vaccine can cause several other immune-related disorders in addition to ITP. MMR increases the risk of atopic dermatitis (eczema).[39,40] The following disorders, though probably very rare, have been reported after MMR vaccination: inflammation of the nerve behind the eye leading to a loss of vision, usually temporary (optic neuritis), painful inflammation of the large pancreas gland situated beneath the stomach (pancreatitis), Guillain-Barré Syndrome, an immune disorder of the nerves causing (temporary) paralysis and acute disseminated encephalomyelitis (ADEM), a disorder causing symptoms similar to MS.[41,42,43,59]

Another rare side-effect of the MMR is a gait disturbance, in which the child becomes unsteady, walks into doors, bumps into tables and falls more than normal. This probably occurs in about one in 10,000 doses of MMR. Though most children recover within a few days, it may last for several weeks.[44]

More common reactions are a fever (high temperature), rash, conjunctivitis (sticky eyes), drowsiness, irritability and arthritis (inflammation of joints). Side-effects are much more common in one-year-olds (receiving their first dose of vaccine) than in four-year-olds (receiving their booster). One in six toddlers will suffer some form of side-effect, with one in twenty getting a high fever of over 39.5° C.[45]

Side-effect:	Proportion of toddlers affected:
Fever	18%
High Fever (over 39.5° C)	5%
Diarrhoea	9%
Rash	9%

Finally, more convulsions (fits) occur after the MMR vaccine than any other vaccine routinely used in the UK. An original manufacturer's data sheet for MMR had cautioned against giving the vaccine to any children who had suffered convulsions. The JCVI had been unhappy with this, and had asked for the wording to be amended.[46] One or two out of every thousand children are hospitalised with convulsions after receiving the MMR vaccine, and are at an increased risk of going on to suffer further febrile convulsions. Children who have had a febrile convulsion before receiving the MMR have a one in fifty chance of a further convulsion after having the vaccine.[47,48]

Though the measles vaccine is live, there were never any cases reported of transmission of the single measles vaccine virus from a vaccinated child to another person. However, there have now been a handful of reports of this happening with the measles component of the MMR, such that health professionals should think twice before giving the MMR to a child with a sibling with impaired immunity.[61, 62]

Private patients

The government appears not to have truly believed its rhetoric on the single vaccines. Though it vocally put out the message that they were bad, they have never been banned. In fact, a significant minority of senior medical advisors in the government felt that the department's support for the MMR was over-confident, and that single vaccines should be made available, at least until further research was done. There was far less certainty in the Department of Health about the safety of the MMR than it admitted in public. There were concerns about the lack of robust safety trials. It was finally decided to fully back the vaccine and not allow the option of single vaccines — with cost being a factor in the decision.

Single vaccines were merely no longer 'licensed' for use. It meant that they weren't readily available through the National Health Service. Though their importation had been 'restricted', they could still be imported by doctors for National Health Service patients or, more commonly, for their private patients.

In this case, licensing is mainly an administrative issue. It means the single vaccines have to be ordered by the doctor on a 'named patient' basis. This requires that each vaccine be ordered for an individual named child, with the clinical reasons that the vaccine is needed. Not having a license does mean that these vaccines haven't passed through the Department of Health's quality control procedures. The significance of this is perhaps best illustrated by what happened in 2005. Because of a shortage of licensed MMR vaccine the government had to import unlicensed MMR vaccines from Germany and the USA.

We live in a free market society. Where there is demand, there is usually supply — at a price. Many parents wanted the single vaccines for their children after 1998. If they couldn't get them in this country, those that had the time and money went to France or other European countries, like the government, where they were more readily available. Doctors and private clinics started to import the vaccines into the UK. A thriving private market grew.

Whilst most providers were offering a good service, it was inevitable that a few less scrupulous providers emerged. I was told of one doctor who offered all three vaccines on the same day, rather undermining the point of giving them separately. Another was given a nine-month jail sentence, and struck off the medical register, for forging the results of blood tests on children to whom he had given single vaccines. A very few of us provided this choice to our National Health Service patients which, contrary to popular belief, we were, and still are, allowed to do.

Obtaining and importing the single vaccines was far from easy. Supplies were often difficult to obtain, particularly when manufacturers learned they were to be imported into the UK. This led to shortages and it was especially frustrating for parents to embark on a course of single vaccines for their child, only to be told that one or more was unobtainable. Over time the single vaccines started to become unavailable as the few large multinational manufacturers stopped producing them in favour of the more lucrative triple MMR vaccine. The single mumps vaccine has not been available since

2009, and single rubella since 2015.

Who believes whom?

Family doctors interpret medical knowledge for their patients. In order to try to stay one step ahead of the game, the Department of Health regularly surveys parents to find out the climate of opinion on vaccinations. Mothers steadily lost confidence in the safety of MMR throughout the 1990s, accompanied by an increasing belief that the vaccine could be more of a threat to their children than the diseases it's aimed to protect against. (Low parental confidence in the MMR is not confined to the UK. Uptake of the vaccine by two years of age in 2014 was only 76% in Austria; and in the USA, where vaccination is compulsory for schooling, uptake was 91%, well below the WHO target).[60] It means that, despite the avalanche of public information, fewer parents than ever before believe the propaganda the government has put out for the past twenty years.

The government blames health professionals for not being supportive enough in pushing the MMR — despite the financial control it has on doctors' budgets through immunisation targets.[49]

Do health professionals themselves no longer believe what the government puts out to justify what happens in their surgeries? There have been several surveys of the attitudes of health professionals' views towards the MMR vaccine. The majority of doctors continue to support the government's policy on the MMR vaccine. But the statistics reveal that trust is fading rapidly.

1998:   Full confidence in the MMR by HPs* fell from 59% to 41% after research first suggested a possible link with bowel disease and autism

1998:   Fewer than half of all HPs were convinced of the necessity of the second dose of the MMR vaccine[50]

1998:   16% of HPs felt a link between MMR and autism was 'very likely or possible'[51]

2001:   Over a quarter (26%) of family doctors felt the government had failed to prove there was no link between MMR and autism and bowel disease[52]

2002:   28% of Scottish family doctors were either 'very concerned' or 'fairly concerned' about the side-effects of the MMR[52]

2003:   A third of HPs wouldn't advise giving MMR to a child with a close family history of autism[53]

HPs refers here to health professionals such as doctors, practice nurses and health visitors — that is, all those most directly involved in giving children vaccinations.

Significantly, many doctors have refused to give their own children MMR and have opted to give them the single vaccines instead. I have given the single vaccines to many doctors' children. At the same time, vital and accepted information about the vaccine does not seem to be reaching health professionals. In 2004 a survey revealed that doctors' and nurses' knowledge of side-effects of the MMR was very poor.[54] There are now even some signs of the rot spreading beyond MMR. Researchers who performed a survey in May 2004 wrote: 'The high level of concern about the safety of the [MMR] vaccine expressed even by parents who had immunised their children is worrying in its implications for public confidence and trust in health care.'[55]

Personal view

Since starting to offer the single vaccines in 2001, I have not heard from the government or health officials any compelling reason to stop the procedure. On the other hand, the numbers of parents convinced that their child's autism has occurred as a result of the MMR vaccine has grown. There are now many thousands. Some of these parents will, inevitably, be wrong. But can all of them really be mistaken? My experience as a doctor has taught me to think long and hard before disputing what parents tell me about their children. I find it implausible that all these parents are wrong.

It's not known for sure from this still anecdotal evidence which children are at risk, but a pattern appears to be emerging. The MMR vaccine is unlikely, in many, to be the only cause of harm. It is likely to work in conjunction with other factors. Many of the affected children:

- Suffer from asthma, eczema or hay fever.
- Have had recurrent coughs, colds and ear infections, often requiring treatment with antibiotics.
- Have family members who suffer from one of the auto-immune disorders such as diabetes, multiple sclerosis or thyroid disease.[56]

As one female doctor observed, 'I continue to feel that in certain vulnerable groups there may be some risks attached to MMR... I do not feel this has been adequately studied.'[52]

Dr Andrew Wakefield's research was dismissed as flawed and junk science, and following a two and a half year General Medical Council disciplinary hearing — the longest in GMC history — Dr Wakefield was found guilty of 'serious professional misconduct' and was struck off the medical register, barring him from practicing as a doctor. The case is far too complicated to discuss in any detail here. However, one of the key findings against him was that he performed unnecessary and distressing investigations on children in pursuit of his own agenda of proving that the MMR vaccine caused autism and bowel disease. He was found to have been 'dishonest, irresponsible and showed callous disregard for the distress and pain of children.'[57] What is extraordinary, and would appear to contradict this damning verdict, is that not one parent of a child investigated by Dr Wakefield complained about his investigations and treatments; indeed many of them were standing outside the GMC making quite clear their support for him. The GMC felt it had no option but to strike Dr Wakefield off the register because 'it is the only sanction that is appropriate to protect patients and is in the wider public interest.' Following the GMC verdict the *Lancet* formally retracted the 1998 paper that sparked the whole furore.

Did Dr Wakefield deserve to be struck off? If we were all to have our actions examined in minute detail over two and a half years, I doubt if any of us would come out without a blemish. I have no doubt that he made errors of judgment. But I do believe that he was acting in the best interests of the children he saw and treated. His main crime would appear to have been to criticise vaccines. This made him extremely unpopular with the vaccine manufacturers, the government and those who depended on funding from the large pharmaceutical companies. The medical establishment has made it absolutely clear to all of us that it will not tolerate criticism of its vaccine policies. The obstacles to doctors attempting to conduct research into the safety of vaccines bear testimony to this.

You might reasonably think that the striking off of Dr Wakefield would be sufficient for the authorities, but not a bit of it. The British Medical Journal published a series of articles in 2010 by the journalist Brian Deer in which it claimed that Dr Wakefield fabricated the test results in a case of deliberate fraud. This would have required the collusion of all his 12 co-authors, all of whom stand by the published findings, though most have distanced themselves from the link with autism.

Others who have questioned the safety of the MMR vaccine have also experienced unreasonable pressure to keep quiet. A researcher at a top autism research unit at Cambridge University was concerned that there might be a link between the MMR vaccine and autism. She was, however, discouraged to do any further research in this area. A senior colleague told her that doing so would be 'sawing off the branch we are all sitting on', a reference to the substantial funding received by the department from a manufacturer of the MMR.

One senior doctor, who was in the Department of Health at the time of the introduction of the MMR, was made to sign the Official Secrets Act. He had the consequences of discussing certain sensitive issues spelled out to him on his retirement. He says that he should really speak out, but fears for the security and safety of his family were he to do so. He has suggested that relevant documents in the Department of Health may have been illegally shredded. Many others have told lawyers they'd like to help but felt unable to risk their careers or to jeopardise funding.[58]

Despite the obstruction, the research into the safety of the MMR continues.

The facts are as follows: the measles vaccine virus (the most potent of the three) has now been found in the bowel of many children affected with autism and bowel disease. The same vaccine strain virus has been found in the fluid surrounding the brain of some of these children. This does not prove that this causes the problems, but they are not the places where one would expect the virus to be. It's hard to explain what it's doing there if it's not contributing to the disease.

The MMR vaccine contains three live viruses. It's the first vaccine ever used on a large scale to contain more than one live virus. Live viruses will interact with each other, both qualitatively and quantitatively. This doesn't necessarily mean the vaccine will cause harm; but it does mean that this interaction could cause side-effects that no one had predicted.

Like any medicine, MMR may act in different ways in different children. But there are three possible methods by which MMR could be causing autism:

- Direct invasion of the measles vaccine virus into the brain.
- The MMR vaccine may cause an abnormal immune reaction in susceptible children. This may result in an auto-immune reaction (similar to other auto-immune diseases) in which the body's immune system attacks itself, in this case the brain. Abnormal MMR antibodies have been found in autistic children.
- It's possible the measles virus invades the gut, where it causes inflammation, resulting in a 'leaky' gut. This results in the absorption of heroin-like (opioid), and other, toxic substances that then travel into, and damage, the brain.

The government's response to any new published research is as follows. If it supports the official claim that the MMR is 'safe', then the research is described with words such as 'exemplary' or 'a clean and elegant piece of work.' Any piece of research that challenges the safety of the MMR is invariably 'fatally flawed'.

We live, supposedly, in a free and open society. This makes it all the more strange why it has been impossible to have a rational discussion about the risks — and benefits — of the MMR vaccine, without personal attacks and accusations of putting children's lives at risk.

Amanda's first baby, Alfie, was born on September 9th, 2008. His first year of life went well. He received all the recommended NHS vaccines and was developing normally. On November 1st, 2009, at the age of 13 months, Alfie was given the MMR vaccine. He was out of sorts for a few days, which Mum thought nothing of as she had been warned that he may not be himself for a short while after receiving the vaccine. But then he started behaving unusually, becoming strangely angry and frustrated — something his mother had never seen in him before. On November 10th, nine days after Alfie's jab, Amanda went to work as usual and Alfie was looked after by his father. When she got home Alfie had a temperature of 39.3°c. She called her GP and was reassured, as this is a common time to develop a fever after the MMR vaccine, and was advised to give paracetamol and to put him to bed. Alfie's temperature went down a little after the paracetamol but he was very drowsy and went to sleep immediately when Amanda put him to bed at 7pm. She went to check him half an hour later and found him curled up in the corner of his cot. She went to feel his temperature but saw that his face was blue and that he was not breathing. Paramedics arrived five minutes later but were unable to resuscitate Alfie. The MMR was never blamed for his death.

I write about Alfie because his tragic story is one of several I have heard where babies have died seven to ten days after being given the MMR vaccine (the most common time for a feverish reaction to the vaccine) but where the death certificates or coroners' reports have never implicated the vaccine. Alfie's death was categorised as 'sudden unexplained death', as were other similar deaths. This is strange, to say the least, as it is well recognized that reactions, including febrile convulsions, commonly occur a week or so after being given the vaccine. I suspect that there is pressure not to implicate the vaccine in any of these deaths, however plausible it is that the vaccine may have contributed, for fear of causing a 'scare' and putting parents off giving the MMR to their babies.

Italian court case

In April 2012, a court in the Italian city of Rimini, on independent medical advice, ruled that a boy's autism had been caused by the MMR vaccine he had received. Valentino Bocca had been given the MMR vaccine in 2004 when he was one year old. Within hours of receiving the triple jab he developed diarrhoea and went off his food. Two days later he started to regress, losing skills he had previously acquired and lost all interest in his surroundings. He stopped sleeping at night, waking several times screaming in pain. For years, despite his parents' suspicions, doctors told them that the vaccine could not possibly have been causing his symptoms. Valentino's story is similar to thousands of other children who received the MMR vaccine and whose parents have also been told that the vaccine was not – and could not have been – the cause of their child's regression. Valentino's case is the first in which the authorities – both medical and legal – have acknowledged that the triple live vaccine can cause autism. It is worrying that the MMR vaccine given to Valentino has exactly the same active ingredients as one of the two MMRs used routinely in the UK.

Deceit and cover up

In 2004 the USA CDC published a paper that appeared to show that there is no link between the age at which a child is vaccinated with the MMR and the subsequent risk of developing autism. Ten years later one of the paper's co-authors, William Thompson, confessed that some information had been deliberately left out of the paper as they had, in actual fact, found a link but that this was suppressed and evidence shredded. When their data was reanalysed, it emerges that boys who received the MMR vaccine before 36 months of age were 69% more likely to develop autism than those vaccinated after 36 months. The difference was even more marked in African American boys, who were over three times more likely to develop autism if they were given the vaccine before 36 months of age.[63]

19
Hib

A Spectacular Retreat

Four years after the introduction of the MMR in 1988, the government embarked on yet another addition to the national immunisation schedule with a novel vaccine. In 1992, it introduced a new type of vaccine called a 'conjugated' vaccine to immunise the population against Hib. 'Conjugated' means that the outer coating of the vaccine bacterium is attached to a protein in order to make immunisation more effective, much like the addition of aluminium. The protein stimulates the immune system to produce a greater reaction than the vaccine would have done on its own. The protein in Hib vaccines used in Britain is the tetanus 'poison-made-safe' (toxoid), similar to what is used in the tetanus vaccine.

Hib is a bacterium* that lives up the nose of many people without doing any harm at all. But it can be a dangerous bug. Unlike the measles virus that causes measles, or the whooping cough bacterium that causes whooping cough, Hib can cause many different illnesses, many of them mild such as ear infections. But Hib diseases usually refer to serious or 'invasive' Hib such as meningitis, blood poisoning, pneumonia and inflammation of a part of the throat (epiglottitis).

Before 1992, a Hib vaccine had been available but it didn't work in children under eighteen months. As the disease is most serious in very young children, they are the ones you would need to immunise.

But there was also a large question mark over whether there was any need for national immunisation of children. A child that is fundamentally well, has been breastfed and lives in healthy surroundings is far less likely to become ill, or die, from Hib disease than a sickly child living in an overcrowded and unhealthy environment.¹

Before vaccination, every year around one thousand children under five became ill with invasive Hib. Of these over nine hundred made a complete recovery, but thirty-five died, and seventy became permanently disabled. The chance of a child under five catching one of the potentially serious forms of 'invasive' Hib infection was, therefore, around one in three and a half thousand, the risk of dying one in a hundred thousand, and of getting disabled one in fifty thousand every year. However, the risk was greatest in the first two years of life — with a peak risk between six and twelve months. The disease was rare in children over 5 years of age.

The cases of invasive Hib split out as follows. Over half are (bacterial) meningitis; most children can be successfully treated with antibiotics, but a little fewer than 3% of victims will die. The second most common condition caused by Hib is an inflammation of part of the back of the throat (epiglottitis), which occurs in one tenth of cases in children under five, and which can be fatal (in 3-4% of children) if not treated quickly. Cellulitis (an infection of the skin) is the result of 9% of Hib infections in young children. Blood poisoning occurs in 7%; though rare, this is the most dangerous form of Hib disease, with one in seven sufferers dying. (Other diseases occasionally caused by Hib include pneumonia and bone and joint infections.)

These are serious figures, but there are many factors that affect a child's resistance to infections other than protection by vaccination. In the case of death from invasive Hib, half of the children who died from the disease were already suffering from underlying health problems such as cancer, prematurity or congenital abnormality — emphasizing the risk of any infection to chronically ill children.[2] The question was whether Hib immunisation would actually protect the small proportion of unfortunate sufferers, without causing an increased risk to the majority.

Undeterred, the Department of Health charged ahead. Trials of various Hib vaccines, before their introduction into the UK, had suggested that they were somewhere between 75% and 95% effective. These trials followed up the children for only a year or two.[3,4] Trials to look at the long-term effectiveness of the vaccine before its introduction were simply not done; this is now commonplace in the Department of Health's enthusiasm to introduce new vaccines quickly. Emboldened by the precedent set by the MMR, it seemed intent on creating an exception for vaccines that was afforded to no other medicine. A new policy appeared to have emerged that, because we 'know' that they are so effective, vaccines don't need to be tested with the same rigour as other drugs and medical interventions. Even in the '50s and '60s, when belief in medical progress was at its highest, such a view did not exist.

The campaign

In 1992 the Hib vaccine was added to the baby vaccine schedule at two, three and four months, in addition to vaccines against diphtheria, tetanus, whooping cough and polio. At the time of the vaccine's introduction, all children between one and four years of age were offered a single 'catch-up' dose in the hope of producing a large and immediate population effect. To coincide with the vaccine's launch, the government ran a high profile national television advertising campaign.

The campaign was a resounding success. Within two years of the introduction of the vaccine, serious Hib infections in children had fallen by over 90% in England and Wales. The dramatic fall in numbers of Hib cases was even better than many had expected. Scotland also reported a spectacular 92% fall in invasive Hib disease.

The results in Britain were doubly impressive because they resulted from giving only three doses of the vaccine — in the first few months of life. Though all other countries that had introduced the Hib vaccine were also reporting a huge drop in cases, most of these were using a four-dose schedule that included a booster dose, usually given in the second year of life.

A self-congratulatory study, part-funded by the drug company Pasteur-Merieux, a manufacturer of the Hib vaccine creating such good business, was published in the prestigious medical journal *Lancet:* 'Hib disease is now close to elimination in the UK,' trumpeted the authors, 'and we suggest that a booster is not necessary in the second year of life.'[5] It contained claims that the vaccine could be 98% effective. The authors would soon be eating their words.

The end of the honeymoon

Then something unexpected happened. Cases of Hib stopped falling in 1998 and started rising again. By 2002 cases were in the two hundreds, higher than anything seen since the vaccine was introduced ten years previously.

So what was going on? Uptake of the Hib vaccine had remained consistently high (between 93% and 95%) since 1994, so the increase did not appear to be due to a fall in the numbers of children receiving the vaccine. The Department of Health, ever inventive, publicly suggested three possible reasons for the setback:[6]

Department of Health: the effect of the initial 'catch-up' campaign (immunising all children under 4 when the vaccine was first introduced) had now worn off.

  Fact: this was unconvincing. The largest rise in cases was in the one to four years age group. The catch-up campaign shouldn't have mattered if the protection received by babies from their three jabs had lasted until their fifth birthday, as the vast majority of Hib infections occur in the first five years of life. The facts suggested that the vaccine had not being doing its job as well as expected.

Department of Health: during 2000-1 a different four-in-one DTP-Hib vaccine had been used, which may have interacted with, and decreased the effectiveness of, the Hib vaccine.

  Fact: this was possible, but as the rise in Hib cases started before this vaccine was in use, it could, at most, have only been part of the cause of the rise.

Department of Health: there was a small decline in the numbers of children being immunised.

  Fact: this was far-fetched. The vaccination rate had actually remained consistently high. It is true that the coverage had fallen very slightly from 95% in 1995 to 93% in 2001. Nevertheless, it is unlikely that a fall of only 2% would have much impact on the number of cases.

In reality, the vaccine just wasn't up to its rosy praise. In 1999, Mary

Ramsay was one of several government-funded doctors who reported that the vaccine was over 98% effective.[7] She was, it turned out, way off the mark. After the rise in Hib cases, she had to backtrack rapidly in 2003, conceding that actually the vaccine was only 57% effective – a shocking figure.[8]

Even more worrying was her discovery that the protection the vaccine gave to babies was only short-lived. Babies receiving the Hib vaccine in the standard UK schedule at two, three and four months were only 60% protected for two years, after which the protection fell to 27% – hardly any protection at all.

This should have been discovered through proper trials before the vaccine was introduced, not after the vaccine had been in routine use for ten years. Though not publicly, even the Joint Committee on Vaccination and Immunisation (JCVI), the expert body that advises the government, admitted in 2002 that one probable reason for the increase in cases was 'waning immunity', or a fall off in protection over a rather shorter timescale than had been expected.[9]

Other possible causes for the dramatic drop in invasive Hib were discovered.[10] The figures only included children with Hib disease confirmed by a laboratory. Laboratories had to report these cases to the government's central surveillance centre in London. However, the laboratories were being less efficient at reporting Hib cases after the introduction of vaccination than they were before.[11] If cases were not being reported, then that means that children were still having the disease, but were not being counted in the statistics.

The conclusion was inevitable: the success of the three-dose vaccination was wilting visibly.

The response of the Department of Health to the increasing numbers of invasive Hib cases was straightforward: if the enemy is resisting the attack, use more firepower. A second Hib catch-up campaign (the first one happened at the time of its introduction in 1992) started on Monday 12 May 2003. All children aged between six months and four years were offered a further dose of Hib vaccine, even if they had completed their full course of three doses as a baby.

It was hoped that the campaign would be completed within four months, but administering extra vaccines at times when children do not normally receive them is organisationally difficult, and the campaign dragged on into 2004. The campaign succeeded in reducing cases, especially in the under-five age group. The Chief Medical Officer, Sir Liam Donaldson, told doctors in his December 2004 newsletter that the rate of Hib disease in children under five had plummeted due to the recent campaign and further congratulations were in order. 'We were able,' he said, 'to act quickly to nip this problem in the bud.'[12]

But the catch-up campaign only postponed the inevitable need for an additional Hib booster vaccination in the increasingly congested childhood schedule. The retreat had begun. The JCVI acknowledged in 2003 the possible need for a booster, and by 2005, it was not a case of 'if', but 'when' it was needed.[13,14] Despite earlier claims that a booster was not necessary, one was finally introduced in September 2006 as a combined jab with Meningitis C given at twelve months.

The result

It is now known that the vaccine does offer reasonable immunity against Hib disease, but that this does not last as long as required. In particular, babies vaccinated at two, three and four months are likely to lose their immunity in the second year of life. This would have been found out had the Hib vaccine undergone adequate trials before introduction in the national schedule. It always was a discoverable flaw, but it remained hidden by the way the vaccine was introduced by the DoH.

Instead a decision to expose every healthy child in Britain to the vaccine was taken on evidence that was incomplete, in the hope, rather than knowledge, that it would achieve its aims. It seems likely that this approach was intentional and not a matter of government inefficiency, oversight or omission. A UK vaccine expert, for example, has recently argued, 'a placebo-controlled trial would have been unethical' in the case of Hib.[15] Such trials are considered the gold standard, and non-negotiable, in the case of all other medical interventions.

Indeed we now know that giving two doses in the first year of life is just as effective as three doses (though the UK gives three doses as it is part of the 6-in-1 vaccine), but a booster is still required in the second year of life to prolong protection.[29]

Worryingly, it also looks as though the fall in Hib disease may be countered by a rise in another, equally serious, infection. This has already happened in Finland and Sweden, where pneumococcal infections (for which a vaccine has now also been introduced) have partially replaced Hib infections since the introduction of the Hib vaccine.[16]

Other thought-provoking research suggests that the Hib vaccine may reduce deaths from Hib, but not necessarily the overall death rate in children.[17] It's all very well reducing deaths from one infection, but if these were to be replaced by deaths from another disease, then children would be no better off.

The side-effects in vaccinated children

The safety trials performed before introduction of the vaccine showed no major safety problems, but these trials were all either very small or actively followed up the children for no more than a short period of time, so that only very common, or very serious, reactions occurring shortly after vaccination would have been detected.

One of the concerns about adding increasing numbers of vaccines to the vaccine schedule is the damaging effect they may have, either alone or in combination, on the baby's developing immune system. There have been huge rises in the numbers of people affected by immune disorders in recent years, one of the most common of which is diabetes.

The number of young diabetic children has been growing dramatically in recent years as new vaccines have been added to the schedule. Of course, this does not necessarily mean the vaccines are causing the rise but, as it is known that vaccines, including Hib, can affect the immune system in a way that could make these diseases more likely, vaccines have to be one possible suspect.[18] Controversial research suggests that the Hib vaccine, in particular, may be contributing to the increasing number of children getting diabetes.[19]

Studies in three areas of England have looked at the number of children getting diabetes during the 1980s and 1990s. In all areas the rate of children under five (the group that receives the most vaccines) newly diagnosed with diabetes has been increasing.

Increases in numbers of young diabetic children have occurred throughout the UK since the introduction of the Hib vaccine. But as the numbers were already rising prior to its introduction, there must be uncertainty over the exact contribution − if any − of the Hib vaccine. There is currently no conclusive evidence that vaccines are contributing to the huge rise in diabetes; indeed some published papers refute the link, but these have, in turn, been criticised. One of the papers challenging a link between vaccines and diabetes did, in fact, demonstrate a 14% rise in diabetes in children who had received the Hib vaccine, though it is possible that this increase occurred by chance.[20]

The Hib vaccine has also been associated with an increased risk of asthma, allergies and a rare paralysing disorder of the nerves called Guillain-Barré syndrome, all of which are disorders of the immune system.[21,22,23]

Adults

Though invasive Hib is primarily a disease of children, it can affect adults. After the introduction of the vaccine, there was a rise in adult cases up to a peak in 2003, after which numbers started to fall; the concern about adults getting invasive Hib disease is that they are far more likely to die from it than children are. Over 10% of adults, and 30% of the elderly, who get Hib disease will die.[24,25]

The probable explanation for this rise in adult cases is that, before immunisation, everyone used to come across the Hib bug, which was widespread in the community, with only a tiny proportion becoming ill. Most developed antibodies and became immune. This immunity was boosted naturally every time contact was made with the Hib bacterium.

Since the introduction of Hib vaccination in 1992, fewer people come across Hib in the community, because the vaccine has been so 'successful'. The problem may be that when an adult now comes across the Hib bacterium, there is much less likelihood that he or she has sufficient natural immunity to protect against invasive Hib disease. So the introduction of the vaccine for children may have caused the rise in Hib disease in adults.

As the doctors working for the government's 'Health Protection Agency', responsible for vaccination, rather sheepishly concluded,

'Childhood vaccination programmes may have unanticipated effects on the epidemiology of disease in older age groups.'[26] In other words, mass vaccination of children can change the way a disease behaves so that it causes more, rather than less, problems – at least in one age group.

The same government-funded doctors were hopeful that the 2003/4 'catch-up' campaign would induce 'herd immunity', resulting in a decrease in Hib disease of all age groups including adults. There has been a fall in adult Hib disease following the booster campaign, but the same phenomenon of a rise in adult cases has also been reported in the Netherlands where the vaccine programme already contained a regular booster given in the second year of life, so the decline might be short-lived. However, since 2010 the number of confirmed cases of Hib has remained very low, at below 30 a year, with the majority being in adults.

Before vaccination, though, one in twenty healthy children co-habited with the Hib bacterium in their noses and throats, yet only 0.2% succumbed to the disease.[27,28] As with all diseases, the 'resistance' of the body, both genetically and from the way children live and are brought up, appears to be more important than the 'virulence', or strength, of the infection. Instead of focusing on these aspects, we have now replaced this situation with mass immunisation and a dependency on the Hib vaccine. Against the benefit of fewer children catching Hib, we have to set the side-effects of the vaccine, and the risk of increasing the disease in older people – in whom it is more serious. One study has even found that children fully vaccinated against Hib were six times more likely to carry potentially dangerous Hib bacteria in their noses than unvaccinated children. The study's authors were unable to explain this but it provides yet more evidence that vaccinations can change our relationship with bugs in ways that may not be favourable.[30]

20
Meningitis C

A Nation of Guinea Pigs

Fresh from its bruising experience with the Hib vaccine, the Department of Health drew few lessons from the blinkered enthusiasm with which it had introduced the vaccine. In 1999, only one year after major safety issues had been raised about the MMR vaccine, it proved it was willing to go even further. The idea for the new vaccine was fuelled by terrifying news headlines during the late 1990s: 'Killer Disease Claims More Victims', 'Brain Bug Kills More Babies', and 'Meningitis Scare as Student Dies'. It was against a backdrop of headlines like these that the government announced the bold and ambitious plan, in 1999, to immunise all fourteen million children in the UK against the disease. New vaccines provide good news among the barrage of criticism directed at British governments.

The government teamed up with three commercial drug companies to fast-track a vaccine onto the market. Britain was to be the first country in the world to introduce the new life-saving vaccine into the child vaccination programme. Like the Hib vaccine it was one of the newer, high-tech 'conjugated' vaccines in which the shell, or outer coat, of the bacterium is attached to a 'carrier' such as the diphtheria or tetanus 'poison-made-safe'.

There was one minor issue. There are several types of meningococcal bacteria — one of the smallest living organisms — all of which can cause serious illnesses, including meningitis and blood poisoning. Most infections in the UK (around 59%) at that time were Men B, caused by the B strain of the bug, whereas the C strain caused about 39% of infections. But there was to be no vaccine against the B strain for a further fifteen years. So the proposed vaccine could only be a humbler part of the solution.

This was but a small blemish on the ambitious plans. The government's Chief Medical Officer argued that Meningitis C had been killing an increasing number of children over the previous years and had become 'one of the foremost causes of death in children and young people.'[1]

The government was undoubtedly right about the seriousness of the disease. Even though it caused only 39% of the infections, Meningitis C is a scary illness. This type is the nasty one that can cause a rash that doesn't go away when pressed with a glass. It can cause blood poisoning and meningitis. More importantly, it can progress very rapidly, and even kill, within twenty-four hours. Around one in ten children who get the illness die, and a further three in twenty suffer from permanent problems including scarring, hearing loss and amputation because of the blood poisoning.

The launch

The Department of Health had put pressure on all three companies to provide the vaccines as quickly as possible. This resulted in a uniquely short development period of only five years.[2] Three Meningitis C vaccines were used in the UK campaign. The first one to be licensed, in October 1999, was Meningitec, manufactured by Wyeth; Menjugate, made by Chiron, was licensed in March 2000, followed in July 2000 by Baxter's Neusvac-C.

Whereas the government had not been unduly held up by safety trials of the Hib vaccine seven years earlier, it took a real gamble with this one.

The risk of Meningitis C disease was perceived to be so great that it took the unprecedented step of introducing the new Meningitis C vaccine without any evidence that it actually worked.[3] The Department of Health's head of immunisation, Dr David Salisbury, would later be unrepentant, stating two years after the introduction, 'We saw no place for a randomised controlled trial,'[2] which, though necessary to test the true effectiveness of the vaccine, may have delayed its introduction by three to five years.[4] Some small trials had been done, but only to test children's antibody responses, or probable immunity, with blood tests. Finding that children did produce antibodies against Meningitis C after vaccination, it was decided that it was likely to work. After all, it was manufactured in a similar way to the Hib vaccine.

The only large (19,000 children) safety study performed before the vaccine was licensed and introduced into the UK was designed primarily to look at another vaccine, and was based in the USA on their two, four and six-month schedule. The second largest study, which was only half way through at the time the vaccine was licensed, was performed in the UK and involved 2,796 children. Four 'serious adverse events' were considered to be possibly related to the vaccine.[5] In other small studies, many children had redness at the site of the injection but no serious side-effects were reported. None of the safety studies compared vaccinated children with unimmunised children, called 'controls,' and they were therefore unable to provide any conclusive information on side-effects caused by Meningitis C vaccines. Apart from the two studies already mentioned, none involved more than three hundred or so children and were therefore incapable of detecting uncommon but serious reactions.[6]

Interestingly, at one JCVI (Joint Committee on Vaccination and Immunisation – the body that advises the Department of Health) meeting five months before the introduction, at which the main agenda item was the new Meningitis C vaccine, no fewer than three of the eleven members present were involved in drug companies' trials of the new vaccines. It was a sign how intertwined the pharmaceutical companies, the Department of Health, and 'independent expert committees' such as the JCVI had become.

Nonetheless, this usually pro-vaccine committee 'felt it was not well informed regarding the protection the vaccine offered,' and 'expressed caution in a number of areas.'[4]

The campaign started hurriedly on 1 November 1999, accompanied by a £2 million advertising campaign. The logistical nightmare of vaccinating fourteen million children in one year was a huge challenge. Fifteen to seventeen year olds were the first to be vaccinated, for two good reasons, firstly the death rate of Meningitis C disease was highest in adolescents, and secondly for PR purposes. The JCVI had advised before the vaccine's introduction that it 'felt that the public image was of adolescents dying,'[4]

Babies were the next to be vaccinated, with three doses as part of their routine vaccination schedule. It was given as a two-dose course to children aged four to twelve months, and a single dose to all children from one year old upwards. In all, during the following twelve months, over eleven million British children were given the new vaccine.

Despite the concerns that had been voiced by government advisors, and the decision taken to do without three to five years of trials, the public was reassured that the Meningitis C vaccines had undergone 'extensive testing,' had an 'excellent...safety profile at all ages,' and were 'highly effective.'[1,7] They were expected to be 'about 98%' effective — an impressively high figure for any vaccine and not dissimilar to the short-lived hopes for the Hib vaccine.

On 1 November 1999, the day the campaign began, the government's Chief Medical Officer (CMO), Professor Liam Donaldson, declared the campaign a 'tremendous success.'[8] To do this before the first vaccination had been given might have seemed somewhat premature. But it appeared that the government had backed the right horse.

Initial assessments seemed very promising. The effectiveness of the vaccine in the first nine months of use was calculated as between 93% and 97%. Even though this was not quite as high as the original 98% hoped for, they were good figures by any standards. The Department of Health had every right to publish a paper with the words 'A Success Story' in the title.'[3] Another article by government-funded doctors published in the Lancet detailed a vaccine effectiveness of 97% in adolescents, and 92% in toddlers.[9]

The government's boasts appeared to be vindicated when confirmed cases of Meningitis C fell from a high of 983 in 1999 to 320 in 2001.

The vaccine programme was extended in January 2002 to include all those up to twenty-four years of age. In the same year the Department of Health published a paper describing the vaccination campaign in detail. The paper described an 'overall 81% reduction' in Meningitis C infections in children following the campaign.[3]

The Department of Health doctors were doubly delighted when it was shown that those who had not been vaccinated had a 67% reduced attack rate of Meningitis C. They explained this by a bonus effect of the vaccine: it was increasing the 'herd immunity'. The vaccine was doing this, it was suggested, by decreasing the rate of carriage of the Meningitis C bug in the noses of those who had been vaccinated, thereby making it less likely that they would transmit the infection to unvaccinated contacts.

The academic credentials of the writers of these papers could not be bettered. One of them, Doctor Elizabeth Miller, for example, became a professor and was awarded an OBE in 2004, 'in recognition of her services to Public Health Medicine.'

Alarm Bells

Alarm bells started ringing, however, when a follow-up study on vaccinated children was reported in the medical journal, Lancet, in the summer of 2004. It was now four years on and a more considered view could be taken of the vaccine's medium term effectiveness. Had there been trials, instead of mass immunisation, such information would have been used to consider whether introducing the vaccine offered compelling benefits rather than review the vaccination itself.

Though sliding away from the original 98% prediction, things looked reasonable in all the children from five months to eighteen years of age who had been vaccinated in the one-off catch-up campaign; for these children the vaccine was now calculated as being at least 83% effective.

Nonetheless, fifty-three children who had been vaccinated had gone on to develop Meningitis C disease, and four of these children had died. Of those fifty-three 'vaccine failures,' twenty-one were in children who had been routinely vaccinated at two, three and four months of age. For this age group, the vaccine effectiveness was estimated at 66%, which is not good enough. Whilst the vaccine appears to give good protection to babies for the first year after vaccination (93% effective), this falls to zero protection after a year.

The figures speak for themselves: of nineteen cases of Meningitis C disease that occurred in children more than one year after routine immunisation, at two, three and four months, eighteen occurred in children who had been fully vaccinated against the disease. The policy of vaccinating babies for Meningitis C at two, three and four months was providing them with protection lasting no longer than one year.[10]

It soon became clear that a booster dose was going to be necessary if children were to remain protected into their second year of life, an inevitability acknowledged by the JCVI in early 2005. As part of the Department of Health's overhaul of the immunisation schedule in September 2006, a booster was added at twelve months of age, as a combined Hib/Meningitis C vaccine.

There has been much tinkering with the meningitis C vaccine schedule since its introduction. Two years after the introduction of a booster dose, the infant schedule was reduced from three to two doses in order to make way for the new pneumococcal vaccine. Then in 2015 the infant schedule was cut back further to just one dose at 3 months of age, still with a booster at 12 months, this time to make space for the new meningitis B vaccine, while at the same time adding in a Meningitis ACWY vaccine as a teenage booster. Finally, in 2016, the primary dose was removed altogether with young children now receiving only the 'booster' dose at 12 months. Time will tell whether this will be sufficient to give sufficient protection prior to their receiving the Men ACWY shot as teenagers. The evidence for the effectiveness of these different schedules is based on antibody studies. But antibody studies have already proved unreliable predictors of the effectiveness of this vaccine.[11]

The figures

There is little point in vaccinating millions of healthy children if the disease, however serious, is only going to affect very few. Every medical intervention, and that includes all vaccinations, has side-effects. There is always a trade-off between benefit and risk that must be assessed with every vaccine. The disease must be sufficiently common to justify a national vaccination programme. How common was Meningitis C?

It is often difficult to estimate how widespread an illness is — for various reasons. First, the doctor has to make the correct diagnosis, which is not as easy as one might think. Doctors are more likely to diagnose an illness that is in the public eye simply because they are more likely to think of it. If you don't think of an illness, you can't diagnose it. So diseases that are being talked about a lot (as meningitis was in the 1990s) are likely to be over-diagnosed.

The government's CMO, Professor Donaldson, had written in 1999 that Meningitis C was 'one of the foremost causes of death in children and young people.' The official figures for total laboratory confirmed cases (in other words those that we can be sure what they are — no estimating) of Meningitis C in England and Wales certainly support that the number of cases was on the rise. They were decreasing in the early 1990s from 467 in 1990 to 290 in 1994. But then the number of confirmed cases of Meningitis C started going up rather steeply up to a peak of 983 by 1999.

The Department of Health estimated — there are no laboratory-confirmed reports of this — that somewhere between eighty and a hundred and fifty people (mostly under twenty years of age) were dying every year in England and Wales from Meningitis C. It argued that this justified vaccinating the whole population.

But not all researchers have since agreed with the official figures. For example, the number of cases of Meningitis C in Scotland had been declining from the mid-1980s to the mid-1990s.[12] In addition, a study from Birmingham reported that 'meningococcal disease was being over-diagnosed' (as usually happens when an illness hits the headlines) and that, at least in Birmingham, they had not seen the rise in Meningitis C cases that the official figures were showing.[13] A falling death rate from the disease, despite an increase in cases, supports the argument that more, possibly milder, cases were being diagnosed. This, interestingly, was mooted by the JCVI as early as May 1997.[14]

Age (Years)	Catching Meningitis C*	Dying from Meningitis C*	Permanent damage from Meningitis C*
0-1	1 in 6,600	1 in 66,000	1 in 44,000
1-4	1 in 15,500	1 in 155,000	1 in 100,000
5-9	1 in 34,000	1 in 340,000	1 in 227,000
10-14	1 in 45,700	1 in 457,000	1 in 300,000
15-19	1 in 19,000	1 in 190,000	1 in 130,000
20-24	1 in 70,000	1 in 700,000	1 in 470,000
25+	1 in 60,000	1 in 1,600,000	1 in 1,000,000

* Yearly risk of...

So whether the numbers were increasing in England and Wales because of a real increase in the disease, or because we looked harder and got better at finding it, is in some doubt. It has been suggested that the increase in numbers of cases was a consequence, at least in part, of two other developments: firstly new improved lab tests for Meningitis C, which were introduced during the 1990s, shortly before the introduction of the vaccine, and secondly 'enhanced surveillance,' or looking harder for the illness, that had started in January 1998.

What matters, crucially, is what the risk is of a child catching this type of meningitis, and what happens if they do?

The age group at highest risk from catching Meningitis C is under one year. Before vaccination started a maximum of one hundred children under one year of age were catching Meningitis C in England and Wales annually. This gave every child under one year old a 1 in 6,600 chance of catching the disease. For every ten children that catch Meningitis C, one will die and one or two will suffer a permanent problem such as a hearing loss, scarring or even amputation of a leg or arm. The remaining seven or eight will make a full recovery. That means that every child under one has a 1 in 66,000 chance of dying from Meningitis C and a 1 in 44,000 chance of a permanent disability from it.

These calculations (see above) are based on the government's own figures which may be on the high side.[15] It is also important to bear in mind that every child's risk is not the same. For example, children from 'deprived' backgrounds (for example in areas with high unemployment and overcrowding) are up to twice as likely to get meningitis as those from better-off environments.

So, whilst Meningitis C is undoubtedly a serious disease, a child's chance of actually catching it is small.

Against this should be set the side-effects of the vaccine. Because of the hurried introduction of the vaccine, partly as a result of political pressure, not only was there no proper trial of effectiveness, but there was also little research into safety.

Following the start of the massive immunisation campaign doctors and nurses were encouraged to report any side-effects to the Department of

Health using the 'yellow card' system, as is normal practice with the introduction of any new drug or vaccine.[16] At the end of the campaign after
fifteen months, the department had received 12,880 reports of 26,682
suspected reactions.[17] It is likely that many of these reactions were coincidental and had nothing to do with the vaccine. But, as they were all
reported by doctors who 'suspected' an adverse reaction, it is probable that
many were vaccine-related. As a result of these reports, adverse reactions
including headache, nausea, vomiting, rash, dizziness, faints, malaise,
enlarged glands, and allergic reactions including anaphylaxis (a severe and
life-threatening allergic reaction) and seizures, were added to the vaccines'
data sheets. The occurrence of these side-effects, though concerning, is not
surprising. However, it confirms the inadequacy of the safety trials before
introduction of the vaccines.

There were 291 reports of convulsions, half occurring on the day of
vaccination. Though an initial report by the Department of Health felt that
the data 'supported a causal relationship between Meningitec (one of the
Men C vaccines) and convulsions,'[18] a later report backtracked, concluding,
'the most difficult part of this and previous safety assessments has been the
assessment of causality with convulsions.'[17] The vaccines' data sheets now
refer to 'very rare reports of seizures.'

Most worrying of all, eighteen deaths were suspected by doctors or
nurses to have been caused by the vaccine. Eight of these were classified as
SIDS (sudden infant death syndrome) and a further three were 'unascertained'. This means that no cause was discovered for eleven of the deaths,
though the vaccine had been suspected by a health professional.

There has been considerable controversy over the possible link between
vaccines and SIDS, and the Department of Health published a paper on the
relationship between the Meningitis C vaccine and SIDS. The paper was
headed 'Restricted commercial' and 'Not for publication,' which I obtained
under freedom of information legislation.[19]

The research compared the numbers of children dying from SIDS in the
days following vaccination with expected numbers of children dying from
SIDS had they not been vaccinated. One problem is that those children not
being vaccinated, whether for social reasons or because they were unwell,
are the very children that are more likely to die from SIDS. The authors of
the paper did attempt to allow for this in their calculations. Another
problem was that it was not known at exactly what age the children had
received their vaccinations. This is important because the likelihood of dying
from SIDS is at a maximum in the second and third months of life, after
which the risk falls off rapidly.

The authors had to make 'guesstimates' of the ages at which the children
were vaccinated. They also performed intricate mathematical calculations,
and made numerous other assumptions, before concluding that there was
no evidence that the vaccine caused any cases of SIDS. However, even apart
from the many assumptions that were made, there are difficulties in
accepting the report's conclusion.

The figures of the numbers of children dying from SIDS after vaccination relied on the reporting of these to the Department of Health as suspected adverse reactions. If the doctor involved felt that a baby's death was not caused by the vaccine then it would not have been reported. As most doctors believe that vaccines do not cause SIDS, it is probable that cases went unreported. It was noted in an accompanying paper that several of the babies had risk factors for SIDS, though that should not preclude the vaccine from being a contributory factor. The report did not look into the three other 'unascertained' deaths.

On balance some, if not most, of the deaths may not have been caused by the vaccine. However, from its introduction until September 2005, a total of thirty deaths have been suspected by doctors to have been caused by the vaccine, of which fourteen have been classified as sudden unexplained deaths. This is a higher number of suspected deaths per dose than any other widely used vaccine.[20]

Other problems have also been noted. There have been reports in the medical literature of adverse reactions following Meningitis C and similar meningococcal vaccinations including a disorder of the immune system called Henoch-Schönlein purpura, which has also been associated with other vaccinations.[21] The vaccine can cause a relapse in children with the serious kidney disorder called nephrotic syndrome, also believed to be caused by a disturbance of the immune system. In children with this disorder, the vaccine may do more harm than good.[22]

The combined high-tech vaccine of Hib and Meningitis C (Menitorix – now given routinely to children at twelve months), also first used in the UK, has undergone only very limited safety studies; at the time of its introduction into the UK, there were no published scientific papers on the vaccine's safety or effectiveness. However, information obtained from GSK, the manufacturer, states that common side-effects, occurring in over one in ten of children, include irritability, drowsiness, loss of appetite, pain, redness, swelling and fever.[23]

Following the apparently successful mass introduction of the Meningitis C vaccine into the UK market, other countries soon followed suit. The majority of European countries have added the Men C vaccine to their national schedules, most preferring just a single dose given between 12 and 15 months. Most countries have reported sharp falls in cases in the years following the vaccine's introduction.

Trial and error

Before coming to any conclusions on the Meningitis C vaccine it is necessary to consider two further points. Many organisms such as the meningococcus (of which one type is Meningitis C) spend most of their time living harmlessly in, or at least on, many people. In the case of the meningococcus, it lives innocuously in the noses or throats of at least one in ten, possibly up to one in two, of us.[24,25] So millions of people in the UK are walking around with bacteria that can kill within twenty-four hours.

But extremely few of us become ill as a result of our close relationship with this bug. If we live healthily and keep our immune system in good shape then it is very unlikely that we will fall prey to this bacterium. We must all inevitably come across the meningococcus on many occasions, yet very few of us become ill.

One might question whether it would be more profitable to look at why 99.9% of us never succumb to the infection, rather than vaccinating 100% of us against it. Meningitis C actually causes less disease than its more troublesome relative Meningitis B, against which a vaccine was finally marketed in 2013, after decades of research.

Replacement of one group of bugs with another

A worrying phenomenon that is being increasingly seen with the introduction of more vaccines is that the type of bug targeted by the vaccine is then replaced by another type of the same bug. The meningococcal bug comes in many different forms: by far the most common is the B group, though annual cases decreased dramatically from 1,296 in 1998 to 418 in 2015 despite the absence of any B group vaccine during this period. However, cases caused by the relatively uncommon Y group increased from 22 in 1998 to 93 in 2015 and the W group from a low of 19 cases in 2008 to 176 in 2015. These rises caused sufficient concern for a Men ACWY booster to be introduced in 2015 for teenagers. Whether these changes are related to vaccination against the C group is currently uncertain. There is greater evidence for vaccine-induced 'sero-group replacement' with the pneumococcal bug.

Meningitis C is rare but serious. It is certainly serious enough (with a one in ten death rate) to qualify for vaccination, but whether it is common enough to justify vaccinating everyone is less certain. One vaccine expert wrote in 1998: 'Generally speaking, the incidence of meningococcal disease [in industrialised countries] is too low to indicate vaccinations for the whole population, or even children, but some risk groups and epidemics are important exceptions.'[26]

The government clearly disagreed and has, in effect, conducted the world's largest ever clinical trial on every child in the UK. A multinational group of doctors commented, 'As the first nation in the world to embark on such a programme [Meningitis C vaccination], the safety and efficacy of this approach will be watched with great interest.'[27] In the absence of clinical studies into the vaccine's effectiveness, the question is whether the government is now making its decisions on the use of vaccines on a basis of trial and error.

21
The '5-in-1' & '6-in-1'

Less and less choice

If further evidence were needed that the government's vaccine policy is dominated by vested interests, the introduction in 2004 of the first '5-in-1' vaccine would be a good example. The first vaccine to be used was Pediacel, manufactured by Aventis Pasteur, later to be replaced by GSK's Infanrix-IPV-Hib. This new vaccine for babies aged two, three and four months was launched in October 2004 in a flurry of media controversy. Babies were to be vaccinated for exactly the same diseases with the new vaccine as they were before. But the new vaccine combined the following components in one:

1. Diphtheria
2. Tetanus
3. Whooping cough
4. Polio
5. Hib

In August 2004, doctors at the Department of Health were preparing for the launch of Pediacel, along with two other vaccines for older children, when the *Daily Telegraph* swept the carpet from under their feet. The lead story on its front page on Saturday 7 August was entitled 'Sweeping Changes to Baby Vaccines.'

A leak was the last thing the Department of Health wanted, as it took the initiative away from its own doctors and PR department. Parents were already mistrustful of doctors, and particularly the government, over the MMR furore. The Telegraph story implied that the main reason for the new vaccine was to remove the mercury, a view apparently supported by Dr Peter English, a government-funded doctor, who listed one of the primary objectives as 'to do away with Thiomersal [mercury] vaccines.'[1] He was to be contradicted by the DoH, which played down the removal of mercury. Doctors were unimpressed that the first they heard of the new vaccine was through the media, rather than from the Department's letter that was due to arrive in their surgeries the following week.

By the next day things got worse: 'Alarm Grows over Multiple Jabs for Babies,' proclaimed *The Observer*. Parents were now confused. They were being told that the new vaccine was 'safer',[2] but that the old vaccine was 'extremely safe.'[3] That may be so, but many of my patients were asking: if the new vaccine is 'safer', then mustn't the older one be less safe? What's more, the new 'safer' vaccine would not be available for over two months.

Some parents, who were concerned about the presence of mercury in vaccines, asked their doctors if they could wait until the new mercury-free vaccines arrived before immunising their babies. The reply was often reassurance that they were worrying about nothing. In addition, the parents were warned in no uncertain terms of the dangers of waiting, even for a few weeks, to have their babies vaccinated.

On Monday 9th August, the Department of Health started a damage limitation exercise amid concerns that a '5-in-1 vaccine' might overload the immune system. More negative headlines appeared including 'Chaos Over 5-in-1 Baby Vaccines' and 'Patient Fury at New Super Vaccine for 8-Week-Olds.' Whether or not multiple vaccinations can have harmful effects on the immune system, it seemed to have gone unnoticed in the press that babies were still being vaccinated against the same number of diseases as they were previously. Some doctors were at pains to point out that the introduction of the new 'purer' whooping cough vaccine meant that the overall load on the baby's immune system was actually less. 'Health Bosses Calm Fears over Baby Jab,' said Tuesday's *Mirror*.

By Wednesday, a little late to have been able to reassure parents, doctors finally received official notification of the new jabs from the DoH.

The government's problems didn't end there. It was revealed, on the following weekend, that Professor Michael Langman, the chairman of the committee that advises the government on immunisations, was receiving funds from MSD (Merck Sharp & Dohme) for research in his department at Birmingham University.[4]

MSD manufactured the three newly-introduced vaccines, in its partnership with Aventis, as Aventis Pasteur MSD. This does not imply any wrongdoing by Professor Langman, but it did not inspire confidence in the independence of some important medical decisions. It also brought attention to a new phenomenon: how the powerful pharmaceutical industry has become entangled with the medical establishment. Several of the doctors on the vaccination committee (JCVI) have commercial links with vaccine manufacturers.

The whole introduction of the new '5-in-1' vaccine was a fiasco. As one doctor said of the Department of Health, 'It's botched it up again.'[5]

Paradoxically, the department that had been so skilled in launching the new MMR, Hib and Meningitis C vaccines on a cloud of superlative expectations had bungled the introduction of the one vaccine where it could make a good medical case for its need. By contradicting its own doctors, it had merely eroded its trust among the population even further and emphasised the Kremlin-like atmosphere surrounding vaccines.

The Pediacel vaccine was virtually no different in respect of the diphtheria, tetanus and Hib elements. But in three important ways it corrected the vaccine mistakes of the past that many doctors had been worried about.

First, the 5-in-1 replaced the old whole-cell whooping cough vaccine that can, occasionally, cause brain damage that can be permanent (for years accepted by the Department of Health, but since denied). The new vaccine was the safer acellular one. Though available for over twenty years, the delay in its introduction was, we were told, because we were waiting for a vaccine that was as effective as the whole-cell vaccine. The department claims, correctly, that the new whooping cough vaccine 'tend[s] to cause fewer adverse reactions.'[6] It does, indeed, cause fewer seizures (fits) and floppy babies, as well as less fever, fussiness, pain, drowsiness, anorexia, redness and swelling. A new safer acellular vaccine had been licensed and available for years through the National Health Service. The department had recommended its use during 2000 and 2001 when there were supply problems with the old vaccine.

Second, the live polio vaccine was at last removed from the schedule. In its place came the safer but more expensive killed, or inactivated, polio vaccine. For the past decades more people in the UK had been paralysed from the live polio vaccine than from the disease itself. The killed vaccine had been available since 1956 (when it was in use in Britain until 1962). The DoH has always claimed that the live polio vaccine provided better 'community protection.'[7]

Third, the 5-in-1 vaccine contained no mercury. Compared to the introduction of the other improvements which took the department decades, the government acted to remove mercury relatively quickly, in a matter of years. Officially, there is no safety concern over mercury. The switch to a mercury-free vaccine was merely a happy coincidence.

At an additional cost of over £5 per patient per dose (for Pediacel), the government had not sacrificed safety for cost. Two booster vaccines were introduced as well. Repevax (later Boostrix-IPV) is the same as Pediacel except that it does not contain Hib; also some of the other components, particularly the diphtheria, are in a lower strength more suited to boosting immunity. It is given as a pre-school booster, along with the second MMR, to children 3-5 years old. Revaxis is similar to Repevax but only contains the diphtheria, tetanus and polio vaccines. It is used as a booster for teenagers.

Does the combined vaccine work?

There has been no research into the effectiveness of Pediacel itself as a multi-component vaccine.[8] The vaccine stimulates good antibody production to all five diseases in children, with the exception of the Hib component that appears not to work so well in premature babies born under 32 weeks.[9] However, testing for antibodies can only provide a guide as to whether a vaccine can be expected to work. The only real test of whether a vaccine works is whether it prevents children from getting a disease they would otherwise contract.

The only effectiveness research that had been done was in Canada with a very similar vaccine to Pediacel, called 'Pentacel' — in use since 1997. In this study the number of children getting Hib disease (meningitis, blood poisoning or throat inflammation) over 1998 and 1999 was studied. A total of eighteen children contracted invasive (serious) Hib disease. Half of the eighteen children had received at least one Hib vaccine and five had been fully vaccinated with three or four doses.[10] Whilst the type of Hib vaccine was not known in all the children, the majority had received either Pentacel or a similar Hib vaccine. It is not a ringing endorsement of the Hib component of Pediacel.

It is possible that the side-effects of a multiple '5-in-1' vaccine like Pediacel may be more than the sum of its individual components, were they all to be given separately. There is evidence that a greater number of vaccine components increases side-effects such as fever and fretfulness.[11] The lack of attention being paid to this problem was acknowledged at the First International Symposium on Vaccine Safety in 2002, 'The safety of combined vaccines, for example, requires to be evaluated as most of the available information is derived from studies evaluating the various components separately.'[12] Every vaccine combination should be tested for safety in its own right — something that is not happening.

At the time of the introduction of Pediacel into the routine childhood immunisation schedule in the UK in October 2004, there had been only one published study on its safety. This involved five hundred children, given a nearly identical vaccine, who were only followed up for 3 days after vaccination, unless they had a 'severe' reaction in which case they would be followed up for longer. Not all the children were given the Pediacel-like vaccine. Of those who were, two 'serious' reactions were reported: one had two periods of strange head movements and the other had several brief episodes of apnoea (stopping breathing). The doctors in the study felt that the vaccine was unlikely to be the cause of either problem, though did not explain how they came to this conclusion.[13]

Since its introduction it has been confirmed that the vaccine can cause: crying, feeding problems, convulsions (a fit or seizure) and episodes of apnoea, slow heart rate (bradycardia) and low blood oxygen after receiving combination vaccines similar to Pediacel. Episodes of apnoea and bradycardia are especially common in premature babies in whom they can be life-threatening.[14,15]

A further UK trial involved Pediacel itself, which was given along with the Meningitis C vaccine at two, three and four months, like in the routine UK schedule at the time. Published over a year after the vaccine's launch, this study confirmed that the vaccine caused fewer reactions than the vaccine it was replacing, which contained the whole-cell whooping cough vaccine. But a high proportion of babies still showed reactions such as irritability and crying.[16]

Pediacel was given at the same time as a Meningitis C vaccine, and so some of the reactions reported may be due to either or both of the vaccines. Also, the figures include all reactions occurring within a week of the vaccine, so it is most unlikely that all the problems were caused by the vaccine in all the children. Babies who suffered a severe local reaction (redness, swelling or tenderness) after the first dose were more likely to suffer similar reactions after subsequent doses. However, these are the only details of reactions that the study — sponsored by the manufacturer of the vaccine — provides. It is clear that side-effects were frequent. However, less common, but possibly serious, reactions could easily have been missed because of the small numbers of children involved.

The reactions reported with Pediacel

	Proportion of children affected after each vaccination:
Local redness	38%
Local swelling	25%
Local tenderness	18%
Fever (higher than 37.5°C)	12%
Irritability	48%
Crying	39%
Less active	23%
Eating less	26%
Vomiting	26%
Diarrhoea	24%

Whilst most side-effects are more common in vaccines containing the old 'whole cell' whooping-cough vaccine, there is one that occurs more often with the newer 'acellular' vaccine. The more of these vaccines that a child receives, the more likely it is that pain or swelling will occur at the site of the injection. Though rarely serious, this can be very uncomfortable.

There is some evidence that large combination vaccines may not be as effective as single or smaller combinations but that they cause more side-efects.[19]

The amount of aluminium in Pediacel is less than that in Infanrix-IPV-Hib which is now also used.

Parental views

Though the uptake of the 5-in1 vaccine has been consistently high, at well over 90%, parents have expressed concern at the large quantity of vaccines given to very young babies and a significant minority would feel more comfortable if they were able to give their child single vaccines. Some feel forced into giving the baby the vaccine. [17] A survey of parents in the USA in 2009 found that over half had concerns about the serious side—effects of vaccines, and a quarter believed that vaccines could cause autism in healthy children. This corroborates my personal experience in my immunisation clinic where I have heard many parents tell of the relentless pressure they are put under by health professional to comply with national immunisation schedules and the reluctance of these same professionals to enter into any rational discussion on the subject. In reality doctors are not as confident about vaccines as they make out. Not only do doctors regularly bring their children to my immunisation clinic, but also a survey of health professionals in 2008 found that 1 in 6 GPs had concerns about immunisation, with the most common concern being that babies were being given too many vaccines. A 2011 survey of rural primary care doctors in Oregon, USA, found that a third had some concern about the safety of vaccines.[18] More recently, a 2014 survey of 1,712 French GPs found that 254 (16%) had seen a patient with a serious health problem possibly related to vaccination and 314 (1 in 5) had reservations about vaccination.[34] Doctors are not as unanimously pro-vaccine as you might think.

6-in-1 vaccine

Two 6-in-1 vaccines were granted European licenses in October 2000: Hexavac, made by Aventis Pasteur MSD and Infanrix Hexa from GSK. Both contain vaccines against diphtheria, tetanus, polio, whooping cough and Hib (like the 5-in-1 currently used in the UK) with the addition of hepatitis B. One study showed that side-effects were over six times as likely to occur after Hexavac than after Infanrix Hexa.[20] A review of the two vaccines found very little evidence of safety or effectiveness for Hexavac and criticised the manufacturer for its 'secrecy' and 'reluctance to share important information about its products.'[21]

Meanwhile, in Italy, doctors were alerted to reports of children being taken to a local hospital within a few hours of receiving Hexavac, typically with symptoms of fever, irritability, drowsiness and unusual crying. Things were to get worse as reports emerged from Germany of babies dying suddenly within 48 hours of receiving the 6-in-1 jab.[22,23] It is often difficult to know whether the tragic unexplained death of a baby shortly after vaccination is caused by the vaccine or is merely a coincidence. However, an analysis of deaths in one year old babies within 48 hours of receiving a 6-in-1 jab in Germany found three deaths when none, or possibly one at most, would have been expected – a difference most unlikely to have been caused by chance.[24] This increased risk was only found with Hexavac and prompted a call for 'immediate action by the authorities' to study this in depth.[25] The European Drug Agency (EMEA), based in London, gave out a mixed message. It said that a 'possible signal has been generated' (in other words the vaccine may have caused the deaths), but that 'this does not currently constitute a risk to public health.'[26] It is interesting to ponder on the conflict between a risk to public health, that is the large majority of children, and the risk to a few susceptible children – a conflict that, at least with vaccines, comes down with increasing frequency in favour of public health.

On September 20, 2005, the EMEA announced it was recommending, 'as a precautionary measure the suspension of the market authorisation for Hexavac.' Intriguingly, the reason given for taking the vaccine off the market was not the reported deaths, but decreased effectiveness of the hepatitis B component of the vaccine. Presumably the agency was determined not to cause any alarm or scare amongst parents. However, it demanded that all

Hexavac vaccines be recalled and that the distribution of the vaccine be suspended, extreme measures if the concern really was the reduced effectiveness of a single component.[27] The suggestion that the 6-in-1 vaccine could be killing even a tiny number of children triggered an acrimonious debate in the letters pages of the journal *Vaccine*. The doctors who had raised the concern were personally criticized, and accused of creating inappropriate anxiety and fuel for the so-called 'anti-vaccine movement'.[28,29,30] They retorted by defending their report, accusing vaccine specialists of failing for decades to look effectively for adverse reactions to vaccines.[31] A German study later found that the risk of a baby dying more than doubles in the two days after receiving one of the 6-in-1 vaccines. However, because this finding was not 'statistically significant', or could have happened by chance, the study authors felt able to conclude that, 'no increased risk was seen.'[32]

In 2013, an Italian court ruled that a hexavalent vaccine caused the death of a six-month-old baby girl in 2003. The court ordered the public release of a confidential report submitted by GSK on its 6-in-1 vaccine Infanrix Hexa (the vaccine now used in the UK) to the EMEA in 2011. The report included an analysis of sudden deaths in children under one year of age after receiving the vaccine. There were 65 deaths in the first 10 days after vaccination and only 2 deaths in the subsequent ten days. These figures are at first sight alarming and suggest the vaccine as being a cause of death. However, the manufacturer pointed out that the numbers of sudden deaths were well below the 'background' rate expected and that reports are far more likely to be made when they occur shortly after receiving a vaccine. Nevertheless the figures are not reassuring and the report also contains case histories of deaths that were possibly related to the vaccine.[33]

The 6-in-1 vaccine, now including hepatitis B, was introduced into the UK in the autumn of 2017. This is a hugely regressive step as it includes hepatitis B, a vaccine that is completely unnecessary in nearly all children and, at the same time, makes it very difficult for parents to leave out the vaccine as it is bundled together with five others. It also increases the number of vaccines given to babies by four months of age to 24.

Age	Vaccine	No Vaccs	No Jabs
2 months	DTaP/IPV/Hib/Hep B (6-in-1)	9	3 plus drops
	Pneumococcal, Meningitis B		
	Rotavirus		
3 months	DTaP/IPV/Hib/Hep B (6-in-1)	7	1 plus drops
	Rotavirus		
4 months	DTaP/IPV/Hib/Hep B (6-in-1)	8	3
	Pneumococcal, Meningitis B		
12 months	Hib/Men C booster	7	4
	Pneumococcal, Meningitis B		
	MMR		

22
Pneumococcus

Ever More Optimism

In the space of a few years, yet another new vaccine was introduced in Britain into the, by now crowded, childhood immunisation schedule. It was introduced in September 2006 and raised the total number of vaccinations to twenty-five before the fifteenth month. Like the Hib and Meningitis C, it, too, was a high-tech 'conjugate' vaccine based on attaching the outer coating of the bug to a protein carrier. The vaccine aims to immunise against a bug called pneumococcus. Like so many potentially dangerous bugs, it lives harmlessly in the noses of many children, most of whom develop natural immunity to the bug, but can cause pneumonia (hence its name) and meningitis or even death on occasion.

The new conjugated vaccine was called Prevenar and was developed by Wyeth. An older and relatively ineffective vaccine against the bug had been available for some years (the polysaccharide vaccine). It was routinely given to elderly people, as well as adults and those children over two considered to be 'at risk' in the UK, but without any good evidence that it actually worked in preventing illness or death.[1,2]

Prevenar works better than the older vaccine, but the experience with Hib and Men C shows that it is easy to overestimate the effectiveness, and safety, of conjugated vaccines. Even the robustly pro-vaccine Joint Committee on Vaccination and Immunisation (JCVI) that advises the government, wasn't initially convinced that mass immunisation with Prevenar was necessary.

Its members had been considering the introduction of the new conjugate vaccine into the UK schedule for some years. But as recently as 2004, they advised against introducing the vaccine.[3] They felt there was a lack of crucial information on the vaccine as they didn't know how many doses were needed to offer protection. Importantly, there was no clear indication of how many children were affected by the disease. Nor did they know if the vaccine would offer any 'herd immunity'. (One member, Professor Brent Taylor, was reported as saying that he suspected that the vaccine would have been introduced earlier had it not been for the public hysteria over the MMR vaccine; though he conceded that the effectiveness of the new vaccine was still uncertain.[4])

These concerns are real enough on their own. But the generally pro-vaccine JCVI was also concerned about the disease the vaccine sought to combat. A particular problem with this bug is that of serotype replacement – the substitution of one type of pneumococcus with another. If the vaccine successfully stops children either getting ill from, or carrying in their noses, certain bugs, a likely consequence is that these are simply replaced by others. These replacement types could be just as, or even more, harmful.

Serotype replacement is a potential problem for many vaccines, but the pneumococcus bacterium is especially good at transforming its make-up so that it is no longer recognised by the antibodies created by the vaccine. This would result in less, or even no, reduction in overall pneumococcal disease. Nor was it an academic problem. Prevenar had been introduced into the USA childhood vaccination schedule in 2000, as a four-dose course given at two, four, six and twelve to fifteen months. The phenomenon was already being seen in the USA.[5,6,7]

Miraculously, however, in October 2004, less than four months after expressing several reservations over the immediate introduction of the vaccine, the JCVI agreed 'in principle to the introduction of pneumococcal vaccine for children.'

It still didn't sound very convinced. Somewhat limply the committee concluded, 'there were no medical reasons not to offer the pneumococcal vaccine alongside the other primary immunisations,' despite precious little evidence that it could be safely used as part of the UK schedule, or presumably any positive medical reasons for doing so. It also 'recognised that some parents may have concerns' and the experts themselves were still unsure of the number of doses required or when they should be given.[8]

Determination

Prevenar had been licensed for use in Europe in 2001. In early 2002, the Chief Medical Officer advised doctors that this new vaccine should be given to the few children under two years of age who were in certain 'at-risk' groups; this included children with heart, lung, liver or kidney disease but this only applied to a very few children. In 2004 this was changed to include all 'at risk' children aged under five.

As would be expected of a highly profitable product, the manufacturer vigorously promoted the vaccine. It's often difficult to distinguish between lobbying by pharmaceutical companies and that done by 'independent' pressure groups. In Australia, Wyeth allegedly helped fund a lobbying campaign by a supposedly independent group to get the Federal government to introduce universal pneumococcal immunisation.[9]

The UK Department of Health announced the introduction of the pneumococcal vaccine in February 2006, though it was not until 4 September that it was finally launched. By early 2007, it was recommended for all children in eleven European countries, including the UK. At a cost of £34.50 a dose (but negotiated for an undisclosed lower price for the NHS), it was then the most expensive routinely used childhood vaccine, and became the most profitable vaccine ever – until it was usurped by Gardasil, the 'cervical cancer vaccine'.

Determined to add the vaccine to its schedule, the DoH was happy to introduce a complex shake-up of the national vaccination schedule in order to accommodate the vaccine. Most countries that use the vaccine give it as a primary course of three vaccinations followed by a booster in the second year of life. This would have necessitated giving three injections at each of the two, three and four month attendances, which would not have been popular with babies or their parents.

The DoH got its way by, uniquely, offering both the Meningitis C and pneumococcal vaccines as a two-dose course followed by a twelve-to-thirteen month booster. The necessary addition of a Hib booster resulted in the most complicated vaccination schedule anywhere in the world.

The convoluted arrangement necessitates children receiving different combinations of vaccines at every attendance – a situation that still exists today in 2017 after the introduction of two additional vaccines. A leading vaccine expert expressed particular concern that the three injections required at four months were 'a danger to patient and doctor.'[10] The Department of Health pressed on regardless of the increased risk of mistakes being made, resulting in children being given the wrong vaccines.

The new schedule was approved by the JCVI even though, again, it gave half-hearted support pointing out major reservations:

- There is increasing evidence of interactions between vaccines when administered in combinations or simultaneously during infant immunisation
- The effectiveness of the Meningitis C vaccine may be reduced when given with the 5-in-1 vaccine alone or in combination with the pneumococcal vaccine
- There is an increased risk of side-effects from the combination of pneumococcal and 5-in-1 vaccines compared to the 5-in-1 vaccine alone[11]

The increased complexity of the new schedule, along with the necessity of two or three injections at every visit, was also likely to result in a lower uptake by parents.[12]

Flexible figures
As with the Hib and Meningitis C bugs, it is only serious illnesses caused by the pneumococcus bacterium that are of concern here. It is a common cause of middle ear infections (otitis media) in children. These are troublesome diseases for a child, but generally minor ailments. It's only when the bug invades the body that it becomes a major problem. So the chief concern is serious, or 'invasive', pneumococcal disease (IPD).

IPD manifests itself in three main ways: meningitis, pneumonia and blood poisoning, in roughly equal proportions. These are serious illnesses, though the death rate in children (2-10%) is much lower than in the elderly (25%).

As with other serious infections, healthy children have a much smaller chance of dying than children who already have a serious ongoing medical condition. Children with diabetes and, especially, asthma, have been found to be more susceptible to IPD.[38] So the illness is certainly serious, though much more so in children who already have health problems.

At the time of the introduction of the vaccine there were around 5,000 cases of IPD in England and Wales every year. But only around 700 of these were in children. Over half were in the elderly, over sixty-five years of age, who are also far more likely to die from the disease.[13]

Official data showed that the number of cases in children was small and stable. That is, until new figures were released by the Department of Health. It then appeared that the number of cases in children had been increasing steadily over the ten years before the introduction of the vaccine, though at a far slower rate than for older age groups.[14]

It's interesting to observe how rates of an infection always seem to be on the increase at the time a new vaccine is introduced. Researchers would certainly have been looking harder for cases prior to vaccination to ensure accurate figures — 'enhanced surveillance' for pneumococcus began in 1996. But that doesn't explain why official figures going back ten years were adjusted from showing no increase to showing a rise over time.

Whichever figures are used, there is plenty of common ground. The risk is greatest in early childhood (especially under one year of age) and in later life (particularly over seventy-five years). Those aged between five and sixty-five have an extremely low risk of getting IPD.

The risk is also greater in children with other health problems, not only of dying from the disease, but also of catching it in the first place. Over a third of children catching the disease suffer from a serious underlying disease of some sort or another (anything from cancer to congenital heart disease).[15] Children living in deprived and overcrowded conditions are over twice as vulnerable to the disease.[16]

Well over half of all children admitted to hospital with IPD have one or more other diagnoses, suggesting that they were at increased risk because they had other medical conditions.[17] The disease doesn't strike randomly. As with most other infections, the risk to a child varies greatly, depending on the child's health and social circumstances. So though the overall annual risk of a child under five catching the illness is around one in 5,000, the risk to a healthy child is nearer one in 10,000, whereas the risk to a child with ongoing health problems is much greater.

Research from Hertfordshire found that 86% of all children under three carried the pneumococcus bacterium in their nose or throat at some stage over a ten-month period — without getting ill.[16] Why do so many live healthily in such close proximity to a potentially lethal germ, whilst so few become ill? It seems that it may not be the bug itself that is the primary cause of the problem, but the susceptibility of the child. In fact, the close association with the microbe can be helpful, as in most children it stimulates immunity against future infection. It's possible that the eradication of the bacteria from the noses of children renders them more susceptible to serious infection in later life.

Finally, looking at deaths from IPD, before immunisation around twenty children under five years of age certainly died from IPD every year. Two doctors published a paper in September 2005 challenging these figures and suggesting that the number of deaths in children under five caused by IPD is 'at least as high as 43.' Their 'estimate' may be correct, but one of these doctors was an employee of, and the other a paid consultant to, Wyeth, the drug company that makes Prevenar, the pneumococcal vaccine; they could, at the very least, be accused of a conflict of interest.[18] By the time of its press release to accompany the launch of the vaccine, the Department of Health was claiming that no fewer than fifty children died every year from IPD.[19]

If one assumes that as many as thirty children under five died from IPD every year, this would mean that the disease is serious, but the risk of catching it is small. The risk of catching IPD is so much less in western European countries compared to the USA that an expert review has questioned the value of vaccinating all children against such a rare disease.[20]

Does the vaccine work?
Routine pneumococcal vaccination was introduced in the USA in 2000. Since then there's been a large fall in the number of children going to hospital with IPD, suggesting the vaccine is working well. But recent figures suggest that, after a large drop in the number of cases, the number of children with IPD may now be on the rise again, as this adaptable bug adapts to the challenge of a vaccine.[21]

A closer look at the research shows that, in children under two years old (the 'at-risk' age group), the vaccine prevents 85-90% of all IPD caused by the subgroups (serotypes) of bug covered by the vaccine, but appears to be less effective in children with chronic health problems — the very children whom it is more important to protect.[22,23]

This effectiveness is based on four doses of vaccine; it was introduced into the UK in a unique three-dose schedule, comprising an initial two-dose course (at two and four months) followed by a booster at 13 months. A study done after the vaccine was introduced suggests that the vaccine is likely to be effective when given this way, provided the third (booster) dose is given in the second year of life; but that it probably works better when the first two doses are given a little later, at three and five months.[34, 37]

The pneumococcal vaccine doesn't protect against all pneumococcal bugs, of which there are many types. It was estimated that the vaccine would result in a two-thirds reduction in IPD in children. However, more recent real-world experience from the USA now suggests the overall reduction in IPD is somewhat less than 60%.[21] Once again, the true effectiveness of a vaccine is found to be less than that originally hoped for.

Another difficulty is that the disease is most common, and most dangerous, in the very first month of life, before any vaccine can be given.[15] The vaccine has only a limited effect on the number of children with 'nasal carriage' of the serotypes of bug that the vaccine protects against.[40] Where the vaccine does reduce the rates of nasal carriage of types covered by the vaccine, these have been replaced by pneumococcal bugs not covered by the vaccine; yet more evidence that the bug successfully adapts to the vaccine. So the disease cannot be totally eradicated, meaning that newborn babies, the most vulnerable group of all, can never be completely protected by vaccination.

However, on the positive side, it appears that vaccinating children has the bonus effect of preventing IPD in older adults living in the same household.[24]

A combination Pneumococcal and Meningitis C vaccine was tested in an attempt to reduce the number of injections given. However, the combination was less effective than when the vaccines were given separately. The combined vaccine also interfered with the effectiveness of other vaccines given at the same time such as diphtheria and Hib, thwarting its possible use in the new vaccine schedule.[25] Giving the pneumococcal vaccine at the same time as Hib — as is done in the UK — may also reduce the effectiveness of the latter vaccine.[26]

Is the vaccine safe?

Like so many modern vaccines, this one was introduced with inadequate safety trials. In those that had been done, the pneumococcal vaccine was usually given with other vaccines, which made it very difficult to know which vaccine may have caused what side-effects. So the only information available is on common reactions that occur shortly after vaccination. Rare side-effects, or those that may not appear until months later, are unlikely to have been uncovered.

However, information is available on local side-effects, that is those occurring at the site of the vaccination. This vaccine causes local reactions, such as pain, redness and swelling, in a high proportion of children — more so than most other vaccines.[27,28]

These 'local' reactions are less frequent in babies, and more common in toddlers who receive the booster. It can cause a fever and drowsiness in some children — probably more often than most vaccines.

Side-effect	Proportion of children affected[29]
Redness	32%
Redness over 2.5cm	17%
Pain	24%
Pain affecting movement	16%
Swelling	30%
Swelling over 2.5cm	10%

The JCVI approved the vaccine in principle for general use in the UK, despite 'some concern that there was a relatively high level of local reactions reported.'[30] Compared to the 5-in-1 vaccine used alone, the pneumococcal vaccine appears to cause more episodes of floppy baby reactions, more inconsolable crying, more convulsions, and more hospital admissions.[11,31]

One study has shown that asthma is more common in children who had received the vaccine compared to those who hadn't.[32] This doesn't prove that the vaccine causes asthma, but suggests it might.

The vaccine has been in use for over twenty years in the USAA, where numerous possible side-effects have been reported. These are reports from both doctors and parents, and clearly not all the problems described will have been caused by the vaccine. However, some reactions recurred in the same child after a further pneumococcal vaccination, which makes them very likely to have been caused by the vaccine; these included fever, irritability, prolonged crying, stomach disturbances and seizures (fits). One hundred and seventeen deaths have been reported as being possibly related to the vaccine in the first two years of its use and, although researchers have concluded that none of these deaths could have been caused by the vaccine, the majority remain 'unexplained.'[33]

Replacement of one bug with another

The biggest problem with the pneumococcal vaccine is that of 'serotype replacement', where types of the bacteria not covered by the vaccine increase to replace the types targeted by the vaccine. In the USA, where the vaccine was introduced in 2000, and being given to over two thirds of children by 2006, there was a drop in pneumococcal meningitis overall. But hidden within the good news was a serious problem: the rate of meningitis caused by serotypes not covered by the vaccine increased by 60% overall and by 275% (or nearly threefold) in children under two years of age. An additional worry is that an increasing number of these strains are becoming resistant to antibiotics — in other words, untreatable.[35] The same thing has been happening in other countries including Australia and the UK, where the number of young children with IPD caused by serotypes not covered by the vaccine has increased rapidly since the vaccine's introduction.

Canada has also suffered from the consequences of serotype replacement. In 2010 Winnipeg experienced a doubling of cases of IPD despite the introduction of the PCV vaccine four years before. The increase in numbers of cases was caused largely by an increase in serotype 12F which had previously been very rare and is not included in the vaccine.[39]

A new vaccine

The solution to the problem was to introduce, in 2010, a 13-valent pneumococcal vaccine (Prevenar 13) increasing the number of serotypes covered from seven to thirteen. This is unlikely to be a long-term solution because the pneumococcal bacterium has 90 known different serotypes. New serotypes, that are not protected by the new 13-valent vaccine, are now emerging as causes of IPD. The number of children under 2 years of age in the UK getting IPD caused by non-vaccine strains has continued to increase year after year.

All the big vaccine giants are currently working on new expanded pneumococcal vaccines.

23
HPV

A Vaccine too Soon?

The HPV vaccine has become a controversial addition to the UK national immunisation schedule. It was introduced for all twelve to thirteen-year-old girls in the autumn of 2008. HPV (Human Papilloma Virus) is the virus that causes genital warts. It is important because genital warts are believed to cause between 80 and 100% of cases of cancer of the cervix (the neck of the womb).

The vaccine was introduced with unprecedented haste and, sadly, it seems that all the mistakes of the past described in previous chapters were repeated. We can look at the same three questions asked throughout this book of each vaccine.

Is the disease common and serious?

There is no question that cervical cancer is serious, though it is not common. Around 3,000 women are diagnosed with cervical cancer every year and under a thousand will die. It is now being described as the second most common cancer in women, but this is somewhat misleading. Cancer of the cervix is indeed the second most common cancer in women worldwide, though this is not the case in the UK.

What some may be calling the second most common cancer in women in the UK is in fact a type called 'CIN 3' (also known as carcinoma-in-situ) which is picked up through screening — which is now routine in Britain. This is not a cancer, but is a precancerous stage; a third of cases will revert to normal without any treatment, and only one in six is likely to progress into cancer.[1] True cervical cancer is much less common, ranking twelfth, and comprising 1.7%, of all female cancers.[2] The figures are from 2010, around the time of the introduction of the vaccine but well before the vaccine could have had any effect on the numbers. In 2015 cervical cancer remained the twelfth most common cancer in women, causing a mere 1.8% of cancers.

Number of female cancers in England in 2010

1	Breast	41,259
2	Lung	15,041
3	Colon	14,628
4	Endometrium (Body of the womb)	6,834
5	Ovary	5,535
6	Melanoma	5,505

7	Lymphoma	5,371
8	Pancreas	3,561
9	Leukaemia	2,934
10	Kidney	2,630
11	Bladder	2,446
12	Cervix	2,305
13	Oesophagous (gullet)	2,286
14	Lip, mouth and throat	2,149
15	Stomach	2,137

Deaths from cervical cancer are, thankfully, even less common, ranking twentieth in frequency and representing only 1.2% of UK female cancer deaths in 2010. Though the vaccine was introduced in 2008, it will not have any impact on deaths for many years. The leading female cancer deaths are as follows.[3] By 2015, before the vaccine could have had any effect on deaths, cervical cancer remained a relatively rare cancer causing 720 deaths, one% of all female deaths from cancer.

Female cancer deaths in England 2010

1	Lung	13,165
2	Breast	10,290
3	Colon	4,280
4	Ovary	3,676
5	Pancreas	3,619
6	Oesophagous (gullet)	2,165
7	Rectum & anus	2,122
8	Lymphoma	1,930
9	Leukaemia	1,776
10	Stomach	1,635
11	Brain	1,422
12	Bladder	1,409
13	Liver	1,371
14	Kidney	1,295
15	Endometrium (Body of the womb)	1,270
16	Other intestine	1,167
17	Multiple myeloma	1,110
18	Mesothelial and soft tissue	951
19	Skin	832
20	Cervix	816

The exaggeration of the severity of an illness is commonplace before the introduction of a new vaccine, in an attempt to bring the public round to support, and take up the vaccine. Over twelve times the number of women die from lung or breast cancer than they do from cervical cancer. Cancers of the brain and kidney each kill hundreds more women every year than cervical cancer. So cervical cancer, the disease that it is ultimately hoped the HPV vaccine will protect against, is certainly extremely serious, but is relatively rare and far from the greatest cancer threat to women.

Does the vaccine work?

Here we have another example of a vaccine being rushed in before we know whether it really does what it says on the packet — prevent cervical cancer. One manufacturer (of the first vaccine to be licensed) announced that its vaccine was '100% effective.'[4] But 100% effective against what? This claim referred to its early trials, showing the vaccine to be 100% effective at preventing pre-cancerous changes associated with only the types of HPV in the vaccine, in a carefully selected group of women aged sixteen to twenty-three years of age. All the women were given a full three-dose course of vaccine, and were followed up for an average of two years only.

In other words, the 100% result:

- Does not apply to girls under sixteen — the age group now given the vaccine routinely
- Only refers to four out of the hundred or so types of HPV; these are associated with 70% of cervical cancers, and not the remaining 30%
- Refers only to pre-cancerous changes, and not cancer itself
- Applies only to a highly selective group of women, and not the population at large
- Requires all three doses of the vaccine to be given
- Only applies to the first two years after receiving the vaccine

Even before the vaccine was recommended for use in the UK, the claims of effectiveness began their usual decline. Research on Gardasil (one of the two HPV vaccines) — undertaken by the manufacturer — was published in May 2007 in the *New England Journal of Medicine*. This study followed up over 12,000 women for three years. The manufacturer now claimed 98% effectiveness (a little down on 100%, but still excellent for a vaccine) in those women who fitted its strict trial protocol. The effectiveness again refers to pre-cancerous changes and not to cancer itself. But a closer look at the study reveals less cause for unrestrained optimism. When all women are included, the vaccine's effectiveness falls to a more modest 44%. But the story doesn't end there; if we look at all pre-cancerous lesions, caused by any type of HPV, in all women, the effectiveness drops to 17%, with no demonstrable effect at all in preventing CIN 3, the most serious precancerous lesion, and the one that is most likely to go on to become cancer.[5]

A four-year follow-up study on 17,599 women showed a 96% effectiveness against CIN 1 in women who adhered to the strict protocol but a more modest 69% effectiveness in a more real-world situation. It is no wonder that an accompanying editorial referred to the 'modest efficacy' of the vaccine, warning that 'a cautious approach may be warranted in light of important unanswered questions about overall vaccine effectiveness, duration of protection, and adverse effects that may emerge over time.'[6] Further research published in the

Lancet confirmed the above figures.[7] Research on Cervarix, the DoH's initial preferred vaccine for the UK, showed a short-term (15 month) effectiveness of 90% against pre-cancerous lesions in a selected group of healthy women aged 15-25.[8] Again, an accompanying editorial urged caution in interpreting the industry-funded study.[9]

However, even if the vaccine were 100% effective against the strains of HPV in the vaccine (which it is not), and even assuming that HPV causes all cervical cancer, the HPV types covered by the two vaccines make up only 75% of all cases of invasive cervical cancer in the UK, leaving a quarter that cannot be covered by the current vaccines.

This is not meant to undermine the potential of this vaccine to save lives, but at the moment that is all it is — potential. Trials are under way to look at whether the vaccine does indeed protect against cervical cancer (to 'guard against guessing' as the researchers call it), but no results are expected before 2020. The results may disentangle the reality from the hype.

The reason that the vaccine showed little benefit in the general population of women aged sixteen to twenty-three who did not fit the strict entry criteria for the manufacturer's trial, was probably because these women were already infected with HPV; this suggests that the vaccine is only likely to work if given to girls before their first sexual encounter. However, up to 5% of virgins may already be infected with HPV — and the vaccine may therefore not work for them.[10,11]

A more recent study of the real-world effectiveness of the vaccine shows 46% effectiveness at preventing high grade cervical abnormalities (we're not even at cancer yet) only a minority of which will go on to become cancer; and the 46% (remember the initial 100% boast by the manufacturer?) only applies to those women who have received the full course of three shots of the vaccine.[22] At the time of writing (2016) not a single cancer has yet been shown to have been prevented by the vaccine. Any real benefit on top of screening programmes against cervical cancer is questionable at this stage.

Is the vaccine safe?

Trials have largely looked at the immediate side-effects of vaccination. Over three quarters of ten to fifteen-year-old girls reported pain at the injection site after receiving Gardasil, and 1 in 10 developed a fever after one or more of the three injections.[12] The manufacturer of Gardasil have followed up over 11,000 women for 4 years after being given their product along with over 9,000 who were given an inactive placebo injection. Nine women who were given the vaccine developed potential auto-immune disorders (AIDs) — mainly arthritis-related — compared to three in the slightly smaller control group. This suggests that the vaccine may increase the risk of AIDs by two and a half times. The total number of women affected was small, and so this difference may have occurred by chance, but the only way of knowing one way or the other is to follow up larger numbers of women over longer periods of time. It is surprising that the regulatory authorities appeared unconcerned by these warning signals which, as time passes, appear to have heralded a real danger.[13]

Ever since the introduction of the vaccine there have been reports of alarming side-effects, from the vaccinated girls, their parents, and doctors. Thousands of teenage girls have described headaches, muscle pains, fatigue, cognitive and sleep disturbances after receiving the vaccine and some parents believe it has resulted in their daughters' death. This would readily be dismissed by the medical establishment if doctors were not also reporting serious and debilitating reactions to the vaccine. What's more, these reactions often followed a similar pattern that had the biological plausibility of being an auto-immune reaction to the vaccine.

Research is now suggesting that traces of viral HPV DNA left in the vaccine from the manufacturing process combines with the aluminium adjuvant to produce a long-lasting compound that cannot be easily broken down and removed by the body. This HPV DNA-aluminium compound can then travel across the blood brain barrier where it may stimulate the immune system in such a way as to cause auto-immune disorders or even death. HPV DNA has been found in the brain of two girls who died after receiving the vaccine.[24] Many of the symptoms described by the girls are similar to those of POTS (postural orthostatic tachycardia syndrome) a rare life-changing and debilitating chronic health condition.

A 12-year-old healthy girl felt unwell with a fever, sore throat and malaise a few days after receiving her first dose of HPV vaccine. Two days after receiving her second shot she fainted and from then on suffered from dizziness, palpitations and often nearly fainting. She suffered from pain in her arms and legs along with a burning sensation in her hands and feet and incapacitating fatigue. She went on to develop chronic severe headaches, loss of memory and difficulty in concentration. She felt nauseous with abdominal pain and lost her appetite. The pain in her arms and legs worsened over time. She is no longer able to attend school and remains socially isolated. She was diagnosed with POTS. Her story is, tragically, echoed by many others.

POTS is an auto-immune disorder of the autonomic nervous system responsible for control of bodily functions such as heart rate, balance, digestion, bladder control and sleep. It causes dizziness, fainting, headaches, nausea, sleep disturbance, abdominal pain, weakness, difficulty in concentrating, shortness of breath and chest pain amongst other symptoms. These symptoms are triggered by standing and relieved by lying down. Doctors have described POTS in numerous girls and women following receipt of the HPV vaccine.[20] Doctors have also described women who have suffered from ovarian failure, ADEM (a rare MS-like auto-immune disease that can cause paralysis and blindness), fibromyalgia, multiple sclerosis (MS), Guillain-Barré syndrome (GBS) and systemic lupus erythematosus (SLE) and even death, all auto-immune disorders believed to be caused by the vaccine.

In Japan, doctors reported a large number of severe neurological and POTS-like reactions to the vaccine. The extent of severe reactions caused by the vaccine in Japanese girls caused the government to suspend recommendation of the vaccination in 2013.

Then, in 2015, a Canadian academic called for a halt of the HPV vaccine programme because of widespread safety concerns. Even more alarmingly, the WHO and other health authorities have been accused of covering up safety concerns, in particular by presenting misleading information to a Japanese government expert enquiry into the vaccine.[25]

A recent study of adverse reactions to the vaccine in the Canadian state of Alberta found that one in ten of all women who received the vaccine visited a hospital emergency department within seven weeks of receiving the vaccine.[26] The study authors make no comment on this remarkable statistic and so it is difficult to draw any conclusions from it, but it is hard to believe that anywhere near one in ten of girls and women aged between nine and 24 years would normally visit a hospital emergency department in any seven-week period.

Replacement of one bug with another

Just as we have seen happening with the PCV, there are already early indications that the strains of HPV targeted by the vaccine will be replaced by equally nasty types that are not covered by the vaccine, resulting in a perpetual catch-up to produce ever-more comprehensive vaccines.[23]

Second rate vaccine for UK

The UK government chose GSK's Cervarix over Merck's Gardasil as its vaccine of choice for UK girls, despite the JCVI's preference for Gardasil, price differences notwithstanding.[15] The decision to offer GSK the contract, estimated to be worth £100 million a year, was greeted with dismay in the UK.

There are specific concerns about Cervarix. Many doctors were disappointed that the opportunity was missed to offer girls protection against HPV types 6 and 11 (present in Gardasil but not Cervarix), which cause 9 out of 10 cases of genital warts.

There are also particular safety concerns over Cervarix, which contains the new adjuvant ASO4, which contains both aluminium and MPL, a substance derived from the coating of a Salmonella bacterium. ASO4 is a potent stimulator of the immune system; this may be useful in triggering immunity, and making the vaccine effective, but the worry is it may be such a powerful immune stimulant that it causes immune-related disorders, something that already occurs with less powerful vaccines. It certainly causes injection reactions of pain, redness and swelling in over three quarters of girls given the vaccine.[16] Preliminary data also warned of the possible risk of auto-immune disease and spontaneous abortions following Cervarix.[17] What's more, there is only a small amount of experience with ASO4, which has only ever previously been used on a small scale in a vaccine used to protect patients with kidney failure from hepatitis B. Once again, we are witnessing a national immunisation campaign serving as a mass experiment to test the safety of a vaccine.

The UK switched from Cervarix to Gardasil in 2012.

Miscarriage

There had been concern that a vaccine given to young women, some of whom would be in the early stage of pregnancy, could cause miscarriages. A study of over 26,000 women aged between 15 and 25 involved in the original trails of Cervarix (GSK's HPV vaccine) concluded reassuringly that, 'there is no evidence *overall* [my italics] for an association between HPV vaccination and risk of miscarriage.' But a closer look at the actual results reveals that women who conceived within 90 days of receiving the vaccine, arguably the most vulnerable period, had an increased risk of miscarriage of 62% compared to women given the 'control' hepatitis A vaccine. A total of 14.7% of pregnancies conceived within 90 days of vaccination were miscarried; 9.1% of these would have occurred anyway, but 5.6% (the 'attributable' risk) may have been a direct consequence of receiving the HPV vaccine. Another way of looking at the figures is that of every 20 pregnancies conceived within 90 days of vaccination, 2 would result in a natural miscarriage and 1 would result in miscarriage caused by the vaccine.

So how did the authors come to their reassuring conclusion in the light of their findings? For two reasons. Firstly, over the total follow up period of two years there was no *overall* increase in miscarriages in women who had received Cervarix; it was only when the pregnancies conceived closest to the vaccine were examined that differences emerged. Secondly, the researchers used a method of statistical analysis requiring a probability of fewer than 1 in 40 ($p<0.025$) that this result could have occurred by chance; the actual probability of a chance association between miscarriage and receiving the vaccine in the previous 90 days was 1 in 32 ($p=0.031$). Therefore, although there was less than 1 in 30 probability of this result happening accidentally, the researchers were able to discount this as statistically insignificant.

The problem for us is that clinically, in the real world, the result is very significant. A 60% increase in miscarriages in pregnancies starting within three months of the jab is an issue, and one that potential recipients of the vaccine need to be told about. Whilst this finding needs to be confirmed in further studies, the way things stand now is that it is possible – if not probable – that this increased risk of miscarriage after receiving Cervarix is real. The least we should be doing is warning potential recipients of the vaccine of this possible risk.[21]

Conclusion

This new vaccine protects some women against some forms of HPV infection that, rarely, lead to pre-cancerous changes in the cervix that may – in a small proportion of women – lead to cervical cancer. All that can be concluded so far – as far as effectiveness is concerned – is that the vaccine looks promising, but we are a long way from knowing whether this vaccine will really help reduce cervical cancer in women. In any event there is little need for a vaccine that may help prevent some cases of a relatively rare cancer – even it is safe. And sadly, after its introduction on a massive scale, it is looking as though it is anything but safe. However, Big Pharma's marketing has won the day at the expense of the health of many girls and women. The reports of disabling side-effects from this vaccine have been alarming. The numerous pleas for caution in introducing this new vaccine were tragically ignored and many girls and women are paying the price.

24
Rotavirus

A Vaccine to save the NHS money

The introduction of the rotavirus vaccine is the latest example of a disturbing pattern of vaccines being introduced into an increasingly congested immunisation schedule for diseases that very rarely cause serious harm.

Rotavirus is a diarrhoea and vomiting bug that hardly ever causes serious illness in children in developed countries such as the UK, Europe and North America. In these countries the worst that is likely to happen is that a child gets sufficiently dehydrated to require overnight admission to hospital to be given fluids, usually by mouth.

It is certainly true that rotavirus causes several hundred thousand deaths a year in underdeveloped countries, though it is probable that many of these would be prevented if resources were concentrated on clean water and adequate sewerage systems rather than simply on vaccination.

So why is the vaccine recommended for children in many developed countries? The answer appears to be to save health services money. The vaccine was introduced into the UK NHS immunisation schedule in July 2013 since when it has been given as a live oral vaccine (drops in the baby's mouth) at two and three months of age.

Withdrawn for safety concerns

The rotavirus vaccine has a chequered history. The first vaccine, Wyeth's RotaShield, was found to cause a rare but serious bowel problem called intussusception and was withdrawn in 1999 after only nine months' use in the USA. Intussusception occurs when part of the bowel folds in on itself and is a life-threatening medical emergency. Nearly half of those affected require surgery, of whom 40% have the affected section of gut removed. In the UK around one child in every 170 who gets intussusception will die.[3,4]

Following the withdrawal of RotaShield the race was on to develop a safer rotavirus vaccine. Two rotavirus vaccines have been available since 2006: Rotarix made by GlaxoSmithKline (used in the UK) and RotaTeq manufactured by Merck. Though both vaccines are live and are administered as drops in the baby's mouth, Rotarix is derived solely from human rotavirus whereas RotaTeq is derived from a combination of human and animal (bovine) rotavirus.

How serious is rotavirus infection?
In the UK cases of rotavirus gastroenteritis peak during the winter and early spring months. It is not known for certain whether any children at all die from rotavirus infection in the UK, but it has been estimated that there may be up to 3 deaths a year.[5] The disease, however, is a significant burden to the NHS, causing an estimated 13,000 hospital admissions (usually for oral rehydration), 27,000 emergency home visits and an estimated 80,000 GP consultations every year. Breastfeeding is as effective as the vaccine in protecting babies against rotavirus and also helps prevent other causes of diarrhoea; breastfed infants have little chance of contracting rotavirus compared to bottle-fed infants.[6]

Perhaps of most importance to the NHS accountants, the introduction of a rotavirus vaccine was estimated to save the NHS £14 million every year.[2] The money men must have been delighted when savings from the first year of use of the vaccine were estimated to have been £7.5 million for secondary healthcare alone.[7]

How effective is the vaccine?
The vaccine is moderately effective. Both rotavirus vaccines prevent around seven out of ten cases of any rotavirus diarrhoea and over eight out of ten cases of severe rotavirus diarrhoea in the first year of life. Rotarix may be more effective than RotaTeq in the second year of life. Both vaccines work rather less well in underdeveloped countries where rotavirus is a much more serious disease.[8]

Intussusception
The first rotavirus vaccine, RotaShield, caused intussusception in between one in 5,000 and one in 10,000 children (and was withdrawn from the market because of this). Subsequent analysis revealed that the risk of intussusception was very much greater when the first dose of vaccine was given after three months of age, and that the risk to babies vaccinated at the recommended age, starting at two months, was between one in 11,000 and one in 16,000 babies.[9] Sadly, it appears that the newer vaccines may be no safer than the withdrawn vaccine. The overall incidence of intussusception in California increased after the introduction of the vaccine.[10] Both currently used rotavirus vaccines increase the risk of intussusception more than fivefold in the seven days after the first dose of vaccine.[11] The risk of intussusception after Rotarix, the rotavirus vaccine used in the UK, is one in 18-19,000 babies – provided they are vaccinated on time (the risk is greater if vaccination is delayed – a common occurrence). So it appears that the vaccine used in the UK may have at least the same, and possibly greater, risk of intussusception than the vaccine that was withdrawn because of this risk.

Intussusception is a medical emergency with around half of those affected requiring surgery and half of those having surgery needing a bowel resection (part of the bowel being removed). One child out of every 200 affected will die.

If all babies in the UK received the rotavirus vaccine on time, we can expect to see 41 cases of intussusception a year caused as a result of the vaccine. 20 of these children will require an operation and 10 will have part of their bowel removed. One baby will die every five years. These figures depend on babies receiving the vaccine in a timely manner and, if they are given the vaccine later than recommended, the risks of intussusception are greater.

In France the rotavirus vaccine was recommended for widespread use in 2013. However, recommendation of the vaccine was suspended in April 2015 following a report by the Technical Committee on Pharmacovigilance after a 'worrying' number of serious side effects including 47 cases of intussusception and the deaths of two babies.

Parents should be warned of the small but serious risk of intussusception before consenting for their baby to receive the vaccine.

Other side-effects

The rotavirus vaccine is a live vaccine and can cause diarrhoea, irritability and, occasionally, abdominal pain. The live vaccine is commonly excreted in the baby's faeces and could, therefore, be transmitted to close contacts. This is unlikely to be dangerous but can rarely cause symptomatic gastroenteritis (diarrhoea and vomiting) which could be dangerous, especially in someone with a compromised immune system.

All live vaccines, by their very nature, run the risk of mutating such that they can cause symptoms of gastroenteritis and there is already evidence to show that this is, albeit rarely, happening with the rotavirus vaccine.[12]

Contamination with pig virus

In 2010 Dr Eric Delwart, a professor in molecular biology at the University of California, San Francisco, analysed a wide range of live viral vaccines with the optimistic intention of demonstrating that they were pure and contained no contamination with any other live material. To his concern, he discovered viral contamination in both brands of rotavirus vaccine. GSK's Rotarix was contaminated with Porcine circovirus (PCV) types 1 and 2. Both these viruses are common in pigs and neither has been known to cause illness in humans though PCV2 can cause illness in pigs. This discovery led the FDA to temporarily suspend the use of Rotarix in the USA. One might wonder how a vaccine derived from a human rotavirus strain could be contaminated with a pig virus! Even though the virus was originally obtained from a child in Cincinnati, it was grown on monkey kidney cells. The probable culprit, however, was an enzyme derived from the pancreas of a pig which was also used to make the initial seed stock. This means that it is likely that the pig viruses were present in all of the doses given to the millions of children since the vaccine came into use.

We have been here before; several decades ago polio vaccines given to tens of millions of children worldwide were contaminated with the monkey SV40 virus which can cause cancer in animals.

Though there is no evidence that PCV1 and 2 can cause harm in humans that does not, of course, mean that they are safe. As both viruses are common in healthy pigs it is likely that humans frequently come across these vaccines by eating pork, but this would be by ingestion and so the virus would come up against the natural defences of the gut which is quite different from having a virus injected directly into the body.

The bottom line

Rotavirus is a common cause of diarrhoea and vomiting in babies in the UK. However, it is extremely rare for it to cause deaths in developed countries. Importantly, the vaccine causes rare, but serious, side-effects. The vaccine is an unnecessary edition to an already congested immunisation schedule. However, if you are going to give your baby the rotavirus vaccine ensure that you give the first dose on time, at eight weeks of age, and certainly by 12 weeks of age in order to minimise the risk of intussusception.

25
Influenza (Flu)

'The influence'

The introduction of the pneumococcal vaccine in 2006, though questionable on a population level, was at least given in order to save children's lives. When it was announced in 2012 that the flu jab was to be given to all children every year from the age of 2 up to 16 years, there was never any pretence that it was the children who were the main beneficiaries.

Epidemics throughout history

Epidemics of flu — or influenza to call it by its full name — have probably afflicted mankind for over two millennia.[1] The first certain pandemic[2] was in 1580. This started, as most have, in Asia, and then spread to Africa, Europe and, subsequently, America. The whole of Europe was affected over a six-month period; 8,000 deaths were reported in Rome and some Spanish cities were decimated.[3] The name 'influenza' originates from Italy: a Florentine family is accredited with using the word 'influence' to describe an unusual conjunction of planets at the time of epidemics, from which the word 'influenza' is derived.

'Russian Flu' hit the United Kingdom between 1889 and 1890, with a third of the adult population falling prey, and London being particularly badly affected. It was not until this late-Victorian epidemic that flu was widely accepted as being infectious.[4] It had previously been attributed to natural phenomena, such as earthquakes or astrological influences. However, even by 1891, some held the belief that the recent pandemic had been caused by a poisonous gas derived from comets in outer space.[5] Official advice for sufferers was to stay in bed, keep warm, drink brandy and take quinine and opium. One doctor wrote to the *Lancet* advising 'champagne or whisky every three hours', and the use of cannabis for any associated cough, headache or backache.[6]

Over the last two hundred years, there have been eight pandemics, now taken to mean a worldwide epidemic, of which by far the largest was the 'Spanish Flu' of 1918-19.

'The greatest medical holocaust in history.'[7]

The 'Spanish Flu' pandemic of 1918-19 ranks with the plague of Justinian in the sixth century, and the Black Death of the fourteenth century, as one of the three most destructive human epidemics ever to occur. There is disagreement over where the pandemic started. What is certain is that the First

World War provided a fertile breeding ground for the virus, which soon mutated to become far more lethal than normal, causing an up to tenfold increase in death rates. The transformed virus spread from Brest, one of the busiest French ports during the war, to the rest of Europe, Africa, North America and Australia. In an attempt to halt the spread of the virus, dance halls, theatres, schools and churches were closed in some American cities, while police in Chicago were asked to arrest anyone who sneezed. It became known as 'Spanish Flu' probably because Spain, as a neutral country during the war, did not censor news of the epidemic. The pandemic, which is estimated to have infected 50% of the world's population, caused more deaths in a few months than all the hostilities of the First World War over four years. Official figures put the global death toll at around 20 million, but it may have been nearer 100 million.[8] The official death toll in England and Wales was 200,000. An unusual feature of the 1918-19 pandemic was its propensity to kill those in the prime of life, aged in their twenties and thirties.

Recent pandemics

The 'Asian Flu' pandemic of 1957-8 caused more than a million deaths worldwide, killing 40,000 in the USA, whilst the 'Hong Kong Flu' of 1967 killed 30,000 in the UK. Well before the swine flu 'pandemic' of 2009/10, experts had been predicting that a pandemic was overdue. We had been told the most likely source would be a mutation arising from the marriage of a 'bird flu' virus and a human flu virus, though when and where this would occur was impossible to predict.

The Swine Flu 'pandemic' of 2009/10

Vested interests and preparation

In 1999 the WHO, spurred on by the Hong King bird flu outbreak of 1997, started to prepare for the next pandemic. Its first preparedness plan pulled no punches over the threat. 'Should a true influenza pandemic virus again appear that behaved as in 1918, even taking into account the advances in medicine since then, unparalleled tolls of illness and death would be expected.' This scary warning was prepared in collaboration with the European Scientific Working Group on Influenza (ESWI). WHO did not inform us that the ESWI was funded entirely by flu-drug and -vaccine manufacturers. Nor did WHO mention that two of the six authors of the plan had links to Roche, the manufacturer of a drug treatment for flu. The ESWI pressed for planning for the anticipated flu pandemic as well and lobbied politicians to 'take measures to encourage the pharmaceutical industry to plan its vaccine/antivirals production capacity in advance'. The ESWI itself admitted that it needed to convince these same politicians that flu vaccines were both beneficial and safe.

In 2002 the ESWI convened a meeting of influenza experts at its headquarters in Geneva, perhaps not coincidentally the same Swiss city that houses the WHO's headquarters. The purpose was to develop WHO's guidelines for the use of vaccines and antivirals during an influenza pandemic. The meeting was attended by representatives from Aventis Pasteur, a manufacturer of a flu vaccine. Two years later the WHO published a key report from that meeting, 'WHO guidelines on the use of vaccines and antivirals during influenza pandemics 2004'. The author of the section relating to Vaccines was Professor Arnold Monto who, at the time of writing the guidelines, was receiving consultancy fees from several pharmaceutical companies including GlaxoSmithKline (GSK), Novartis and Sanofi, all manufacturers of a swine flu vaccine. The WHO made no mention of this conflict of interest. The WHO's lack of openness and transparency extended to the composition of its Emergency Committee formed to advise on how best to manage a pandemic. The identities of its members were kept secret by the WHO until outside pressure forced it to reveal details of the 15 members which included Professor Monto and others whose organisations had financial relationships with swine flu vaccine manufacturers. Professor Monto received $3,000 in speaker fees from GSK alone in a single three-month period in 2009 at the time of the pandemic.

The sole 'advisor' to the committee, Professor Neil Ferguson had acted as a consultant to vaccine manufacturers Novartis and GSK.

Pharmaceutical companies had put around $4 billion (£2.8 billion) into developing the swine flu vaccine. It is understandable that they wanted a return on this investment.[9]

Moving the goalposts

Swine flu contracts worth billions of pounds were triggered by the official declaration by WHO of a pandemic. What is extraordinary is that in the summer of 2009, only weeks before a pandemic was officially declared, WHO changed its definition of what constitutes a pandemic. Previously, WHO stated, 'An influenza pandemic occurs when a new influenza virus appears against which the human population has no immunity, resulting in epidemics worldwide *with enormous numbers of deaths and illness* [my italics].' Immediately before the swine flu pandemic was announced the definition was changed so that now, 'A pandemic is a worldwide epidemic of a disease. An influenza pandemic may occur when a new influenza virus appears against which the human population has no immunity...*Pandemics can be either mild or severe in the illness and death they cause, and the severity of a pandemic can change over the course of that pandemic'* [my italics].

Previously pandemics had to be serious, threatening many lives; now they could be completely harmless, they simply had to be widespread. So swine flu manufacturers must have felt they had won the jackpot when, on 11th June 2009, the WHO officially announced that the world was at the start of an influenza pandemic.

The timeline of the pandemic

March 2009: Reports emerge from Mexico of the outbreak of a new swine flu virus closely followed by media headlines warning that a 'killer pig flu' would sweep the world.

Friday 24th April: The WHO announces that it is 'extremely concerned' about the outbreak. It is reported that 60 people have already died from the virus in Mexico.

Saturday 25th April: The death toll in Mexico rises to 81.

Sunday 26th April: 20 people are reported to have been diagnosed with swine flu in the USA, but none is seriously ill.

Monday 27th April: The death toll in Mexico has risen to 149.

The first cases in the UK are confirmed in two holidaymakers who have returned home from Mexico. Both are only mildly ill.

Tuesday 28th April: Cases are confirmed in the USA, Canada, Spain, Britain, New Zealand and Israel.

Wednesday 29th April

Vials containing samples of the swine flu virus are transported from the USA to a government laboratory in north London. The race for a vaccine is on. A 22-year-old man, recently returned from Mexico, becomes the first Londoner to be diagnosed with swine flu after suffering mild flu-like symptoms.

Thursday 30th April: New cases are diagnosed in Europe, Africa and South America; WHO warns that a pandemic is 'imminent'. The number of UK cases reaches 8, though none is seriously ill. Meanwhile in Mexico, the death toll has risen to over 160.

Friday 1st May: WHO director Margaret Chan declares a worldwide alertness level 5 for a danger of pandemic and recommends that all governments declare a national health emergency and activate pandemic emergency plans.

Saturday 2nd May: Something strange happens. Mexico announces that the confirmed death toll is now only 16 (it was 160 only two days ago). The other 'suspected' deaths have probably been caused by the thick polluting smog lying over Mexico City. It is beginning to look as though the swine flu virus is not as virulent, or harmful, as first feared and actually causes a rather mild flu which kills fewer people than normal flu. However, the WHO warns that countries should not lower their guard, even though the outbreak in Mexico appears to be waning with only a handful of deaths.

Sunday 3rd May: The WHO changes its definition of an influenza pandemic so that it no longer has to be serious resulting in many deaths (see *Moving the goalposts* above).

Monday 4th May: Three London schools close down as a result of pupils being diagnosed with the illness. The government appoints a swine flu 'Tsar' to deal with the threatened pandemic.

Thursday 7th May: The number of confirmed deaths in Mexico now stands at 42.

Friday 15th May: Baxter and GSK receive orders from the UK government for 90 million swine flu vaccines — enough for one and a half vaccines for every man, woman and child in the UK (despite signs that the virus appears not to be as dangerous as first thought) at a cost of £239 million.

Friday 22nd May: The total number of cases in the UK reaches 120; all are mild.

Thursday 4th June: 459 cases are confirmed in the UK though nearly all are mild.

Thursday 11th June: The outbreak is now officially a 'pandemic' as Dr Margaret Chan, the director general of the WHO, having taken advice and guidance from its emergency committee, announces 'the world is now at the start of the 2009 influenza pandemic.' The virus has spread to 74 countries, infected nearly 30,000 people and caused 141 deaths globally.

Friday 12th June: The total number of UK cases passes the 1,000 mark, with the vast majority remaining mild. (I was working as a GP in central London at the time and remember the chaos as we were instructed to visit all suspected swine flu cases at home wearing a facemask, plastic apron and gloves. We then had to take two nose and two throat swabs from the patient before starting them on antiviral drugs. More than one patient told me that the side-effects of the treatment were more unpleasant than the symptoms of flu.)

Sunday 14th June: The first swine flu death in the UK, indeed in all Europe, occurs in Scotland as a 38-year-old lady with undisclosed underlying medical problems dies.

Saturday 20th June: The number of UK cases passes the 2,000 mark. Meanwhile, worldwide there have been 231 deaths and 52,160 cases affecting around 100 countries.

Saturday 27th June: A 73-year-old Scottish man with 'very serious underlying health issues' dies.

Friday 26th June: A six-year-old girl, who had serious medical problems, becomes the third person to die from swine flu in the UK.

Friday 3rd July: The fourth death is in a 19 year old man from London; like all the others he had serious underlying health problems.

Monday July 6th: A 9-year-old with 'serious underlying health problems' becomes the fifth person to die on the UK.

Tuesday 9th July: The first apparently 'healthy' person dies from Swine flu in the UK.

Friday 11th July: Eight-year-old Louis Austin, from Manchester, is misdiagnosed over the phone as having swine flu. He dies the following day from severe diabetes and would almost certainly have lived had the correct diagnosis been made.

Thursday 16th July: The UK Chief Medical Officer (CMO), Sir Liam Donaldson, announces the launch of the National Pandemic Flu Service helpline for England. This enables patients to obtain anti-viral drugs without seeing a doctor. At the same time he makes an alarming prediction. Though only 29 people (nearly all with underlying health problems) have died from the epidemic so far, Sir Liam predicts that up to 65,000 people could die in the UK from the pandemic. He stresses that this is a worst-case scenario, but that he expects at least 19,000 deaths. Sir Liam also announces that the government has ordered 132 million doses of the swine flu vaccine –

enough for two shots for every UK citizen. *Within weeks this alarming forecast was downgraded so that 19,000 deaths became the worst case scenario. The usual annual death toll from flu is 6,000 – 8,000.*

Late July: Trials of a swine flu vaccine on healthy volunteers start in Australia as Roche announces a 200% rise in sales of its anti-flu drug Tamiflu.

Thursday 30th July: The number of weekly cases hits a high of 110,000 in England

Friday 31st July: 16-year-old Charlotte Hartey, of Oswestry, Shropshire, dies in Royal Shrewsbury Hospital. She had been diagnosed with swine flu over the phone on 22nd July and prescribed Tamiflu. An inquest later heard that she had died from complications arising from tonsillitis after being misdiagnosed with swine flu and could have been saved had the correct diagnosis been made.

Tuesday 4th August: Two-year-old Georgia Keeling, from Norwich, dies at the Norfolk and Norwich University Hospital with a diagnosis of swine flu. An inquest later conformed that the cause of death was meningitis and that she had been wrongly diagnosed.

Summer 2009: The number of new cases being diagnosed steadily falls.

Thursday 17th September: CMO Sir Liam warns that, after a summer reprieve, swine flu could be on the way back with an estimated 5,000 cases in the previous week in England alone. Nevertheless the benign nature of the pandemic is becoming increasingly clear with the total UK death toll standing at only 79.

September 2009: Two new swine flu vaccines are tested in the UK on children, including babies as young as 6 months.

Friday 25th September: Official approval is given for Pandemrix, GSK's swine flu vaccine, to be used on adults and children from six months of age. The UK government has ordered 60 million doses of the vaccine.

Wednesday 21st October: Nationwide vaccination starts in the UK, initially on those with underlying health problems (who are more likely to become seriously ill or die from swine flu), pregnant women and health professionals.

December 2009: The vaccine is rolled out to all children under 5 years of age.

Mid December: The CMO acknowledges that the swine flu virus is considerably less dangerous than had been feared after it has been calculated that the death rate in the UK so far has been 0.026% or around one in 4,000 of those infected. The rate of new cases has fallen steadily throughout autumn and winter.

As the pandemic looks to be on the way out the government is left with the tricky problem of what to do with the tens of millions of swine flu vaccines it has over-ordered.

Wednesday 10th Feb: The national swine flu helpline is closed down.

April 2010: Swiss pharmaceutical company Novartis announces a rise in profits of nearly 50%, boosted by sales of its flu vaccine made during the swine flu pandemic.

Tuesday 10th August 2010: The WHO officially declares the swine flu pandemic over.

The total number of deaths from swine flu in the UK has come to a little over 450, far fewer than the few thousand who die most years from seasonal flu and way below the government's scariest prediction of 65,000 deaths. The UK government has spent £1.2 billion on preparing and responding to the pandemic, of which £239 million was spent on vaccines. Thursday 19th August 2010: The first 12 cases of narcolepsy occurring in children following vaccination with Pandemrix are reported in Sweden.

The fallout

The Council of Europe Health Committee chairman, Wolfgang Wodarg, was one of the most vocal critics of the response to the so-called 'pandemic'. He claimed experts were unduly influenced by the pharmaceutical industry, and questioned whether a virus that proved to be so mild could really be classed as a pandemic.

Sir Liam Donaldson, the government's chief medical officer and public face of the fight against flu in the UK, had to defend accusations that he had personally over-reacted. At the start of the summer, he released data showing more than 60,000 people could die during the first winter. That was subsequently reduced to 1,000 — and even that figure turned out to be an overestimate.

The WHO has struggled to offer a convincing reason why it changed its definition of a pandemic, partly because of its policy of keeping the identity and the deliberations of its pandemic emergency advisory committee secret. The only known member of the committee is its chairman, Australian flu specialist John MacKenzie. WHO spokesman Gregory Hartl said names of those on the sitting committee had not been made public because of the potential 'for bringing undue pressure on them when they are making decisions which have societal and economic impacts'. Research has since uncovered that six of the nine scientists promoting use of the swine flu vaccine in the UK had potential conflicts of interest, ranging from study funding to directorships of pharmaceutical companies. These conflicts of interest were rarely mentioned when they actively promoted use of the vaccine.[10]

The Parliamentary assembly of the Council of Europe published a damning report on the handling of the swine flu pandemic. With regard to the vaccine, it concluded, 'suspicion of undue influence and pressure put on national authorities by the pharmaceutical industry has been reinforced by other factors, such as the character of contractual arrangements concluded between governments and pharmaceutical groups. Reports from several European countries indicate that there was pressure exerted on national governments to speed up the conclusion of major contracts, that dubious practices were followed concerning prices of vaccines, which were not available under normal market conditions, and that there were attempts to transfer liability of the vaccines and medication, which might not have been tested sufficiently, to national governments.' The report, quite rightly, describes these factors as 'most alarming'. Dr Wodarg, who in 2009 was chair of the Health Committee of the European Council, went further: 'in order to promote their patented drugs and vaccines against flu, pharmaceutical companies have influenced scientists and official agencies responsible for public health standards, to alarm the governments worldwide. They have made them squander tight healthcare resources for inefficient vaccine strategies and needlessly exposed millions of healthy people to the risk of unknown side-effects of insufficiently tested vaccines.' He claimed that the 2009 pandemic was 'one of the greatest medical scandals of the century'.

Government indemnity

The WHO granted four pharmaceutical companies licences to hold exclusive patents for the pandemic flu vaccine. If the threat to the world were as great as the WHO was claiming then why were not all equipped laboratories over the world encouraged to produce the vaccine as swiftly as possible in an attempt to save the millions of threatened lives? The four multinational companies took advantage of their exclusive patented rights and increased the price of their vaccines whilst at the same time preventing the production of generic versions of the vaccine.

Because of concerns over the safety of the vaccines, which had not had time to be adequately tested, manufacturers requested that governments indemnify them from all responsibility for any unexpected side-effects. All governments, with the sole, and admirable, exception of Poland, granted pharmaceutical companies the indemnity they had requested. The Polish government decided not to purchase any vaccines because it felt unable to reassure its population that the vaccines were safe. Polish people were arguably better off than other Europeans. The (small) number of people dying from swine flu in Poland was proportionately the same as in neighbouring countries that carried out mass vaccination.

Big profits

Looking at the balance sheets of the pharmaceutical companies it is clear that many did make a healthy profit out of swine flu. Vaccine producer Novartis, for example, posted an 8% jump in profit in 2009.

The company's annual report cited swine flu vaccine sales as a major reason for the increase — though such a profit is, of course, not proof of any undue influence by the firm.

Sanofi-Aventis, another swine flu vaccine manufacturer, registered net profits in 2009 is 7.8 billion (an 11% increase) due to a 'record year' of flu vaccine sales.

Sales of swine flu vaccines in 2009 were expected to result in overall profits of between $7 billion and $10 billion to the companies producing the vaccines. The manufacturers were in a win–win situation whereby they were able to make huge profits whilst at the same time offloading the financial risks of compensation for any serious adverse reactions to nation governments.

Narcolepsy

The link between the swine flu vaccine and narcolepsy in children was first spotted during the spring and summer of 2010 by Lars Palm, a Swedish neurologist following the massive flu vaccine campaign. 'Usually, it is unlikely that I'd diagnose more than one new narcolepsy patient per year,' said the doctor. 'Suddenly I had six new cases in just a couple of months. It emerged that the narcolepsy symptoms had started within a couple of weeks after the Pandemrix shot.'

Narcolepsy is a chronic and debilitating auto-immune neurological disorder that causes disabling sleep disturbances. Sufferers experience excessive sleepiness during the day such that they might fall asleep in the middle of a conversation or while playing a game. They can also experience sudden loss of muscle control triggered by emotion (cataplexy), sleep paralysis, and disturbing hallucinations. Some children paradoxically also show symptoms of hyperactivity.[ii]There is no effective treatment.

Pandemrix was the most widely used swine flu vaccine in Europe (where it was given to over 30 million people). In the UK it was given to over six million people, including many children. It is made with the novel adjuvant ASO3 containing squalene as well as thiomersal (mercury).

Following Dr Palm's observations in Sweden, cases of narcolepsy following vaccination were reported from over a dozen countries including Finland, France, Germany, Iceland, Ireland, Norway, North America and the UK.

Even after concerns were raised about the link between the vaccine and narcolepsy, the UK Medicines and Healthcare Products Regulatory Agency (MHRA) claimed: 'The Pandemrix vaccine remains available and should continue to be used as recommended. The benefits of vaccination outweigh any risk of a possible side effect.' The Pandemrix vaccine, made by GlaxoSmithKline, had been used in 47 countries following the swine flu outbreak. More than 30 million doses were given across Europe.

Studies found that the risk of a child who received Pandemrix developing narcolepsy is more than ten times the risk of a child who had not been given the vaccine; somewhere between one in 19,000 and one in 54,000 children vaccinated went on to suffer narcolepsy caused by the vaccine.

In June 2015 a 12-year-old boy was the first to be awarded damages after being left severely disabled by narcolepsy caused by the swine flu vaccine. The boy's parents received £120,000 from the UK Vaccine Damage Compensation Programme, which awards the fixed sum of £120,000 to anyone who can prove that they have been severely damaged by a vaccine given as part of the NHS recommended schedule. The threshold for being classified as 'severely damaged' is high and the compensation payment is woefully inadequate to provide the care needed for the damaged child. The families of scores of children suffering from narcolepsy after receiving the swine flu vaccine have launched legal action against the manufacturer

GlaxoSmithKline. However, any financial settlement will be met by the UK taxpayer because the government offered the multinational pharmaceutical company indemnity. The UK government, and thus the UK taxpayer, is also paying for expensive medication costing £12,000 per person per year for 80 children who developed narcolepsy after receiving the vaccine.

Pandemrix

Pandemrix, made by Glaxo Smith Kline (GSK), was the UK's swine flu vaccine of choice. It is not surprising to discover that this vaccine causes serious side-effects since it contains both mercury (as thiomersal) – a poisonous metal that had been removed from all routine childhood vaccines given in the UK – and squalene – a potent stimulator of the immune system. The UK government chose to offer the UK population Pandemrix rather than the probably safer (and mercury and squalene free) Celvepan. One can only assume that it was cheaper. The German government gave the game away by offering Celvepan to politicians, civil servants and the military and giving Pandemrix to the rest of the population.

Concerns about the safety of squalene continue to be published.[12] The safety of using squalene in vaccines has been studied very little and certainly not sufficiently to exclude long-term problems. This is particularly important because animals injected with squalene have developed auto-immune diseases similar to multiple sclerosis (MS), rheumatoid arthritis and systemic lupus erythematosus (SLE). Vaccines have often been associated with auto-immune disorders and it is worrying that a substance has been used that may increase this risk. Reassurances by the WHO and the UK DoH that the use of squalene in vaccines is safe is not based on sound evidence. Squalene should not have been used as an adjuvant in a vaccine given to millions of people including children without substantial evidence of its safety, both in the short and long term.

GPs ran out of regular seasonal flu vaccine in Jan 2011, long after the swine flu 'pandemic'. The DoH instructed doctors to use supplies of the left over swine flu vaccine instead. Not only was swine flu not one of the dominant strains doing the rounds, but in the cavalier fashion that we have seen far too often, the vaccine was recommended despite its by then recognised link to narcolepsy.

Other side effects

It is possible the swine flu vaccine causes an increase risk of Guillain-Barré syndrome (see below), idiopathic thrombocytopaenia purpura (ITP – a rare bleeding disorder) and Bells' Palsy, a paralysis (usually temporary) of the face.

How serious was the Swine Flu Pandemic in children in the UK?

A total of 70 children died in England during the epidemic between June 2009 and March 2010.[13] Two thirds of these children already had medical disorders which put them at much greater risk. The risk to a healthy Caucasian child of dying from swine flu was around one in a million – an exceptionally low risk. Remarkably, children from Pakistani or Bangladeshi families were ten times more likely to die from swine flu than white children, but even then the risk was small. The good news for children with asthma is that this did not increase the risk at all.

Seasonal flu

The main viruses causing flu, influenza types A and B, were discovered in the 1930s and 1940s, with the C-type being discovered later.[14] Though pandemic flu occurs only infrequently, seasonal flu, caused by a variety of one of the three main viruses, is ever-present, though more prevalent in the winter, with localised epidemics occurring every few years. Flu has a very short incubation period of one to three days and causes a high temperature, headache, sore throat, tiredness and aches and pains all over the body.[15] Anyone can be affected but the elderly are generally most vulnerable. It is unpleasant, though rarely serious, in children but, as with all infections, those with underlying medical conditions are more at risk.[16] Treatment involves rest, plenty to drink and medicine such as paracetamol to lower the fever. Most people recover within two weeks. Antibiotics are of no help with flu itself, though may be necessary to treat any 'secondary' infections, typically of the chest or ear.

The vaccine

Vaccinating against flu poses a particular problem. The flu virus is able to mutate rapidly, such that every year different types of flu are likely to predominate. A one-off vaccination can only protect against specific strains, and so is unable to offer long-term protection. Every February, the World Health Organisation (WHO) predicts which strains of flu are most likely to be causing problems during the following winter. Most, but not all, governments follow the WHO's advice when formulating their flu vaccines. Each year a vaccine is made using the whole, or parts, of three or four killed or live flu viruses. As the vaccine is only designed to help protect against one season's flu, yearly vaccinations are required to maintain protection. Natural protection from flu, after an attack, also declines rapidly as the virus mutates. Unlike adults, children under 13 need two separate injections given 4-6 weeks apart if receiving the jab for the first time.[17]

The use of the flu vaccine in children in the UK

Does the vaccine work?

Before 2013 the only children offered routine flu vaccination in the UK were those considered to be particularly at risk, of whom the largest group was those with bad asthma, but also included children with bronchiectasis, cystic fibrosis, congenital heart disease and those receiving drugs that suppress the immune system — such as for cancer. It was assumed that they were more susceptible to chest infections, and that catching flu would be more likely to be serious. The vaccine used, the 'inactivated' or killed vaccine was, on average, 59% effective at preventing proven influenza and 36% effective in preventing any flu-like illness. However, there is no evidence that the vaccine prevented deaths, hospital admissions or serious complications. The effectiveness of the UK 2014/15 vaccine was unimpressive, preventing only one third of cases of flu. But UK children were far better off than Canadian children given the flu vaccine over the same winter, who were twice as likely to catch flu compared to unvaccinated children.[18] The benefit to those children with asthma was questionable as all the evidence suggests that having a flu jab makes no difference at all to a child's asthma, nor does it help prevent flu in these children; one study even found that asthmatic children given the flu jab went on to have worse asthma over the following months than those who were not immunised.[19,20,21] Nor was there any evidence that the vaccine benefitted children with cystic fibrosis.[22] One study found that children who were given the vaccine were *three times more likely* to be hospitalised with a flu-related problem than children who had not received the vaccine.[23]

Yearly flu jabs for all children

In 2013 the UK started to vaccinate all children aged 2 to 16 years with the flu vaccine every year. This is puzzling as flu is rarely a serious or life-threatening disease in the vast majority of children. It is an unpleasant illness, but most people recover from flu within a week or so.

This policy has been described as 'cost-effective' as a result of complex mathematical models that predict the vaccine will reduce the burden of influenza on GPs' work and will reduce the number of deaths and hospital admissions from flu. However, it is not primarily the children who will benefit. Children, especially healthy children, very rarely die from influenza; in fact in some years there are no deaths at all from flu in children under 15 years of age.[24] Nevertheless, the Chief Medical Officer predicted that, even with only 30% uptake of the vaccine, two thousand deaths and eleven thousand hospitalisations from flu would be prevented every year. This is a very suspect prediction and is itself based on no hard evidence but rather extremely complex mathematical modelling relying on many questionable assumptions. If, and it is a big IF, this prediction is correct it is not the children who are being vaccinated, and risking adverse reactions, who are benefiting but rather the frail elderly over 75 years of age who are at risk of catching flu from children. However, three quarters of those over 65 years of age are already given the flu vaccine which makes it questionable what extra benefit vaccinating children might bring even to them. A high proportion of the hypothetical 2,000 deaths saved is likely to be in those who, if spared influenza will, sadly, only go on to die from some other cause in subsequent months. In other words, many, if not most, of the deaths 'saved' are not really saved but merely postponed for a short time.

It has been suggested that vaccinating healthy children against flu may do them more harm than good. Figures from the USA suggest a child is more likely to be hospitalised for vaccine-induced febrile convulsions (fits as a result of a fever) than for complications from flu. Febrile convulsions occur in over 1 in 1,000 vaccinated children.[25] A flu vaccine given to children in Australia was withdrawn in 2009 because of the high incidence of adverse reactions.[26]

At the same time that vaccination was introduced for all children, the type of vaccine was change from the killed 'inactivated' vaccine to the more effective live vaccine, which is up to 80% effective at preventing genuine flu in children over two years of age *provided* the correct flu strains have been picked for the vaccine in the first place. This is not always the case: the 2014/15 vaccine used in the UK was only 35% effective against the predominant strain during that winter.[27] The vaccine is relatively ineffective in children under two years of age.

Pregnant Women
A new recommendation has been for pregnant women to receive the flu vaccine as flu can be more serious in pregnancy. This also gives some protection to the newborn baby (one study suggested 76% effectiveness). Needless to say, the safety of its use in pregnancy has not been adequately tested. One recent study found a sevenfold increased risk of premature delivery in just one of the four years examined; this clearly needs further investigation.[28]

More recent research has found that children born to mothers given the flu vaccine in pregnancy may be at increased risk of developing autism. In particular, children born to mothers who received a flu jab in the first trimester (first three months) of pregnancy may have a 20% increased risk of developing autism.[43]

Vaccination policy in North America
Both Canada and the USA recommend yearly vaccination of all children.

European policy
Though many European countries recommend flu jabs for high-risk children over six months of age, at the time of writing (2016) only Austria and Poland vaccinate all healthy children as in the UK.

Is the illness serious and common enough to warrant vaccination?
It is very difficult to know exactly how much illness, or even how many deaths, flu causes because it is not easy to distinguish real flu from the other illnesses. Doctors often make the diagnosis of a 'flu-like illness'; in other words it is like flu — high temperature, sore throat, muscle aches — but there is no certainty that the illness is caused by the influenza virus rather than one of the many other viruses that can also cause similar symptoms. It is, therefore, difficult to answer the question with any accuracy. But some facts are available.

The cause of death is one of the more (though not totally) reliable statistics. The number of flu deaths varies from year to year but is typically 200-300. However, these are nearly all in those over 70 years of age. It is extremely rare for a child to have a diagnosis of influenza on a death certificate.[29]

It has been estimated that the total number of deaths attributable to influenza is actually much higher, numbering many thousands, because, for example, many of the deaths due to pneumonia may have been a result of catching flu in the first place. Whatever, deaths in children remain very low.

Government doctors estimated that, during the winter of 2003/4, there were 2,000 additional deaths as a result of flu.[30] Even if that were so, very few of them would have been children. Sixteen children did die directly from flu during the 2003/4 winter – more than in any winter for the last twenty years. They were affected by a particularly nasty strain of flu called the H3N2 Fujian-like strain. The paradox is that even if they had all been vaccinated, they were still likely to have died because the flu jab given that year did not cover the strain of flu virus that killed them. Other scientists have estimated, by mathematical modelling, that there are an average of forty four deaths per year from flu in children under 15 years of age in the UK.[31]

Is the vaccine safe?

The flu vaccine can cause the usual side effects of most vaccinations, including fever, rash and mild flu-like symptoms. Alarmingly, there have been virtually no safety studies on the inactivated (killed) flu vaccine in children under two – the very age that healthy children are given it in some countries. In 1976, five deaths were suspected by doctors to have been caused by the flu jab, though the JCVI felt that only one was likely to have been caused by the vaccine.[32] Authors of a Cochrane review were concerned at the lack of safety trials: 'We were astonished to find only one safety study of inactivated vaccine in children under two years carried out nearly 30 years ago in 35 children.'[33] When these same authors attempted to obtain further unpublished safety data, this was denied because the manufacturer did not want to share the information.[34] This begs the question why a vaccine manufacturer would want to withhold safety data on one of their vaccines. The total lack of safety information on a vaccination given to millions of healthy children under two years of age every year is both remarkable and disturbing.

Other very rare side effects, likely to be caused by the vaccine, include Bell's Palsy – a paralysis, usually temporary, but sometimes permanent, of one side of the face.[35,36]

The live vaccine now used in the UK causes a headache in up to 46%, fever in up to 26% of children, vomiting in up to 13%, muscle ache in up to 13%, abdominal pain in up to 2%, nasal congestion in over half, and bronchitis in 3% of those given the vaccine. The vaccine also risks exacerbating asthma in children under three years of age. It has been reported to cause optic neuritis (resulting in temporary blindness).[37] Some authorities recommend the live vaccine should not be given to children with asthma at any age.[38] The live vaccine has one more effect which could have more serious long-term consequences. It changes the make-up of bugs occurring naturally in the nose, causing harmless bugs to be replaced with bacteria that may cause more serious disease. Only time will tell whether interfering with the natural balance will backfire.[39]

Guillain-Barré Syndrome (GBS)

This rare disease keeps cropping up in lists of vaccine side effects. It is an auto-immune disorder that causes paralysis of the arms, legs or, occasionally, the whole body, and has been associated with polio, hepatitis B, Hib, MMR, tetanus and diphtheria vaccines. Some suffer a permanent weakness after GBS, and a few die, though complete recovery is usual. GBS was first connected with the use of a 'swine flu' vaccine in 1976, resulting in the suspension of the vaccine programme in the USA before Christmas of that year.[40,41] Recipients of the vaccine were seven times more likely to develop GBS within 6 weeks of vaccination than the unvaccinated. Because GBS is rare anyway, the actual risk of suffering from GBS as a result of the vaccine was still low, at around one in 100,000. There has been much debate over whether this risk applies to all flu vaccines or just that particular one. The conclusion is that all flu vaccines probably roughly double the risk of getting GBS. Because of its rarity, this means that only one or two people would get GBS for every million vaccinated.[42] However, these figures do rely on passive reporting, so the true risk may be higher.

Conclusion

Giving the flu vaccine to all children is unnecessary and of uncertain benefit — at least to the children receiving the vaccine. The JCVI's recommendation for the introduction of the vaccine was based on several unpublished studies and is therefore far from transparent. Last, but not least, all children will be receiving an additional fourteen to twenty-two doses doses of vaccine up to seventeen years of age with unknown long-term effects on the immune system. The decision to vaccinate all children yearly is not only suspect scientifically but is also questionable on moral and ethical grounds.

26
Meningitis B

Lobbying achieves a U-turn

In July 2013 the Joint Committee on Vaccination and Immunisation (JCVI, the expert body that decides which vaccines should be offered on the NHS in the UK) issued a statement concluding that 'routine infant or toddler immunisation using Bexsero (the meningitis B vaccine) is highly unlikely to be cost-effective at any vaccine price… and could not be recommended (for introduction into the NHS childhood immunisation schedule).' In other words, even if the vaccine were free, its introduction would not be cost-effective.[1]

So how was it, that eight months later the JCVI, in an impressive about-turn, recommended that the vaccine should be given to all children at two, four and twelve months of age?

The answer is that they changed the rules to suit their conclusion. Instead of basing their recommendation on the standard recognised method of calculating cost effectiveness they added additional factors that had not been used previously including the following:

Though the number of cases of meningitis B in England and Wales had fallen by half over the previous decade, the committee decided that the numbers could rise again over the coming years and so increased their estimate of the number of cases.

An allowance was made to cover a proportion of litigation costs brought against the NHS relating to meningococcal disease caused by the meningitis B bug;

An allowance was also made for the loss of the quality-of-life of family members of those who died, or became disabled, from meningitis B;

An estimation that the vaccine would be 95% effective, an improbably high estimate when compared with other vaccines;

An upgrading of the estimate of the proportion of meningitis B strains in the UK that the vaccine would cover from 75% to 88%.

These changes prompted the committee to recommend introduction of the meningitis B vaccine into the NHS immunisation schedule, provided a sufficiently low purchase price could be agreed with the manufacturer.[2]

The addition of the meningitis B and hepatitis B vaccines has made the UK immunisation schedule by far the most complex of any the world over, and resulted in the administration of 31 vaccines by 12 months of age.

Lobbying from vested interests

What caused the committee to have such a major rethink that led to the rapid U-turn in its recommendation? The answer may lie in the commercial value of blockbuster vaccines.

Following its recommendation that the vaccine should not be added to the immunisation programme, the JCVI was subjected to intense lobbying from interested parties including medical experts (some with financial ties to the pharmaceutical industry) and meningitis charities, which are often funded by pharmaceutical companies. Parents of children who had died from meningitis B appeared on national television pleading for the introduction of the vaccine so that other parents should not suffer the same fate. There is nothing that pulls the emotional heartstrings more effectively than a child dying or becoming disabled, especially if the cause is preventable.

We do not know the extent of the lobbying or what influence it had on the committee's recommendation. However, it is surprising that eight months after voicing concerns about the vaccine's effectiveness and safety, it felt able to recommend its nationwide introduction.

Conflict of interests

Professor Andrew Pollard heads up the Oxford Vaccine Group, which developed the meningitis B vaccine and stands to gain financially from its use. He was not a member of the JCVI when it made its original decision not to recommend the use the meningitis B vaccine. Shortly after he joined the committee, as chair, in October 2013 the JCVI changed its mind and recommended that every baby in the country receive three doses of the vaccine.

How common and serious is Meningitis B?

Meningitis B was the last remaining significant cause of life-threatening meningitis in children in the UK for which there was not yet a vaccine. The meningitis B bug (Group B meningococcus) causes meningitis and blood poisoning. One in ten who contract the disease will die and another one in ten will suffer a permanent disability such as brain damage, chronic pain, scarring or hearing loss. The majority of all cases of serious meningitis B disease occur in children under five years of age. It is clearly a nasty disease.[3]

However, it appears to be on the decline, at least in recent years. Following a peak in number of cases in 2000/01 the number of people suffering meningitis B infections halved in England and Wales over the subsequent decade from 1,200 a year to 600 a year with over half the cases occurring in babies and young children. After five years of age the disease is very rare; it does makes a recurrence in late teenage years and early adulthood though it remains less common at this age than in early childhood. Around one in two thousand unimmunised children will contract meningitis B disease between birth and the age of five. Between 2006 and 2010, 250 children under the age of five contracted meningitis B, of which 25 died, every year.[4]

The meningitis B bug, in common with the other main causes of meningitis in the UK (Haemophilus influenzae type B, pneumococcus and meningitis C) commonly lives in the nose and throat (in up to a third) of healthy people. This means that it will be difficult, if not impossible, to eradicate the bugs with vaccination and that herd immunity cannot be relied upon to prevent the disease.

How effective is the vaccine?

Bexsero was first approved by European regulatory agencies in January 2013. The UK was the first country to introduce the vaccine nationally. At the time of writing (2017), the vaccine is also publicly funded in Italy and has been recommended for use in several other countries, mainly in Europe.

There had been attempts to develop a vaccine against meningitis B for many years, but this proved remarkably difficult. One reason is that the outside coating of the bug, against which any vaccine is directed, is similar to substances present in humans (including compounds found in foetal brain tissue) raising concern about the possible development of auto-immune disease in people given the vaccine. The meningitis B vaccine was made using a method called 'reverse vaccinology', a technique never previously used to make vaccines.

The vaccine does not prevent all strains of meningitis B. Current estimates suggest that Bexsero is able to prevent infections from between three quarters and four fifths of the meningitis B strains in the UK.[5,6] In common with many new vaccines recently introduced, estimates of effectiveness are based on antibody blood tests following receipt of the vaccine and the true effectiveness in the real world is unknown. A fall in the number of cases of meningitis B in babies in the months following the introduction of the vaccine suggests it is working. It is also possible that the vaccine may protect against the very rare Men W strain that appears to be on the increase in the UK.[7]

How safe is it?

In July 2013 the JCVI had a number of concerns about Bexsero's safety that contributed to its decision not to recommend the vaccine at that time. The vaccine is likely to cause a fever in six out of every seven babies given the vaccine, far more frequently than with any other vaccine in routine use. Six out of every seven babies are tender at the injection site, and in one of three of those affected the tenderness is severe, resulting in crying when the injected limb is moved. Two out of every three babies develop a fever of 38.5°C or more when given Bexsero along with other routine infant vaccines. It is less likely to cause a fever when given on its own. Other very common side-effects include sleepiness, irritability, unusual crying and going off feeds. It can probably cause convulsions, with or without a fever. It is possible that it can cause Kawasaki disease (a rare, but serious, auto-immune disease affecting the blood vessels) in around one in one thousand babies given the vaccine.[5]

By the time the committee got round to recommending the introduction of the vaccine, its safety concerns appeared to have receded into the background. It simply advised that paracetamol ('Calpol') should routinely be given to babies at the time of vaccination despite evidence that this may reduce the effectiveness of vaccines given at the same time.[2]

It is early days of experience with this vaccine and so it is probable that other side effects may yet come to light. Doctors in Germany have already described a five-month-old girl who was unable to use the arm in which Bexsero was given for weeks after receiving the vaccine and had not fully recovered two months later. They advised that when given along with other vaccines (as usually happens) the Men B vaccine should be given in the leg because of its greater likelihood to cause local reactions.[8]

The bottom line
Meningitis B is a serious life-threatening disease. However, it is rare in the UK and the numbers contracting the disease were steadily decreasing over the 10 years prior to the introduction of the vaccine. The vaccine is new and does appear to cause more side-effects than nearly all other routinely-used vaccines. It is tempting and understandable for parents to want to protect their children against a life-threatening disease such as meningitis. Nonetheless, I would urge caution in giving a vaccine about which so little is known and about which there are ongoing safety concerns.

27
Hepatitis B
Another doubtful vaccine

The hepatitis B vaccine was added to the UK national immunisation schedule on 26 September 2017 as part of a new 6-in-1 vaccine. Hepatitis B (hep B) is different to most of the diseases discussed in this book. A child cannot catch it simply by being in contact with someone with the disease. It is contracted through blood or sexual contact. It is an uncommon disease in the UK and extremely rare in children in this country. So why was the vaccine introduced?

Who wanted the vaccine?
Back in 1996 the drug company SmithKlineBeecham (SKB — now GlaxoSmithKline), the largest manufacturer of the hep B vaccine, tried to get their vaccine more widely used by convening a consensus panel of 'top medical experts' which advocated vaccination of all babies in the UK. SKB paid Shire Hall Communications to launch its report, and the PR company did this most successfully. The result was that no fewer than 26 national and local broadcast bulletins reported that 'top medical experts' were advocating a strategy of universal immunisation in infancy. It was an object lesson in how the media is used.[1] Nevertheless, SKB were unsuccessful at that time in getting their vaccine given to all infants in the UK, and the issue remained dormant until 2004, when the British Liver Trust (which receives funding from vaccine manufacturers) issued a report, which said that hepatitis B 'lurks in the shadows', and called for 'universal [hepatitis B] vaccination…as a matter of urgency'.[2,3]

Though SKB had failed to get the vaccine introduced in the UK, it succeeded elsewhere in Europe with a similar strategy. 'Beecham's business manager claimed with outrageous cynicism, 'We started increasing the awareness of the European Experts of the World Health Organisation about hepatitis B in 1988. From then to 1991, we financed epidemiological studies on the subject to create a scientific consensus about hepatitis being a major public health problem. We were successful because in 1991, WHO published new recommendations about hepatitis B vaccination.' When the immunisation campaign was in full swing, the French official 'experts'…did not hesitate to participate in the hype under the form of 'medical' publications co-authored with salesman.'[5]

The World Health Organisation has for many years been pushing for all countries to give everyone at least three doses of the vaccine irrespective of the need in any particular country.

The British Medical Association (BMA) has repeatedly called for all children to be vaccinated against hep B.[4] The BMA has highlighted the worldwide nature of the problem and the increase in international travel. It produced a report emphasizing that the disease is highly infectious and causes one million deaths worldwide.[5] No mention was made of the fact that there is a negligible chance of catching the disease in the UK unless you have sex with, or come into contact with the blood of, someone infected with the hep B virus. The BMA's call has been backed by the Royal College of GPs.[6] An editorial in the *BMJ* in 2006 again argued in favour of vaccination of all children, pointing out the increasing numbers of UK residents with the disease, but this is largely due to immigration from areas where hep B is common.

Various patients' groups, often part-funded by pharmaceutical companies, have called for universal hep B vaccination as has, unsurprisingly, the Association of the British Pharmaceutical Industry (ABPI).

The argument for mass vaccination is easily understood in those countries where most of the population are likely to become infected with hep B. It is difficult to fathom in countries such as the UK where the disease is uncommon, and especially rare in children.

Reasons not to vaccinate all children

These are straightforward. The UK has one of the lowest rates of hep B of any country in the world. It is extremely rare in children, fewer than ten of whom are infected with the virus every year. Most new carriers of the virus are immigrants, which vaccinating babies cannot prevent. At-risk groups can be offered the vaccine selectively. The hep B vaccine has been associated with serious side-effects (see below).

The change in policy

Up until 2017, the UK had a policy of selective immunisation of those at highest risk (including injecting drug uses, sex workers, those with multiple sexual partners and close family contacts of someone infected) and universal antenatal screening and immunisation of babies born to infected mothers.

There has been continued debate over how successful the policy of targeting at-risk groups has been, and whether all children should be vaccinated. Some argue that many people at risk, particularly injecting drug users, sex workers and prisoners, are not being vaccinated. Vaccinating all children would offer greater protection to all, including these at-risk groups. It has been argued that it would be more 'cost-effective' than 'selective' vaccination; it is, after all, much simpler to vaccinate everyone, especially in childhood, than to go out and try to find those at risk.[7]

The Department of Health (DoH) defended its eminently sensible policy for many years but eventually succumbed to the drive to mass vaccination, in line with WHO wishes. Despite recommending against routine 'universal immunisation' in both 1997 and 2000, the JCVI, by 2005, was becoming enthusiastic about introducing hep B vaccination into the childhood programme.[8,9] The 'cost-effective' option of a 6-in-1 vaccine was finally decided upon.

What is hepatitis B?

Hepatitis means inflammation of the liver. There are a number of viruses that can infect the liver and cause it to become diseased. As these viruses were discovered so they were named A, B, C etc. Hepatitis A is the commonest in many countries, including the UK. It is caught by eating contaminated food or water.[10]

Hepatitis B is different. It is only caught from intimate contact with an infected person. It is nearly always transmitted by blood or sex, but can very rarely be caught through saliva. However, it is a more serious disease than hepatitis A. Some people who become infected go on to become long-term carriers of the virus, often remaining infectious. The hepatitis B virus can, after many years, cause severe liver damage and even liver cancer in some sufferers.

The global picture

In much of the world hepatitis B is a major problem. In many poor areas of the world, including most of Africa and Asia, the majority of children become infected with the virus. Up to half of these children remain persistently infected (though usually quite well in themselves for many years), and some will eventually die from liver cancer or liver failure as a result of their hepatitis B infection. Over the world there are around 400 million people infected with the virus and each year it causes over half a million deaths.[11]

The UK picture

The picture in the UK is very different. Here, hepatitis B is not a common disease, and is particularly rare in children. Between six and nine children in England contract hepatitis B every year. The main risk factors for contracting the virus are injecting drug use and homosexual intercourse.

How is hepatitis B transmitted?

There are two main ways that hep B can be caught — through blood and sex.[12]

Blood

By far the most common form of transmission in the UK is by injecting drugs and sharing a needle with someone with the disease. Blood given in hospital has for many years been tested for hep B and so should not now be a cause of the disease. It is possible to catch the disease if the blood of someone infected gets into direct contact with another person's blood, such as in a needle-stick injury, but this is rare. The largest single group of those contracting hep B in the UK is injecting drug users.

Sex

Sex is the second most common method of catching hep B. The risk is higher for sex between gay men and for unprotected sex.

So, if nearly all hep B is caught from sex or blood (and that mainly through drug users' needles), why are children at risk from the disease?

Well they're not — at least in the UK. However, a very few children do get infected with the hep B virus every year. So how do they catch it?

How do children catch hepatitis B?
By close contact with someone else in the family who carries the infection. This could be by sharing toothbrushes or cutlery, especially if there are any sores or ulcers in the mouth, or if the gums are bleeding. The disease can probably, though extremely rarely, be caught through saliva so it may be possible for a child to catch hep B from another child by playing with the same toy in their mouths.[13,14] However, infected children have shared nurseries, and played with the same toys, with other children, without their catching the disease, so if infection through saliva does occur it is certainly very rare, at least in the UK.[15]

By infection from the mother around birth: If the mother is a carrier of the hep B virus, then she can infect her baby either in the womb or, more commonly, at the time of birth. This is a common method of infection in much of the world but is extremely rare in the UK, occurring in about two babies a year.

The consequences of catching hepatitis B
Most people who catch hep B will, some weeks or even months after becoming infected, start to feel unwell, lose their appetite, feel sick and maybe suffer from abdominal pain. Some will become jaundiced, causing their skin (and especially the white of the eyes) to turn yellow. The vast majority (over 95%) will then make a complete recovery.[16] However, and this is the problem, a small number (2 to 5%) do not eliminate the virus and remain infectious.[17] They remain 'carriers'. Though they are likely to remain well in themselves for many years, they are able to pass the virus on to others via sex or blood. Eventually, maybe after between 20 and 40 years, between a quarter and a third will develop serious liver disease (cirrhosis) or liver cancer from which they are likely to die.[18]

Newborn babies have a hugely variable chance of catching the disease from their mothers at birth, ranging from 10% to 90% depending on how infectious their mother is.[19] However, many will become long-term carriers of the virus. Though most will remain well for decades, some will succumb to liver disease or cancer at some stage in their adult lives.[20] But, even though this is a large problem worldwide, only one or two babies a year are born with the virus in the UK.

Treatment for hep B has progressed over recent years and there are now reasonably effective treatments available for those with progressive disease.

The vaccine
The first hep B vaccine was made from the blood of people infected with hep B. This was introduced in the early 1980s. Being made from blood, it had the disadvantage that it could occasionally transmit infections, from the person from whom the blood was obtained, to the recipient of the vaccine. This was replaced after a few years by a vaccine made from part of the hep B virus grown on yeast — the first genetically engineered vaccine.[21]

Both sides claim the moral high ground
Both those who are for, and those who are against, vaccination of all children

claim to have a strong moral or ethical argument to support their case. The BMA argues that 'where a potentially devastating disease is easily preventable, those at potential risk should be protected' and then state that immunisation of all children is the only way to do this. It has also been argued that the current policy is stigmatising because it focuses on at-risk groups who are already marginalised in our society.[5] Others argue that a vaccine with known side effects should not be given to all children in order to protect the few who put themselves at risk, by choosing risky lifestyle behaviours such as injecting drug use and unsafe sexual practices. What's more, very few of all the children vaccinated will ever be at risk from catching the disease themselves.

Is the illness serious and common enough to warrant vaccination?

This section does not apply those countries where the disease is common such as much of Asia, Africa and the Middle East. It applies to the UK and other areas where the disease is uncommon, such as Western Europe, North America, Australia and New Zealand.

Is the illness serious?

It can be. For those catching the illness, there is a chance, ranging from around 1% in adults to 90% in children born with highly infectious mothers, of becoming a long-term 'carrier'. This, in turn, carries a 25-30% risk of developing liver failure (because of cirrhosis) or liver cancer, usually some decades later.

Is the illness common?

In the UK – most definitely no. The UK has one of the lowest rates of hep B of anywhere in the world, and most of those who do catch the illness are confined to high-risk groups.

There are between four and five hundred new cases in England every year, but fewer than ten of these are children.

Catching the disease is one thing, but as the vast majority of people catching hep B make a complete recovery, how many die or become seriously ill from the disease? The number of deaths from hep B (the ultimate outcome if severe cirrhosis, liver failure or cancer develop) is around 60 a year. However, the time lag between catching the disease and dying from it is, usually, several decades.

Does the vaccine work?

Widely varying claims of effectiveness have been made for the hep B vaccine, as they have for so many vaccines. The effectiveness of a course of three injections in preventing hep B has been claimed to be as high as 95%, whilst one study found it to be as low as 63%. The vaccine's effectiveness is likely to vary between countries – hep B is widespread in many, which will enable 'natural' boosting of immunity after vaccination. The age at which the vaccine is given may also affect its benefit. On average, it is a moderately effective vaccine of about 80% effectiveness, that is protecting 4 out of every 5 people vaccinated.[22,23,24,25] However, none of the trials performed necessarily apply to UK children living in a very low-risk environment. But how long does this protection last?

To boost or not to boost?

There is a great deal of debate in medical circles about whether a booster dose (or even several booster doses) of the vaccine is needed to maintain protection. The debate hinges on how long protection from an immunisation course lasts. Since the protective effect of every other vaccine falls off over time, it would be most surprising if this did not happen with the hep B vaccine as well. It is especially likely to happen in an area such as the UK where the disease is rare and so the opportunity for 'natural' boosting, by coming across the disease, is very small. Studies have given conflicting results. Different countries have different policies with regard to a booster dose: some give one and some don't. The UK currently plan a course of three doses only, given to babies, with no booster.

Is the vaccine safe?

This is yet another vaccine that was initially introduced with a remarkable lack of long-term safety trials. Most of the studies followed up recipients of the vaccine for only a matter of days, and so were unable to detect any of the longer-term problems, such as multiple sclerosis, which has become a particular concern with this vaccine. In 1997, the JCVI noted that the rate of reporting of adverse reactions, compared with other vaccines, was relatively high, but felt that this may have been because many of those vaccinated were health care workers, including doctors and nurses, who, they felt, would have reported reactions more readily.[8] However, there have been many published case reports of adverse reactions to the hep B vaccine, and it has been described by one vaccine expert as being 'remarkable by the unusual frequency, severity and variety of its hazards.'[26]

Guillain-Barré Syndrome

Guillain-Barré Syndrome (GBS) is a rare auto-immune disorder that causes weakness and paralysis, from which most, but not all, sufferers make a good recovery. It is a suspected side-effect of several vaccines. The hep B vaccine can almost certainly cause GBS in a small number of people.[27,28]

Multiple Sclerosis

The biggest area of concern surrounding the hep B vaccine is its probable association with multiple sclerosis (MS), an uncommon but serious auto-immune disease causing progressive weakness, unsteadiness and, sometimes, paralysis. Concern was first raised in France where doctors reported about 200 cases of MS following hep B vaccination in 1996.[29] This caused the French government to stop vaccinating schoolchildren in 1998.[30] Though the vaccine has not been reinstated for schoolchildren, France continues to recommend hep B vaccination for young children soon after birth but take-up by parents has been low. There are numerous research papers examining the possible link between the vaccine and MS; two French studies found a 50% increase in the risk of MS during the two months after hep B vaccination.[31,32] However, other studies did not show any link,[33,34] possibly because of poor study design.[35,36,37] A large study based on UK general practice records is one of the most thorough to date. One feature of this study is that it looks at the date that someone first developed any symptoms of MS, rather than the date the diagnosis was made — which can be many months later. It showed that people vaccinated against hep B were three times more likely to develop MS in the three years after vaccination than those who had not been given the vaccine. This study showed the increased risk in adults (who have been the main recipients of the vaccine in the UK) rather than children, at whom the vaccine is now being targeted. However, if the vaccine is causing this sort of problem in adults, it would be negligent to assume that something similar may not happen in children with their less mature immune systems.[38] However, to add to the confusion, a more recent study was not able to find a link between the vaccine and MS.[39] Two people have been awarded damages in the USA vaccine damage claims court for having had MS caused by the hep B vaccine.

Around 5,000 people are diagnosed with MS every year in the UK.[40] Around a third of these will eventually die from the disease. It is possible that vaccinating every child could cause many more cases.

It has been suggested that neurologists have been reluctant to diagnose MS in anyone who has been given a hep B vaccination.[49]

'Before GPs and practice nurses rush off in droves to cover themselves against hepatitis B litigation, and before doctors give the say-so for the next cleaner / childminder / classroom assistant to have hepatitis B vaccination as a condition of employment, they may wish to consider that I was a perfectly fit, active and well GP before what subsequently proved to be my first attack of MS in 1989, 10 days after my second hep B jab.'
Dr F M Cogan, GP in Oldham[41]

Other side-effects

The hep B vaccine also appears to cause several other immune-related disorders, other than GBS and MS, in susceptible people: these include juvenile diabetes, thrombocytopaenia purpura (a rare bleeding disorder, also caused by the MMR vaccine), optic neuritis (an inflammation of the optic nerve at the back of the eye, causing temporary or permanent blindness, and the most common first sign of MS), rheumatoid arthritis (a chronic, and potentially debilitating, inflammatory arthritis) and SLE (systemic lupus erythematosus).[45,43,44,45] The vaccine can also cause a skin disorder called lichen planus that has also been reported in children receiving the vaccine.[46] It may be a cause of chronic fatigue.[47] Doctors of a twelve-year-old girl who suffered seizures and died after her third dose of the vaccine have warned that, 'vaccination may be the triggering factor for auto-immune and neurological disturbances in genetically predisposed individuals and physicians should be aware of this possible association.'[48] It is possible that auto-immune disease occurring following receipt of the hep B vaccine falls into the recently described 'Auto-immune Syndrome induced by

Adjuvants' (ASIA).[49]

Alarmingly, a study in the impoverished western African country of Guinea-Bissau showed that children who were given hep B vaccination, in addition to measles vaccine, were five times more likely to die between 9 and 12 months compared to those children who only received the measles vaccine.[50] This has disturbing implications as to what this vaccine might be doing to these malnourished children with their inevitably weakened immune systems. It is also a warning about what it could do to our children.

Part of a 6-in-1 vaccine

The new hepatitis B vaccine is given in the UK as part of a combined 6-in-1 vaccine, increasing the number of vaccines given to babies by four months of age to 24. This means that parents who do not wish to give this vaccine to their babies must forgo all the other five vaccines in the combination shot or pay to have some or all of the remaining five vaccines given in smaller doses privately. They are not able simply to leave out this one vaccine, as they can, for example, with the rotavirus vaccine, another vaccine I believe to be unnecessary for the vast majority of children. This is a big problem. A vaccine that is completely irrelevant to nearly all children is in effect being forced onto them, because there is no other easily available option.

Conclusion

The vast majority of the UK population is at very low risk of becoming infected with hepatitis B. As the disease is contracted though blood or sexual contact the risk is particularly small for young children. There are a few groups of people in the UK, nearly all adults, who are at much greater risk of contracting hep B. They include injecting drug users, those with a sexually promiscuous lifestyle (especially gay men), and babies born to infected mothers; all these people should be offered the hep B vaccine. All women should be screened for hepatitis B in pregnancy so that the vaccine, with or without anti-hep B immunoglobulin, can be offered to their babies at birth. There is also a case for vaccinating close family contacts of a hep B carrier, haemophiliacs (who require frequent blood transfusions, even though all blood given in the UK is screened for hep B) and health care workers who come into frequent contact with blood.

The rest of the population, including nearly all children, are at very low risk of getting the disease and do not require vaccination.

The hep B vaccine causes more reactions, some of which are serious, than most vaccines.

It is nonsensical to vaccinate all babies against a disease fewer than ten children in the UK contract a year. The vaccine should be offered to those who need it — not to those who don't.

28
Vaccines and Big Pharma

Profit ahead of the Public Good

Vaccines were regarded for many years as bad business for the pharmaceutical industry. In 1990, the British company, Wellcome, announced it was stopping research into, and manufacture of, vaccines because there was, 'too much litigation and too little profit'.[1] The change over recent decades has been astounding, and today the story is very different: vaccines have become big business, and are now the fastest growing sector of Big Pharma (the pharmaceutical industry).

Billion-dollar vaccine
Prevenar, the pneumococcal vaccine made by Wyeth, became the world's first blockbuster vaccine; it generated over $1 billion in annual sales in 2004, rising to $3 billion by 2009 when Wyeth was taken over by drug giant Pfizer who aggressively marketed the vaccine around the world. Pfizer's revamped Prevenar 13 went on to reach sales of over $6 billion by 2015.

The profitability of vaccines has not been limited to blockbusters like Prevenar. All the major multinational vaccine manufacturers reported large increases in income from vaccines in their 2007 annual reports, with vaccines being their fastest growing products. By 2014 the global vaccines market had grown to $33 billion and is projected to grow to $41 billion by 2021.

The Race to Market Supremacy
The Human Papilloma Virus (HPV) causes nearly all cases of cancer of the cervix (neck of the womb) in women. The discovery of a HPV vaccine promised the first ever vaccine to prevent cancer — and the potential of huge profits for the successful manufacturer. Two of the world's pharmaceutical giants, the USA's Merck and the UK's GlaxoSmithKline (GSK), went head to head in the race to get the largest market share for the new HPV vaccine. Though cervical cancer is relatively uncommon in the developed countries that can afford the vaccine, it has been put at the top of the female health agenda, thanks to publicity largely generated by Big Pharma.

Not since the polio vaccine was trialled in 1954, has there been so much hype over the introduction of a new vaccine. However, unlike polio in the 1950s, HPV is neither an emergency nor a crisis. Another difference is that the polio vaccine had an immediate effect in preventing children dying and becoming paralysed, whereas we will not know the true benefits — or risks — of the HPV vaccine for many years, as cervical cancer develops over a long period of time.

Merck won a crucial battle in the race to get a HPV vaccine onto the market when, in July 2006, it became the first to get its vaccine, Gardasil, licensed in the USA; this was followed by a European license in September of the same year. The vaccine was approved for use in countries throughout the world at unprecedented speed. It was quickly incorporated into national immunisation schedules, despite being one of the most expensive vaccines ever made, costing $125 per dose ($375 for a course); the new meningitis B vaccine, Bexsero, is only slightly less expensive.

GSK had to play catch-up, being granted a European license for its rival vaccine, Cervarix, in September 2007, a year after its rivals; GSK have so far been unable to get Cervarix licensed for use in the USA, where it was not approved until late 2009.

Merck was the clear winner in the early sales battle. In 2007, sales for Gardasil were $1.5 billion compared to Cervarix's £10 million ($18 million).

Merck pursued an aggressive marketing campaign for Gardasil, lobbying state legislatures across the USA in an attempt to have the use of its vaccine made compulsory. During 2007, 24 USA states introduced legislation to mandate the vaccine as a condition for school entry; however by the end of the year only Virginia and Washington DC had passed the laws, with a provision for opt out.

Women in Government, a non-partisan organisation of female legislators across the USA that receives corporate donations from Merck, lobbied lawmakers on HPV vaccination.

Merck's award-winning advertising has promoted the vaccine. Before the film 'Sex and the City,' some moviegoers in the United States saw ads for Gardasil. On YouTube, and in advertisements on popular TV shows, a multi-ethnic cast of young professionals urged girls to become 'one less statistic' by getting vaccinated.

The vaccine makers have brought attention to cervical cancer by providing money for activities by patients' and women's groups, doctors and medical experts, lobbyists and political organisations interested in the disease. There has been a proliferation of cervical cancer awareness conferences and campaigns, sponsored by scientific and patient groups financed by Merck and GSK. It is not always apparent that supposedly expert advice has been paid for by the vaccine manufacturers.[2]

A campaign fronted by doctors and celebrities to persuade European governments, including the UK, to vaccinate all girls against HPV was entirely funded by Sanofi Pasteur MSD, the company that markets Gardasil in Europe. The company spent millions on what was billed 'the first global summit against cervical cancer', which was held in Paris. The organizers, the Club Européen de la Santé, agreed to participate only on condition that Sanofi Pasteur paid.

The summit, which resembled a political rally, called for country-wide vaccination programmes.[3]

Marketing was no less aggressive in Canada, where Merck lobbyists with connections to both the prime minister and the Ontario health minister were working behind the scenes to get the vaccine paid for out of the public purse. The Canadian government promised $C300 million ($258m, £131m) to fund HPV vaccination programmes across the country. The decision was praised by the Society of Obstetricians and Gynaecologists of Canada, itself a recipient of a $1.5 million grant from Merck.[4]

GSK was guilty of promoting its vaccine, Cervarix, before it had been approved by the regulators. After lagging behind Merck in most of the world, GSK received a boost in June 2008 when the UK bucked the trend and chose the UK company's Cervarix for its national immunisation campaign, which started in September 2008.

Leap of faith

What has been happening with HPV is that the drug companies have been investing huge amounts of money marketing a vaccine that no-one will know for 20 years whether it does what it is meant to – that is, protect against cervical cancer. Never before has a vaccine been introduced around the world on such a large scale with so little testing of the vaccine's safety and effectiveness. The vaccine was introduced without knowing how long any protection will last; whether one or more booster doses will be needed – generating further profit for the manufacturers; whether it will ultimately prevent cases of cervical cancer; and with little knowledge about long-term safety. Cervical cancer is not a pandemic sweeping the world, requiring immediate and urgent attention; the 900 or so deaths caused by cervical cancer every year in the UK are, of course, important, but are dwarfed by the 39,000 women who die every year in the UK from heart disease, the 31,00 who die from strokes, and over 11,000 who die from each of lung cancer, breast cancer and lung disease.

In addition, the UK already has a highly effective screening programme for cervical cancer, and the alleged added benefit of the HPV vaccine in preventing cervical cancer, when compared to high-coverage regular screening, is questionable.[5,6] Indeed, the rushed introduction of the vaccine may actually worsen HPV-related illness by undermining the successful screening programme, leaving women less, rather than more, protected.'The manufacturers know this,' claims Dr Angela Raffle, a consultant responsible for the screening of a million women in the West Country, 'so, to sell the vaccination in countries such as the UK, they are busily branding HPV as a new disease, undermining national policymaking by running promotional 'stakeholder' meetings in every locality, planting press stories to create a smoke screen – implying that the real barrier to protecting our daughters is unjustified prudishness – and securing promotional articles in prestigious journals such as the *Lancet*. Rushed policymaking will have disastrous consequences; we must use these vaccines wisely.'[7]

But nothing could stop the hype; an editorial in the prestigious *Lancet* even went as far as to call for compulsory vaccination for all 11-12 year old girls throughout the European Union.[8]

The importance of testing for long-term safety has been forgotten in the perceived urgency to introduce the vaccine: 'We have to take a leap of faith that the vaccine will be safe,' said the Royal College of GPs spokeswoman on women's health.[9] The introduction of new vaccines is best done scientifically with good research — not leaps of faith.

Latest blockbuster

The vaccine widely tipped to be the next blockbuster is GSK's Bexsero, the prohibitively expensive meningitis B vaccine. The UK JCVI originally recommended that the vaccine would not be cost-effective at any price for inclusion in the children's immunization schedule. After extensive lobbying by interest groups supported by the vaccine's manufacturer, the JVCI performed a U-turn and agreed to recommend the vaccine for all children in the UK. Other countries are likely to follow suit and it is predicted that yearly sales for the vaccine will rise to over $350million a year.

Opinion leaders

'Key opinion leaders' are important to pharmaceutical companies; these are senior and influential doctors who help drug companies sell their products. They are engaged by the industry to help boost sales, and are paid large fees to peddle their influence in the medical community. These respected doctors are paid over one thousand pounds for a single lecture, often largely based on slides provided by the company; some earn over £13,000 a year in advisory fees. Dr Angela Raffle, a public health specialist who oversaw screening in the west of England was asked to be an 'opinion leader' to help promote the HPV vaccine, being offered £1,000 to attend meetings. She declined, appalled at the lobbying tactics of the pharmaceutical companies in Britain. Many other doctors were happy to accept payments to promote the vaccine.

There was no justification for the rushed introduction of the widespread use of the HPV vaccine into so many countries; the only reason for this was the race between the two competing manufacturers to win the majority of the billions of dollars a year that these vaccines bring in income. The unseemly haste with which these vaccines were introduced is at the price of inadequate knowledge about their safety and effectiveness. The greed for profit has triumphed over the public good.

The pervasiveness of Big Pharma

Opinion leaders are just the tip of the iceberg. Many of the doctors working on powerful committees that influence government policy have links with the vaccine manufacturers.

The Joint Committee on Vaccination and Immunisation (JCVI) is a committee of experts who advise the government on vaccination policy. The committee is extremely influential, as its recommendations are usually adopted. Commercial organisations — most likely vaccine manufacturers — have attempted to influence the committee's decisions.[10] Several of its members have financial interests, either personally or through their work, with vaccine manufacturers. More specifically, a majority of members of the HPV subcommittee, that recommended the widespread introduction of the HPV vaccine, had financial ties with either or both of the two manufacturers of the vaccine.

Scientists depend on funding to pursue their research, and this financial support is difficult to attract from public sources. The wealthy pharmaceutical companies fund a large proportion of medical research done in the UK and other developed countries. There have been disturbing stories of drug companies keeping unfavourable research under wraps for fear that its release would endanger sales. Doctors who do research on behalf of drug companies are aware that unwelcome results may make the drug company think twice about channelling further funds in the same direction.[11] Much of the research demonstrating vaccine safety has been funded by the drug companies themselves; whilst much of this research will be honestly and appropriately undertaken, it is known that research funded by industry is more likely to reach conclusions favourable to the drug companies.[12]

Speak out at your peril

Dr Andrew Gunn is a doctor who works at the University of Queensland in Australia. He criticised the promotion of Gardasil on radio, describing it as a 'marketing juggernaut'.[13] The problem was that Dr Gunn was an employee of the University of Queensland that had worked jointly with drug company Commonwealth Serum Laboratories (CSL) to develop the HPV vaccine. The vaccine brings in millions of Australian dollars annually to the university. CSL took offence to Dr Gunn's comments and wrote to the University's Vice Chancellor to complain. Instead of defending the doctor's academic freedom to express himself, the University wrote to Dr Gunn, asking him to apologise to CSL. Following strong criticism from academics in Australia and around the world, the University withdrew its demand for an apology. The real issue here is money, and Peter Brooks, the university's dean of health sciences, admitted as much. 'If you've got very large amounts of money changing hands, then it's very difficult, I think, not to let that influence you to some extent,' he said. 'It's a dilemma that universities have'. The problem is that many, if not most, large universities around the globe receive substantial funding from drug companies, making it difficult for all of them not to be influenced by Big Pharma.

*

New markets

Large developing countries like India, China and Brazil are viewed as fertile ground for the marketing of vaccines. However, doctors from the developing world resent being recipients of a scheme imposed, as they see it, by wealthy nations which will result in their being dependent on a technological fix (vaccinations) largely controlled by powerful western multinational companies. Though this approach may be suited to developed nations, it is not necessarily appropriate for poorer countries. They argue that true primary health care, in which people are cared for locally, using socioculturally acceptable and sustainable technology, with health care decisions being made locally,[14] is undermined by a 'prepacked overpriced inappropriate and irrelevant package of medical technologies and thrusting them on the people.'[15]

The vaccine manufacturers cannot be trusted to promote the most appropriate or suitable vaccines. GSK has been accused of inappropriately and unethically marketing their chickenpox vaccine (not promoted by GAVI or WHO) in India. Radio advertisements implied that not giving children the vaccine would lead to significant school absenteeism and thus poor academic performance, and that parents would be negligent not to vaccinate their children.[16]

A profitable future

In the financial markets, vaccines are 'hot'. The vaccine market is already the fastest growing sector in the pharmaceutical business, and the future looks even rosier. The global vaccine market trebled from $6 billion in 2000 to $17 billion in 2008 and continued to grow rapidly to $33 billion in 2014. It is expected to rise to well over $40 billion by 2021. The sales of children's and adolescent vaccines are expected to grow fourfold over the next decade. The success of 'premium priced products' such as Prevenar and the HPV vaccines has shown that the drug companies can charge high prices for vaccines and still sell them in vast quantities. There will be no looking back while vaccine manufacturers are private companies whose remit is to make profit. Under these circumstances we can expect commercial decisions to be made that will not necessarily be in the public interest. There is an argument for vaccine development and manufacture to be state owned. Perhaps only then will the needs of the public's health be placed ahead of the drive for profit.

29
The Developing World

Death by Vaccination

Guinea-Bissau is a small country in West Africa about the size of Belgium. It became independent from its Portuguese colonisers in 1974, since when it's undergone more than its share of military coups and civil wars. Fighting and social upheaval have caused Guinea-Bissau to become one of the world's poorest countries. The average life expectancy is little more than fifty years, and one in five children dies before reaching five years of age. It would appear to be a country crying out for the benefits of immunisation.

The world vaccine community was shaken in 2000, when research was published which showed that children in Guinea-Bissau, given routine vaccinations, were more, rather than less, likely to die over the subsequent six months. Some of the vaccines they received were clearly doing good. The measles vaccine appeared to be hugely beneficial, halving the chance of dying, whilst receiving a TB vaccine also reduced the chance of a baby dying by 28% during the six-month period following vaccination. But receiving either the triple DTP jab, or polio drops, increased the likelihood of death by between 38% and 84%.[1]

Taking into account that vaccinated children were already likely to be better nourished, and living in more sanitary conditions, these findings become even more alarming. The results of this study threatened to undermine the global DTP vaccination programme, which the World Health Organisation (WHO) describes as 'one of the most successful and cost-effective health interventions ever.'[2]

The WHO sent out two experts to Guinea-Bissau to investigate, but they were unable to find anything to invalidate the study. Instead they concluded that the results 'demand an immediate response.'[3] Despite this, WHO remained highly critical of the study, and defended its vaccination policy.[4] The study's Danish authors stood by their results, calling for urgent research into the effect of vaccinations on child mortality.[5]

Some further research has since been undertaken — in Guinea-Bissau, Senegal, Gambia, the Congo, Benin and Malawi — all of which verifies the increase in death rate of children who have been given the triple DTP vaccine.[6,7,8,9,10] The problem appears to be particularly severe for baby girls born with a low birthweight: those given the triple DTP vaccine early, who were <u>better</u> nourished than the baby girls who did not receive the early vaccine (and therefore less likely to die), were <u>five times</u> more likely to be dead by 6 months compared to the less well-nourished baby girls who received the vaccine at the normal time.[46] The only consolation was the confirmation that the measles vaccine was saving lives beyond what one would have expected from preventing measles alone. WHO has continued to defend the DTP vaccine, hoping to 'set the matter aside'.[11]

Further disturbing news surfaced in 2004, with the publication of research into the effects of hepatitis B vaccine given to babies in Guinea-Bissau where, like in many other developing countries, the disease is a big health problem. Babies given the vaccine were twice as likely to die before their first birthday than children not given the vaccine.[12] DTP and hep B are two of the most widely used vaccines around the world. But if they're causing more deaths in the developing world than they're preventing, something is going seriously wrong.

A world without vaccines

A group of people with vested interests in vaccines that has occasionally been mentioned is the international health community, and in particular the World Health Organisation (WHO). The organisation was founded after the Second World War in 1948 on a wave of post-war optimism and the desire to do great works with the new technology and wealth that the Western countries were accumulating ahead of the developing world. Vaccines have always been one of its most popular forms of medical intervention in the developing world, as they offer an appealing technological fix that can be centrally controlled. Now nearly seventy years old, it is an organisation whose importance has grown throughout the world. Its finest hour was in 1979 when it declared smallpox eradicated as a result of its aggressive vaccination policy. It is no wonder that it has since tried to replicate this success.

The WHO rightly refers repeatedly in its published aims to the necessity of an 'evidence base' to guide its policies and strategies.[2] It is often argued that vaccines are more important and of greater benefit in the developing world than in the West. Whereas infections result in relatively few deaths in the West, they are a major cause of death elsewhere. Vaccines, the argument goes, are able to stem the haemorrhaging death rates.

What does the evidence say after more than half a century?

Nearly half of all deaths worldwide of children under five years old occur in babies less than four weeks old. The majority of these are caused by premature births, breathing difficulties, or severe infection. Respiratory infections (mainly pneumonia) are the second most common cause of death in children under five, closely followed by diarrhoeal illnesses. The most common cause of death, for which a vaccine is widely available, is measles which caused 1% of all deaths of children under five in 2015 despite widespread vaccination.

Of all the deaths caused by infections, there are six potentially 'vaccine-preventable' ones. Though figures are necessarily approximate, because of the difficulty in collecting information throughout much of the world, the six 'vaccine-preventable' diseases cause the deaths of over two and a half million children – around a quarter of all deaths in the under-fives.

There are over one and a half million deaths worldwide caused by vaccine preventable diseases every year, though many have been falling over recent years. There has, for example, been a 79% drop in measles deaths from 2000 to 2015.

'Vaccine-preventable' illness	Number of deaths globally	
Pneumococcal disease	500,000	(2015)
Measles	134,000	(2015)
Rotavirus	215,000	(2013)
Hib	200,000	(2008)
Whooping cough	195,000	(2008)
Neonatal tetanus	180,000	(2012)

If it is true that mass immunisation is introduced in the West without the proper controls that apply to other medication, then this has always been the case for the developing world. There are unproven allegations that a catastrophic measles epidemic was caused in 1968 by inoculating South American Indians with a dangerous vaccine for trialling purposes. Similar allegations exist with regards to the cause of AIDS as a result of a vaccine trial (vociferously denied by the leading doctors involved in the trials); and an epidemic of encephalitis cases occurring in Salvador after the withdrawn Urabe mumps-vaccine was shipped over to Brazil. Whether such stories are true or not, as a rule vaccines have been introduced into developing countries with no proof, in the form of controlled trials, that they save lives, or that they are safe.[13,14,15]

The main evidence for success has come from 'observational' data. If cases, or deaths, from a disease fall after the introduction of a vaccine, it is assumed this has happened because of the vaccine. A recent trial, for example, from the Gambia showed an impressively large and rapid fall in Hib disease after the introduction of, and probably caused by, the vaccine.[16]

A possible problem with this approach is shown by the experience of Nigeria. Following increased vaccination, there was a drop in the numbers of measles and whooping cough cases. But this drop was accompanied by similar falls in cases of chickenpox and dysentery, for which no vaccines were given. This casts doubt on whether the decreases were caused by vaccination, or whether they would have happened anyway.[17]

Another study showed that children who received the triple DTP vaccination in Bangladesh were less likely to die than those children who didn't get the vaccine. It also showed that the more doses of the vaccine that a child received, the greater the chances of survival – convincing stuff.[18] However, the study was vulnerable to the criticism that those babies who were vaccinated were more likely to have come from families with better educated mothers, and were more likely to have had contact with the health care system, making their babies' chances of survival better, irrespective of whether they had received vaccinations or not.[1]

Non-specific effects

Other research shows that some vaccines appear to offer unexpected benefits or harms. This is called 'non-specific effect' of vaccination. Beneficial effects have been seen most often with measles immunisation, which appears to offer children a 30-86% reduction in overall death rate, though those who survived natural measles infection also benefited from better survival than those who didn't catch measles.

Vaccination against TB has also been found to save more lives than expected solely from preventing TB, and that is in addition to its apparent ability to prevent leprosy.

These vaccines, it seems, may offer some extra benefit beyond protection against any specific disease. The effect is so pronounced for measles vaccinations, particularly – but inexplicably – in girls rather than boys, that it's been suggested measles vaccination should continue even if the disease were eradicated. It is noteworthy that both these vaccines are live and so have a tendency to stimulate the immune system in a healthy (Th1) direction and may enhance the child's resistance to other unrelated infections.

However, medical research can be frustratingly contradictory, because, back in Bangladesh, babies given the TB vaccine were twice as likely to die as those not given the vaccine. The problem with much of the research showing extra benefit from vaccination is that it's vulnerable to the same criticism as the research from Bangladesh on the DTP vaccine. Children that receive any vaccines have already got a head start on those who aren't vaccinated. They're more likely to be better nourished; have fewer brothers and sisters; have younger and better educated mothers; come from communities with sanitary toilets.[1]

In other words, even before being vaccinated, these children are the ones most likely to survive, which makes it all but impossible to distinguish between the effects of the vaccines and the results of better social conditions.[19,20,21]

Non-specific effects are not confined to developing countries. The likelihood of a child in Denmark being admitted to hospital for an infection are over 60% higher if the most recent vaccine they received is the 5-in-1 DTaP-IPV-Hib rather than the MMR.[49]

The dangers of mass immunisation in the developing world

Two of the most widely used vaccines around the world, DTP and hep B, both appear to be causing more deaths than they are preventing, highlighting the negative side of 'non-specific effects.' Around twice as many children who receive the DTP vaccine die compared to those who are do not receive it. How could vaccines such as the triple DTP vaccine (used in the UK for over forty years until 2004 when it was replaced by a '5-in-1') actually be causing deaths, instead of saving lives? This question is crucial, because it is, after all, generally assumed that these disadvantaged children are the very ones to benefit most from vaccination.

There are several reasons why giving widespread vaccinations might be problematic in developing countries, and why the success of vaccination varies from country to country, or even between regions within a country.

Malnourishment increases the likelihood of side-effects. Poverty, poor sanitation and inadequate food make children's immune systems more vulnerable to disease, but they may also make them more susceptible to vaccine side-effects. In addition, the conditions in which the vaccines are given (often in mass immunisation campaigns) make it particularly difficult for health workers to check for reasons not to immunise (contra-indications), such as a child having a fever, which increases the risks of reactions.

Twelve billion injections are given annually around the world. Of these, around 5%, or 600 million, are vaccinations. Between 30% and 90% of childhood vaccinations given in developing countries aren't sterile, and are therefore 'unsafe.'[22] This means they may have been contaminated and could transmit diseases such as HIV/AIDS, hepatitis B, hepatitis C or malaria to children. The WHO attributes half a million deaths annually to unsafe injections, though only a proportion of these are vaccinations.[23] Unsafe injections are probably responsible for 8-16 million cases annually of hepatitis B, for which there is a vaccine used in most countries of the world given by...injection.[24] Unsafe injections may be responsible for more transmission of HIV/AIDS in Africa than unsafe sex.[25]

As happened in the fifties in Britain, injections can trigger paralysis in children incubating polio. Around two million children may have developed paralytic polio in India during the 1980s as a direct result of a massive DTP vaccination campaign.[26]

What is also true is that vaccines known to be less safe are still widely used, particularly in the developing world. The live oral polio vaccine (given as drops) which can cause polio paralysis itself is thankfully now being phased out as polio is — hopefully — nearing extinction. The whole-cell pertussis (whooping cough) vaccine, part of the DTP, can cause brain damage, a reaction that may be more common in malnourished, vulnerable children. The safer killed polio and 'acellular' whooping cough vaccines now used in the UK have been prohibitively expensive for use in much of the world. Mercury, for example, has been removed from most routine vaccines used in wealthy countries, but remains a component of vaccines used in the developing world. Also this book has revealed the potential danger of aluminium in vaccines; malnourished children may be more susceptible to this.

It also seems that the DTP vaccine, for no explicable reason, might increase the chances of dying from pneumonia, wound infections and diarrhoea.

These factors don't fully explain the disparity in effects between different vaccinations, but the triple DTP vaccine, used in most of the developing world, does contain mercury, aluminium and the less safe whole-cell whooping cough component.

As with other vaccines, measles immunisation has a similar story of partial success. The WHO has, since 1974, promoted the use of measles vaccination throughout the world. This has contributed to a 79% fall in deaths from measles between 2000 and 2015 by which time 85% of all children were receiving a measles vaccine. During the first few years of the 21st century, massive vaccination campaigns in southern Africa contributed to a large fall in measles cases. This is in addition to the vaccine's 'non-specific' benefits.

However, measles vaccination is not an unqualified success story. Vaccine effectiveness in Uganda was found to be only 74% — rather lower than expected, and a high number of children in Nigeria are still contracting measles despite being vaccinated.[27,50] Researchers in Khartoum, in Sudan, also questioned the effectiveness of measles vaccination after they discovered the disease was widespread in the city, and that 59% of children seen with measles had been vaccinated — a proportion not much less than the estimated 70% of the childhood population that had received the vaccine. They write, 'control and elimination of measles will be especially difficult in East Africa.'[28] These concerns have been reinforced by the discovery that at least one wild African measles virus appears to be becoming resistant to the vaccine.[29] Other experts are also pessimistic: 'Though the measles elimination programmes have been very effective in the Americas... global eradication... is likely to be an insurmountable task in the rest of the world.'[30]

In the meantime, 12 years after they first described the negative 'non-specific' effects of the DTP vaccine, the same Danish researchers were still concerned that the WHO were neglecting to pay sufficient regard to their findings and wrote, despairingly, 'the inconsistency between the evidence and current policy is unacceptable...no official initiative has been taken to resolve the contradictions' — strong words for a scientific paper.[46]

This discovery of 'non-specific effects of vaccines' — both positive, as with the measles vaccine, and negative, with the DTP vaccine — has triggered a major debate amongst vaccine specialists. By 2013 the Danish researchers were becoming increasingly frustrated: 'Non-specific effects of vaccines have been dismissed or ignored because they are difficult to explain biologically', they wrote before pleading, 'In our opinion it is now urgent that we explore the effects of vaccines in a more systematic and open-minded manner.'[48] Everyone appears to agree that further trials need to be done urgently, but no-one is coming up with the money and, in the meantime, children are dying from being vaccinated inappropriately.

One size fits all

Infectious diseases are rarely a major public health problem unless they are able to thrive in conditions of poverty, malnutrition and poor sanitation. An immune system that is in a good condition can cope with many more infections than when it is impaired. This effect is strengthened where a population has few members in a weakened condition. The steep decline in the number of deaths from measles, TB (tuberculosis) and whooping cough in the UK and other developed countries, long before the introduction of vaccination, bears testimony to how improving social conditions makes infectious diseases much less harmful.

Vaccination, therefore, is not the only — or necessarily the best — way to prevent deaths from infectious diseases. In the case of measles, malnutrition in general and vitamin A deficiency in particular, contribute to the high death rate in the developing world. Giving children with measles two doses of vitamin A can reduce the death rate from measles by 82%.[31]

In fact, preventive vitamin A supplementation, with or without zinc, is more cost-effective at reducing deaths from measles than vaccination.[32,33] The cost of vitamin A supplementation, for each life saved from measles in developing countries, is $95 compared with $850 for immunisation.[34] Twice yearly supplementation with vitamin A has the added benefit that it can reduce the death rate of children under five by 23%. Additional research suggests that vitamin A does not merely rectify vitamin A deficiency but also may have a direct effect on the immune system.

There can also be hidden benefits to letting diseases run their course instead of preventing them. Though measles vaccine appears to offer extra benefits, so also, it seems, does getting the illness.[35] In Senegal, children who caught, and survived, measles were subjected to only one fifth of the deaths of children who hadn't had measles. Overall, the benefit from vaccination is greater, because of the risk of dying from measles itself in developing countries. However, for those children who survive, an attack may confer an even greater benefit than vaccination.[36]

The biggest obstacles to children's health are a lack of clean drinking water, unsafe sanitation and inadequate nutrition. Over one billion people lack access to safe drinking water — that is one sixth of the world's inhabitants, or over twice the population of the European Union. More than 2.6 billion people — over 40% of the world's population — don't have access to basic sanitation.

The result is that over three quarters of a million children die from diarrhoea every year — more than die from any 'vaccine-preventable' disease. Unsafe water, sanitation and hygiene cause 95% of the diarrhoeal deaths in children under 5 years of age worldwide. One of the most common of these infections is caused by the rotavirus, for which new vaccines have been developed. However, children around the world are more likely to receive vaccinations than have access to clean water and safe sanitation.[37,38] More children are vaccinated against TB than have access to clean drinking water. In addition, DTP, polio and measles vaccines reach many more families than does safe sanitation.

Providing children with safe water and sanitation would save over three quarters of a million children's lives, more than by increasing the coverage of the WHO's currently recommended vaccines to 100% throughout the world — and without the side-effects. Instead of focusing on one disease at a time, such an approach would aim to improve the general physical condition of children.

Lack of access to clean water by one sixth of the world's population contributes to other problems, too. Though the number of babies dying from tetanus has decreased dramatically from 800,000 in the late 1980s to 180,000 in 2002, it remains an important cause of death in newborn babies in many countries. It's caused by contamination of the baby's umbilical cord with dirt — from unwashed hands or a dirty knife, or from the application of cow dung to the cut cord. Though vaccination can prevent tetanus, so can simple cleanliness — ensuring the hands and instruments used at the birth are properly washed.

Malnutrition itself causes 3.1 million deaths of children under the age of five every year. It is the underlying cause of over half of all deaths in under-five year olds around the world. More than a quarter of all children in developing countries are underweight, and therefore at increased risk of an early death.

All the while there is a scarcity of organisation in the developing world. Even if vaccination were the correct approach, the difficulties of implementing this strategy around the world are summed up by a VSO health development advisor: 'Immunisation requires a degree of organisation that exists only with external input: sterilisation, materials, vehicles and fuel, refrigeration, portable ice boxes, maintenance, trained staff, and vaccines or serum samples. Such operations are intrinsically unsustainable in certain environments.'[39]

A disastrous consequence of a catastrophic mistake made in a chaotic environment was the deaths of at least 15 young children in 2014 in war-torn Syria after being given measles vaccines mixed with atracurium, a deadly muscle relaxant used in surgery, instead of water. Sadly, this kind of mistake happens far too often.

In the developing world scarce resources are now prioritised for vaccination. Intensive vaccination campaigns are being undertaken in attempts to eradicate infectious diseases such as polio. These immunisation drives inevitably disrupt routine health services, from which they divert precious funds and manpower. Vaccines must often compete for public funds with basic necessities such as clean water and sanitation facilities.

Even where vaccination works, it's all very well protecting children from one disease, but unless the root causes of disease — malnutrition and poor sanitation — are addressed, they will surely die from something else instead.

Bill Gates

Into this arena Bill Gates stepped as a force to be reckoned with, along with his own vested interests in vaccination. The founder of Microsoft, and the world's richest man, was instrumental in setting up the Global Alliance for Vaccines and Immunization (GAVI) in 2000, with other organisations, including WHO and the World Bank.

In 2000 the GAVI proclaimed 'a new type of public-private partnership,' with the laudable aim of 'protecting children of all nations and of all socio-economic levels against vaccine-preventable diseases.'[40] In early 2005, Gates gave $750 million (around £400 million) to GAVI followed swiftly by a promise by UK chancellor Gordon Brown of £960 million over fifteen years. The UK has been one of the most generous donors, second only to the Bill and Melinda Gates Foundation. The UK had given nearly $3 billion by the end of 2013, more than any other country including the USA, and donated nearly $1.5 billion from 2011 to 2015 alone. Since its inception in 2000, GAVI has committed grants, totalling nearly $8.3 billion up to 2017, to seventy-seven developing nations to support their vaccine programmes. GAVI claims to have prevented over 7 million deaths.

However, donations from GAVI to support countries' vaccination programmes are not unconditional. They are awarded on performance-based criteria. Not only that, GAVI has also been criticised for offering countries short-term funding without adequately considering the longer-term consequences. There's financial pressure on extremely poor countries to introduce new vaccines that might not be needed and would be expensive for them to continue once funding from GAVI stops. Less than half the cost of the immunisation programmes of forty-two of the world's countries is funded by those countries' governments. Sixteen countries don't contribute a penny to their own vaccination programmes.[38] Unless the supply of vaccines is sustainable, their short-term use could cause more problems than it solves.[41]

In Ghana, the cost of a dose of vaccine in 2000 had been $0.41. By 2002, this had increased to $3.25 a dose because of the introduction of a new '5-in-1' (DTP/HepB/Hib) vaccine. This is an almost 800% increase. It's questionable whether this is in Ghana's long-term interest.[42]

The expansion of the vaccine programme has raised the cost of purchasing a full vaccine course in a GAVI supported country form £1.37 a year in 2001 $38.80 in 2011. This is all well and good if GAVI is paying the lion's share. But what happens when GAVI pulls out? 16 lower-middle income countries are now 'graduating' from GAVI meaning they will no longer benefit from GAVI subsidies. These countries are concerned over how they will be able to afford to pay for all the vaccines, some of which they may not have themselves prioritised, in the long term. A Kenyan Health official has described adding all the GAVI-promoted vaccines into the national immunization programme as 'taking out multiple mortgages'.

Honduras had the dubious distinction of 'graduating' from GAVI support in 2015. The cost of just two of the vaccines introduced by GAVI, the PCV and rotavirus, shot up from $1.09 to $25.50 per child at a stroke, costing the government over $5 million a year, money that may have been better spent elsewhere.[47] Many other countries will be 'graduating' from GAVI over the coming years.

In India, WHO and GAVI have been accused of 'bullying the government to introduce newer (and expensive) vaccines such as Hepatitis B and the Hib into the routine programme of immunisation in the country.'[43] This allegation is substantiated by a WHO report, which confirms GAVI has set 'milestones' for the implementation of both Hepatitis B and Hib vaccination in many of the poorest countries in the world on, it is argued, little evidence of their benefit.[2]

The introduction of a 5-in-1 vaccine covering diphtheria, tetanus, whooping cough, Hib and hepatitis B remains deeply divisive amongst Indian doctors. More recently the debate has centred on the benefits and disadvantages of the hugely expensive HPV vaccine.

The Hepatitis B vaccination that WHO wants India to introduce is expensive; more expensive in fact than the combined cost of the vaccines for all the other six infections covered by the country's current immunisation programme. In addition, the rates of the disease have been grossly over-estimated. Even if vaccination were introduced, most Hepatitis B is acquired at birth, and can only be prevented by vaccination within 12 hours of birth; this is an unrealistic target in a country where most births occur at home, often far removed from medical supplies.[44]

Bribery is also used. Indian doctors are offered new, and often less essential, vaccines at a large discount which enables them to make a large profit by offering these to patients. GAVI has been pushing the expensive pneumo-coccal vaccine in many poor countries despite the fact that accurate figures for the number of cases of invasive pneumococcal disease (IPD) in these countries are unavailable. Indeed it has been argued that 'the current pneumococcal vaccines have limited effectiveness in developing countries and the hype surrounding them is more commercial than scientific.'[46]

GAVI and WHO are also teaming up in other ways. They have encouraged the rapid introduction of the new rotavirus vaccines into the poorest countries, where the disease causes half a million deaths annually. But the disease thrives on unclean water and unsafe sanitation. It is arguable that, to save these lives, and those of an additional million children, one should aim instead at providing them with clean water and safe sanitation.

The future

'Imagine a world without vaccines. Life-threatening diseases would present a daily risk. We would live in fear of deadly strains of diphtheria, tetanus and measles; polio would be a constant danger and in a matter of hours could paralyze a child, and smallpox would continue to scar and kill.' This preface to the WHO's global immunisation strategy for 2006-2015 appears designed to scare rather than to inform. It is very reminiscent of the approach taken by the UK Department of Health.

A press release issued in October 2005 claimed that, 'in 2003 alone, immunisation averted more than two million deaths from vaccine-preventable diseases.' Despite arguing in favour of evidence-based interventions, the WHO provided no evidence for this claim, and continues to promote an expansion in the use of vaccines in the developing world, in the absence of any proof that this saves lives.

Undeterred by evidence that some vaccines may be doing more harm than good, the press release continues, 'Immunisation is at an exciting turning point,' with increased funding offering the opportunity 'to introduce new vaccines to millions of the world's poorest children.'

As in its foundation in 1948, the WHO believes the future, rather than the present, holds the promise. 'A revolution is expected in the next decade in the ways that vaccines are designed, manufactured, financed, delivered and administered. Major breakthroughs are occurring in vaccine development. About twenty new or improved vaccines are anticipated within the next ten years.'[45]

30
Informed Consent

Conclusion

In 1977, a courageous article appeared in the prestigious *New England Journal of Medicine* calling for greater openness over vaccination. The author, Dr David Karzon, called for 'a fuller public disclosure of the costs of disease prevention... Immunisation policy has become a public concern,' he wrote, 'and society has declared its right to know and to participate in decision making.'[1] Sadly Dr Karzon's plea, made many years ago, has fallen on deaf ears everywhere around the world. Instead of deepening our knowledge of all aspects of immunisation, health officials throughout the world seem to be intent on blocking the flow of knowledge.

Those within the government or the medical profession who have dared to express concerns in public, are pressurised not to talk. The story of Dr Andrew Wakefield is told in the chapters on MMR, but I have spoken, for the purposes of this book, to others who have been told that their jobs or pensions would be at risk, or even that they would be in contravention of the Official Secrets Act, should they whistle-blow on controversial issues surrounding childhood vaccination.

It is a shocking story I had no idea I would uncover when I started this investigation at the turn of the century. It runs counter to my long training as a doctor and what I was taught about vaccines. It is accepted by everyone that before any medical intervention a doctor has to inform the patient of all risks and benefits so that a properly informed consent can be given. For example, as recently as 2013, the General Medical Council (GMC) responsible for doctors restated this principle in its publication 'Good Medical Practice'. It requires that doctors 'listen to patients, take account of their views, and respond honestly to their questions'. In addition doctors are required to 'give patients [or parents in the case of children's immunisation] the information they want or need to know in a way they can understand.'[2] In the case of vaccines, this is blatantly not happening; instead this private relationship, built on trust and confidence, between doctor and patient is being undermined at its most fundamental level.

Health officials throughout the world have continued to keep alive an idealistic fantasy surrounding vaccines. For over half a century vaccines have continued to be misrepresented as the panacea of modern health, as if they have had the same medical success as the discovery of aspirin or antibiotics.

In 2007, an expert in childhood infection and immunity at the University of Oxford wrote, 'Immunisation is the key to the health of our children'.3

But it is quite clear from history since the early nineteenth century that even the lauded smallpox vaccine never had the massive beneficial effect that is ascribed to it. The reality is that vaccination was only one contributing factor to the disappearance of smallpox, and has played only a small role in the fall in deaths from most infectious diseases in this country.

The perpetuation of the idea of immunisation as the blockbuster protective choice is a deception. It creates expectations that cannot be met by vaccines or health officials and it explains the extraordinary controversies that have always flared up around this type of medical intervention. Though vaccines do work under defined circumstances, they cannot bear the weight of the hopes health officials have been holding out for them for so long. Whenever this gap in effectiveness is found out, a cover up is likely to follow, with the government showing extreme economy with the truth. As in the case of mercury (Thiomersal) in vaccines, health officials deny the suggestion that vaccines could have been fallible. The confusion creates anxiety in parents that can only be met by health officials using isolated facts, out of context, to strike more fear into parents' hearts about what would happen without vaccines. Hence, a vicious circle is created that is hard to break. It is an approach that seems to bypass any 'views' parents may have.

Golden hopes

The golden hopes of scientific medicine have, with some notable exceptions, failed to deliver the promise of a disease-free passage into an ever-youthful old-age. Nor have the hopes for high-tech conjugated vaccines materialised, as the equivocal experiences with Hib, Meningitis C and Pneumococcus show.

The killer infectious diseases of yesteryear have been replaced with chronic ill-health. Over seventeen million adults in Britain suffer from chronic diseases such as arthritis, diabetes and asthma. Modern drugs, for all their benefit, are not the panacea either when they directly cause one in seventeen of all hospital admissions in this country.

In such a climate, doctors become disillusioned, patients desert orthodox medicine for complementary therapies, and all the while health costs soar astronomically. It is no wonder that governments are desperate to cling to whatever apparent successes they have achieved. Immunisation seems to offer a solution at a modest price with central budgetary and administrative control. Doctors who advise the government on vaccination policies have often spent their whole careers working with vaccines and immunisation. Inevitably many are involved in vaccine research and have close ties to the vaccine manufacturers. Conflicts of interest are unavoidable. It would be unacceptable for them to learn that their lives' work were of less value than they had hoped.

None of this is to say that vaccines are of no use at all, or to urge parents to be anti-vaccine. There is no doubt that they have an important role in the protection of children. It is just that this function is not as important or as powerful as we are led to believe. This means that the real doubt starts with mass immunisation. To justify mass immunisation of the whole population three fundamental questions must be answered. First, is the illness serious and common enough to warrant vaccination? If an illness carries a large enough risk of serious harm, or even death, then clearly protection is desirable. However, if an illness rarely causes significant damage, or is very rarely caught in the first place, then mass vaccination cannot be justified. Second, does the vaccine work? A vaccine should be tested to see that it works before its large-scale introduction. Third, and crucially, is the vaccine safe? A vaccine may be very effective — and the illness extremely serious — but it still has to be safe to be acceptable for widespread use. And the less serious the disease, the safer the vaccination must be to justify its use.

All this should be uncontroversial, but that appears not to be the case. Many of those promoting vaccines have a rigid belief system that will allow no criticism or even research that finds problems with vaccines. Despite contradictory, and sometimes clearly conflicting, evidence, the medical establishment is stuck in unshakeable pro-vaccine beliefs. Some of these beliefs are true — at least in part — but the beliefs have far exceeded what the scientific evidence justifies. Paradoxically, it is often these believers who claim to be the most rigorously scientific.

Is the illness serious and common enough?
Doctors in the sixties could be forgiven for unbounded enthusiasm. They had no idea what the next fifty years would bring. However, they cannot be faulted on their scientific rigour. The whooping cough vaccine underwent fifteen years of trials before being widely accepted for use in Britain.

The considerations then were not different from today. In order to introduce widespread vaccination against a disease, that disease should be both serious and relatively common. One hundred years ago, several diseases, including tuberculosis (TB), measles, diphtheria and whooping cough were both common and could also, quite rightly at that time, be described as 'killer diseases.'

The first core question that has been asked of every illness throughout this book has been, 'is the illness serious and common enough to warrant immunisation?' Though the death rates for all the common diseases had been falling dramatically before the introduction of vaccination, diphtheria was still a serious threat in the early 1940s when widespread vaccination began.

It is questionable whether whooping cough was still a 'killer disease' by the time the national vaccination campaign started in 1961. But trials of the whooping cough vaccine had started in the UK back in the 1940s when there were still over a thousand children dying from the disease in epidemic years. So diphtheria and whooping cough vaccines were initially introduced at a time when the diseases were still a real, albeit declining, public health threat.

In November 1967, just months before the introduction of the single measles vaccine to the UK, an article on measles was published in a medical journal. 'There is no doubt that most of these [measles] cases in England today are mild, last only for a short period, are not followed up by complications and are rarely fatal.' Nevertheless, the author, a government doctor, went on to promote 'widespread vaccination' as 'the next logical step in the control of this disease.'[4] An earlier editorial in the *British Medical Journal* reads: 'But the need or desire for a vaccine for the general population of Great Britain is much less certain. Measles is now a mild disease.'[5]

Decades later, this attitude seems to have changed at a time when there have never been fewer deaths from measles. Vaccine expert Dr Nigel Higson said in 2001 that 'Measles is a killer... one of the most rapid killers in the world.'[6] Those of us who were born before 1967 all contracted measles, and our parents were not fearful of this 'killer disease'. It was something all children caught and was rarely serious. During the 1950s and 1960s 'measles parties' were a popular and accepted custom. On hearing that these had regained popularity in the early twenty-first century a Department of Health spokesman said: 'We are extremely concerned that any parent might put the health of their child deliberately at risk in this way.'[7]

Moral dilemma

Every family doctor faces a moral dilemma. Healthy children are at particularly low risk of suffering serious consequences from catching most infectious diseases. Should they all be vaccinated, not so much because it is in their interests, but because they will then afford protection to those vulnerable children who may not be able to receive certain vaccines; children with leukaemia, or those at increased risk, such as the disabled and those with chronic medical conditions? Most information about the risks from both diseases and vaccination refers to average risks to a hypothetical uniform child – a theoretical child that does not exist.

What parents want to know, however, is the exact risk to their particular child – something that is often difficult to calculate. One doctor suggested that 'sending your child to the doctor to be vaccinated is a little like sending your child off to fight in a war. In both cases society asks the parent to accept a small risk for their child to benefit the whole of society.'[8]

Herd immunity

The answer to the dilemma, for some, is the need for 'herd immunity' that will benefit everyone. There remains disagreement, even amongst experts, over what the term actually means. But it is now generally used to mean the protection that non-immune (mainly unvaccinated) people get from mixing with others who are immune (either from vaccination or because they have come across the disease naturally). Paradoxically, it means that if there is herd immunity, this allows a small percentage of parents to choose not to immunise their children and thus avoid the potential side-effects of vaccination while being protected by the herd immunity.

The website of the UK Department of Health describes herd immunity as follows: 'If enough people in a community are immunised against certain diseases, then it is more difficult for that disease to get passed between those who aren't immunised.' One popular way of describing herd immunity (herd 'protection' might be a better name) is to refer to the percentage of children who need to be immune in order to prevent a disease spreading. If a child has not been vaccinated, but nearly all others with whom he comes into contact have, then that child is unlikely to catch the disease.

What proportion of children needs to be vaccinated in order to prevent the spread of a disease in the community? The figure varies and depends on many factors including:

a) the infectiousness of the disease, or how easily it spreads through the community. Measles, for example, is far more infectious than tuberculosis and so requires a greater proportion of the population to be immune to prevent spread;

b) how many other people the infected children come into contact with – diseases spread more easily in crowded cities than in rural areas;

c) the effectiveness of the vaccine.

The 'reproductive rate' of a disease refers to the number of secondary cases that result from a primary infection, or, to put it another way, the number of children that will catch an illness from one infected child. The reproductive rate depends on both its infectiousness and the number of contacts (factors a and b above). There is a big caveat here. Calculations are limited by our poor knowledge of how immunity works, and the differing behaviour patterns of different societies, and different groups within one society.

Measles can be taken as an example. In the 1960s, it was suggested that 55% vaccine coverage would be sufficient to prevent the spread of the disease. This was soon shown to be well short of the mark, and subsequent estimates have varied between 70% and 95%. The Department of Health asserts that at least 90% of children need to be immune to stop the disease being spread.[9] This requires every child to be vaccinated against measles at least once, because the vaccine is, in practice, around 90% effective. There have been repeated warnings of the likelihood of measles outbreaks because of the low uptake of MMR, which has remained low in some areas of London. It is perhaps surprising that there have not been more, and larger, outbreaks than the few there have been.

The Department of Health claims that, 'if 95% of children are protected by MMR, then we can eliminate not just measles, but mumps and rubella as well.'[9] This would require nearly all children to be vaccinated twice and, even then, is an optimistic claim, bearing in mind that outbreaks of these diseases, particularly mumps, have occurred in communities with well over 95% 'protection' from the MMR. Other diseases, such as whooping cough, cannot be eliminated by vaccination because the effectiveness of the vaccine (probably between 50 and 70%) is well below the 95% herd immunity level required to prevent spread of the illness. That is one reason why whooping cough is still widespread in the community. The herd immunity required to eradicate smallpox was only 50-60%, making it a relatively easy disease to wipe out.

Disease:	Herd immunity:*
Diphtheria	85%

Measles	95%
Mumps	90%
Whooping Cough	95%
Polio	85%
German Measles	85%
Tetanus	N/A
Tuberculosis (TB)	The vaccine (BCG) probably does not provide herd immunity

*Estimated proportion of the population required to be immune to prevent outbreaks.

The percentages of the population that need to be immune — which is different from 'vaccinated', as vaccines are not 100% effective — to prevent epidemics vary, though they hover between 85 and 95%.[10,11]

The percentages vary depending on the way of life and social interaction of the community, and are more applicable to developed societies.

Because of the great variation by community, and even country, it is worrying to see plans for European harmonisation being developed. Vaccination policies differ greatly across European countries, not surprisingly, as the needs of different populations vary widely. But there is a growing movement in medicine to standardise everything, ignoring the fact that we are all different.

Europe's top health agency, the European Centres for Disease Protection and Control (ECDC), wants a unified approach to childhood vaccination across Europe. This would probably increase the number of vaccines given and so would be very popular with the continent's large vaccine manufacturers.[12] However, it makes little sense for UK babies to be given exactly the same vaccines, at the same time, as babies from Poland or Greece.

Diminishing returns
The moral dilemma does not stop here. The early vaccines, such as smallpox, diphtheria and whooping cough, were introduced at a time when hundreds of young children were dying every year from the infections. Though the diseases were becoming less harmful before vaccinations were introduced, they were still causing many deaths. In 1941 around 600 children needed to be vaccinated against diphtheria for every life saved; the figure was around 800 for every life saved from whooping cough in 1949.

This situation has changed dramatically. By the time the pneumococcal vaccine was introduced in 2006, around 30,000 children had to be vaccinated in order to save one life. The more recent meningitis B vaccine requires 100,000 children to receive the vaccine to save a single life. It brings sharply into focus the question whether vaccination itself does not create more problems than it is seeking to resolve. This is exactly what is so vexing about the lack of research into MMR and HPV vaccines: if there are side-effects, then they must be set against the benefits of mass immunisation. It is not enough to guess that there are no side-effects merely on the basis that there is inadequate research, and in the absence of follow-up studies. Because the number of deaths prevented is now relatively small, even quite a small risk of side-effects could seriously affect the balance. Even a modest contribution of 10% to the rise in autism would cast a different light on the vaccine.

At the same time, it should be remembered that vaccines are given in the first few months of life because babies, with immature immune systems, are more likely to become very ill from serious infectious diseases at this time. However, they may also be more vulnerable to side-effects from the vaccines in this same early period. Before immunisation, mothers passed on antibodies to their babies in the womb, providing them with protection for the first months of life against illnesses such as measles and mumps. The immunity passed on by vaccinated mothers is both less effective and shorter-lasting.

A potential problem is that, as a vaccine wears off (as all vaccines do) the 'herd immunity' in children could become a 'herd vulnerability' in later life — possibly at ages when complications of the disease are more unpleasant. This is already being seen with whooping cough (which is now a common adult infection) and mumps (which now mainly affects teenagers and young adults).

Vaccination relies on priming the body's immune system to produce antibodies that respond to specific micro-organisms. However, there is a great deal more to immunity. The overall state of health of the immune system is at least as important as the 'virulence' or harmfulness of the infection. It is interesting to consider that doctors and health workers come into contact with infectious diseases every day, yet rarely succumb to the infection. Most of us live in healthy balance with the potentially serious Hib, Meningitis B and C or pneumococcal bugs, resident in our noses, developing natural immunity and never becoming ill from them. Maybe resources should also be directed at researching why most children don't become seriously ill from infections, despite being exposed to them all the time.

While our increasing knowledge of vaccines should enable us to fine-tune this intervention over time, it seems that the reverse is happening, with caution being thrown to the wind.

Vaccines are routinely given to all children at the same time, irrespective of weight, nutritional status, or prematurity. Exactly the same doses of vaccine are given to all children with no attempt to distinguish those that may have a weakness or susceptibility that could make them more vulnerable to side-effects. There is a 'one size fits all' policy which differs utterly from the way all other medicines are prescribed: whereas most drugs are given in a dose proportional to a child's weight, the same strength of vaccine is given to all children, and often adults as well, regardless of size. It may be that ease of administration takes precedence over caution and safety.

Doctors used to be far more cautious about vaccinating. During the 1960s doctors were advising against giving any whooping cough-containing vaccine to a child with a history of fits (including febrile convulsions), asthma, eczema, hay fever or other allergies — in either the child or a near relative.[13,14] With the recent increase in allergic disorders, that would now exclude a large proportion of children from vaccination.

These few 'official' reasons not to vaccinate are subject to a law of shrinkage. In 1996 it was advised in detail that no vaccine should be given to

a child who:
- 'is suffering from an acute illness'. (Most doctors and nurses would take this to mean a child who has a fever or who clearly appears unwell)
- has had a severe reaction to a previous dose of the same vaccine; this included:
- a fever of 39.5°C within 48 hours of being vaccinated
- convulsions within 72 hours of vaccination
- 'prolonged unresponsiveness'
- prolonged screaming for over 4 hours
- severe redness and swelling of the injected limb[15]

In February 2006, following the introduction of the new 5-in-1 vaccine, revised guidelines were issued by the Department of Health. Apart from precautions in a very small number of children with unusual medical histories, vaccination should now only be postponed 'if an individual is acutely unwell'.

What is even more interesting is the reason for this. It has nothing to do with the health of the child. The guidelines explain that it 'is to avoid wrongly attributing any new symptom or the progression of symptoms to the vaccine.'[16] There is no suggestion that vaccination should be delayed as a clinical precaution. USA guidelines have moved a step further, by advising that 'a mild acute illness, with or without fever,' should not prevent a child from being vaccinated.[17] What is clearly happening is that we are becoming less and less careful with regard to immunisation.

Side-effects of vaccination

Though numerous reactions occur after vaccinations, including many reported by parents and those written up by doctors in medical journals, very few are believed by health officials to be 'definitely' caused by vaccines. This raises many interesting questions about the relationship between medical research and medical interventions.

Why do most doctors appear so reluctant to consider that symptoms occurring after vaccinations could be caused by the vaccines themselves? If something untoward happens to a child shortly after a vaccination, the parent may, quite reasonably, blame the vaccine. However, it may well be no more than a coincidence, and unrelated to the vaccine. Many large 'epidemiological' (population based) studies have shown that particular reactions do not occur any more commonly after vaccination than at any other time, supporting the coincidence argument.

However, the argument against this is that most vaccinations are safe most of the time in most people. But all human beings have weaknesses and susceptibilities. As an example, some of us may get indigestion when anxious, whereas others may suffer an aggravation of their asthma or eczema, or get palpitations. So it is plausible, even likely, that different susceptible children will suffer differing side-effects after particular vaccines. These are probably not random events which every child has an equal chance of getting, but more likely related to genetic (inherited) weaknesses and immunological susceptibilities that, as yet, we do not understand. In other words we should not generalise. Every baby, every child, every human being is unique and may react differently to any given vaccine. Reactions occurring in small groups of susceptible children are unlikely to be picked up in large epidemiological studies.

I have talked with parents who are convinced that their children have been damaged by vaccination. They desperately want to know what was different about their children that made them vulnerable to the vaccine. Is there not a way, they ask, for susceptible children to be detected before vaccination, to prevent harm being done? It seems a relatively straightforward request that is not being met by medical science or the health authorities.

There is often debate on what constitutes proof, or evidence, that a particular trigger has caused a specific problem. But lack of evidence of harm is not the same as evidence of safety. The Department of Health said in 2003 that 'there is no evidence of harm from Thiomersal-containing vaccines.' This was because there had been no research into the potential harm of mercury in vaccines, not because any research had been done that had found mercury to be safe.

For something to be proven scientifically (and therefore medically), the connection has to be irrefutable, or beyond any possible doubt. So, to stick with the mercury example, even if it appeared probable that mercury in vaccines caused behavioural disturbances in some children, that would not constitute medical proof. A doctor could still stand up and say, 'there is no evidence that mercury causes behavioural disturbances in children' and strictly speaking, in scientific terms, he would be right. Legal 'proof' is very different and varies from more likely than not (or 'on the balance of probabilities') to 'beyond reasonable doubt'. Many children may, on the balance of probability, have been harmed by vaccination. However, to most doctors, that is not proof that they have been.[18] If vaccines were completely safe, then we wouldn't even be having this debate. However, over the last forty years, one thousand three hundred and eighty-five families have been awarded vaccine damage compensation payments by the UK government as a result of a child being severely damaged by a vaccine.

Doctors themselves give the best indication of the concern there is. Many of the patients in my London clinic who seek alternative vaccine schedules are themselves doctors and nurses. There is a belief amongst those promoting vaccines that once parents have been presented with the 'facts', then they will, by and large, choose to vaccinate their children. This is not always the case. Parents who have the most concerns over vaccinating their children are often the best informed. Dutch parents who were most negative about the introduction of additional vaccines into the childhood vaccination programme were far more likely to be highly educated, and even more likely to be 'health care workers' — presumably including doctors.[19] A vaccine proponent has described this negative attitude as 'pathetic', lamenting that it is exactly this group of the population that 'is expected to set an example for the rest of the community.'

In Saudi Arabia, the hepatitis B vaccine is offered to all health care workers; the more qualified the health worker, the lower the uptake of vaccination.[20]

A study in Switzerland found that better educated mothers were more likely to be 'resistant' to vaccination. The researchers acknowledged that this resistance 'should not be attributed to mothers' ignorance.' Rather, they proposed, it 'could reflect their perplexity towards the choices they are expected to make.'[21] Other studies the world over have confirmed that it is the better educated parents who are questioning vaccines. They simply do not trust those advocating vaccines, and remain concerned about the risks of side-effects that they believe are disregarded by doctors. Offering scientific evidence may make parents even less likely to vaccinate: a group of complementary medicine students were 25% less likely to recommend polio vaccination after either being given evidence supporting vaccination, or seeing a presentation from a polio victim.[22] Contrary to popular belief, doctors are also troubled by childhood vaccination: a 2003 survey commissioned by the Department of Health revealed that a third of family doctors had concerns about the recommended immunisations, which have since increased in number.[23]

Vaccines that may be offered to all children in the UK in the near future include those against chickenpox and hepatitis A. Many other vaccines, including a 7-in-1 combination, are in development. Despite the eager research of pharmaceutical companies, it would be a mistake to add any additional vaccines to the national schedule unless the need is strong, and safety has been adequately demonstrated. This is so far not the case with any of these vaccines. In other words, we should return to the medical caution about loading the immune system of babies and young children that prevailed before the rapid expansion of the vaccination schedule. Furthermore, vaccines should be subjected to the same stringent tests that other medicines are and no longer be treated as if they are in different category.

Future vaccination policy should take greater account of the views of parents. The government needs to invest more in monitoring adverse reactions in response to the increased complexity of today's vaccination schedule. Above all, there needs to be greater openness and honesty, accompanied by a change from the apparent desire of government to 'cover-up' problems, to one where true answers are actively sought. Our children are our future, and deserve nothing less.

ABPI	Association of British Pharmaceutical Industry
ADEM	acute disseminated encephalomyelitis
AID	auto-immune disorder
AIDS	Acquired Immune Deficiency Syndrome
AFP	acute flaccid paralysis
ASD	autistic spectrum disorder
ASIA	Auto-immune Syndrome Induced by Adjuvants
BCG	Bacille Calmette Guérin' (the TB vaccine)
BSE	Bovine Spongiform Encephalopathy ('mad cow disease')
BMJ	*British Medical Journal*
CDC	Centers for Disease Control and Prevention
CFS	chronic fatigue syndrome
vCJD	variant Creutzfeldt-Jakob disease (the human form of BSE)
CMO	Chief Medical Officer
CPS	Chinese paralytic syndrome
CRS	congenital rubella syndrome
CSM	Committee on Safety of Medicines
DoH	Department of Health
DNA	Deoxyribonucleic acid
DTP	diphtheria, tetanus & pertussis (whooping cough)
DTaP	diphtheria, tetanus & acellular pertussis (whooping cough)
EFSA	European Food Safety Authority
EPA	USA Environmental Protection Agency
ESWI	European Scientific Working Group on Influenza
FDA	USA Food and Drug Administration
FSA	UK Food Standards Agency
GAVI	Global Alliance for Vaccines and Immunization
GBS	Guillain Barré Syndrome
GMC	General Medical Council
GP	General Practitioner (family doctor)
GSK	GlaxoSmithKline
Hib	Haemophilus influenzae type B

HIV	Human Immunodeficiency Virus
HMO	health maintenance organization
HPA	Health Protection Agency
HPV	human papillomavirus
ILNH	ileal-lymphoid-nodular hyperplasia
IPD	invasive pneumococcal disease
IPV	inactivated (killed) polio vaccine
ITP	idiopathic thrombocytopaenia purpura
JABS	Justice, Awareness and Basic Support (see Resources)
JCVI	Joint Committee on Vaccination and Immunisation
LSC	Legal Services Commission
MCV	measles containing vaccine
MD	mitochondrial dysfunction
ME	myalgic encephalomyelitis
MHRA	Medicines and Healthcare Products Regulatory Agency
MMF	macrophagic myofasciitis
MMR	measles, mumps and rubella
MS	multiple sclerosis
NCES	national childhood encephalopathy study
OPV	oral polio vaccine (live)
PCV	pneumococcal vaccine
PDD	pervasive developmental disorder
POTS	Postural orthostatic tachycardia syndrome
SKB	Smith Kline Beecham
SKF	Smith Kline French
SLE	systemic lupus erythematosus
SSPE	subacute sclerosing panencephalitis
SV40	Simian virus 40
TB	tuberculosis
UNICEF	United Nations International Children's Emergency Fund
cVDPP	circulating vaccine derived paralytic poliomyelitis
WHO	World Health Organisation

Preface

1 The Hazards of Immunization, The Athlone Press 1967.

2 Martin B. On the Suppression of Vaccination Dissent. Science and Engineering Ethics 2015; 21(1): 143-157

Introduction

1 NHS Immunisation Information, Department of Health. Health Professionals 2003: Childhood Immunisation Survey Report. Available at immunisation.nhs.uk/files/HPSurveyreport.pdf. Accessed March 9, 2006.

A Quick Reference Guide to Vaccines for Parents

1 Siegrist C-A. The Challenges of Vaccine Responses in Early Life: Selected Examples. Journal of Comparative Pathology 2007; 137: S4-S9.

1 Autism and Vaccination

1 Poling JS. Frye RE. Shoffner J. Zimmerman AW. Developmental regression and mitochondrial dysfunction in a child with autism. Journal of Child Neurology. 21(2):170-2, 2006 Feb.

2 Elliott HR. Samuels DC. Eden JA. Relton CL. Chinnery PF. Pathogenic mitochondrial DNA mutations are common in the general population. American Journal of Human Genetics. 83(2):254-60, 2008 Aug.

3 Oliveira G. Ataíde A. Marques C. Miguel TS. Coutinho AM. Mota-Vieira L. Goncalves E. Lopes NM. Rodrigues V. Carmona da Mota H. Vicente AM. Epidemiology of autism spectrum disorder in Portugal: prevalence, clinical characterization, and medical conditions. Developmental Medicine & Child Neurology. 49(10):726-33, 2007 Oct.

4 Shoffner J, Hyams LC, Langley GN. Oxidative Phosphorylation (OXPHOS) Defects in Children with Autistic Spectrum Disorders. Presented at the American Academy of Neurology 60th Annual Meeting: April 13, 2008. Available at abstracts2view.com/aan2008chicago/view.php?nu=AA N08L_INI-1.004

5 Weissman JR et al. Mitochondrial disease in autism spectrum disorder patients: a cohort analysis. PLoS ONE 2008; 3: e3815. Available at plosone.org/article/info:doi%2F10.1371%2Fjournal.pone .0003815;jsessionid=FE6160BB6DD1D9F30C9CC923913 F2D3C

6 Ratajczak HV. Theoretical aspects of autism: Causes—A review. Journal of Immunotoxicology 2011; 8(1): 68-79

7 Bazzano A. Zeldin A. Schuster E. Barrett C. Lehrer D. Vaccine-related beliefs and practices of parents of children with autism spectrum disorders. American Journal on Intellectual and Developmental Disabilities 2012; 117(3): 233-242

8 Hansen S. Schendel D. Parner E. Explaining the increase in the prevalence of autism spectrum disorders. JAMA Pediatrics 2015; 169(1): 56-62

9 Vargas DL. Nascimbene C. Krishnan C. Zimmerman AW. Pardo CA. Neuroglial activation and neuroinflam-mation in the brain of patients with autism. Annals of Neurology 2005; 57(1): 67-81.

10 Jyonouchi H. Sun S. Le H. Proinflammatory and regulatory cytokine production associated with innate and adaptive immune responses in children with autism spectrum disorders and developmental regression. Journal of Neuroimmunology 2001; 120(1-2): 170-9.

11 Sweeten TL. Bowyer SL. Posey DJ. Halberstadt GM. McDougle CJ. Increased prevalence of familial autoim-munity in probands with pervasive developmental disorders. Pediatrics 2003; 112(5): e420.

12 Asher MI, Montefort S, Björkstén B, Lai CKW, Strachan DP, Weiland SK, Williams H. Worldwide time trends in the prevalence of symptoms of asthma, allergic rhinoconjunctivitis, and eczema in childhood: ISAAC Phases One and Three repeat multicountry cross-sectional surveys. Lancet 2006; 38: 733-743.

13 Onkamo P. Vaananen S. Karvonen M. Tuomilehto J. Worldwide increase in incidence of Type I diabetes-the analysis of the data on published incidence trends. Diabetologia 1999; 42(12): 1395-403.

14 Green A. Patterson CC. EURODIAB TIGER Study Group. Europe and Diabetes. Trends in the incidence of childhood-onset diabetes in Europe 1989-1998. Diabetologia 2001; 44 Suppl 3: B3-8.

15 Johnston SL. Openshaw PJ. The protective effect of childhood infections. BMJ 2001; 322(7283): 376-7.

16 Illi S. von Mutius E. Lau S. Bergmann R. Niggemann B. Sommerfeld C. Wahn U. MAS Group. Early childhood infectious diseases and the development of asthma up to school age: a birth cohort study. BMJ 2001; 322(7283): 390-5.

17 Matricardi PM. Rosmini F. Riondino S. Fortini M. Ferrigno L. Rapicetta M. Bonini S. Exposure to foodborne and orofecal microbes versus airborne viruses in relation to atopy and allergic asthma: epi-demiological study. BMJ 2000; 320(7232): 412-7.

18 von Hertzen LC. Puzzling associations between childhood infections and the later occurrence of asthma and atopy. Annals of Medicine 2000; 32(6): 397-400.

19 Silverberg J. Norowitz K. Kleiman E. Silverberg N. Durkin H. Joks R. Smith-Norowitz T. Association between varicella zoster virus infection and atopic dermatitis in early and late childhood: A case-control study. Journal of Allergy and Clinical Immunology 2010; 1126(2): 300-305

20 Rook GA. Stanford JL. Give us this day our daily germs. Immunology Today 1998; 19(3): 113-6.

21 Kemp T. Pearce N. Fitzharris P. Crane J. Fergusson D. St George I. Wickens K. Beasley R. Is infant immunization a risk factor for childhood asthma or allergy? Epidemiology 1997; 8(6): 678-80.

22 Farooqi IS. Hopkin JM. Early childhood infection and atopic disorder. Thorax 1998; 53(11): 927-32.

23 Benke G. Abramson M. Raven J. Thien FC. Walters EH. Asthma and vaccination history in a young adult cohort. Australian & New Zealand Journal of Public

Health 2004; 28(4): 336-8.

24 Yoneyama H. Suzuki M. Fujii K. Odajima Y. [The effect of DPT and BCG vaccinations on atopic disorders]. [Japanese] Arerugi – Japanese Journal of Allergology 2000; 49(7): 585-92.

25 Hurwitz EL. Morgenstern H. Effects of diphtheria-tetanus-pertussis or tetanus vaccination on allergies and allergy-related respiratory symptoms among children and adolescents in the United States. Journal of Manipulative & Physiological Therapeutics 2000; 23(2): 81-90.

26 DeStefano F et al. Vaccine Safety Datalink Research Group. Childhood vaccinations and risk of asthma. Pediatric Infectious Disease Journal 2002; 21(6): 498-504.

27 Olesen AB. Juul S. Thestrup-Pedersen K. Atopic dermatitis is increased following vaccination for measles, mumps and rubella or measles infection. Acta Dermato-Venereologica 2003; 83(6): 445-50.

28 Koppen S. de Groot R. Neijens HJ. Nagelkerke N. van Eden W. Rumke HC. No epidemiological evidence for infant vaccinations to cause allergic disease. Vaccine 2004; 22(25-26): 3375-85.

29 da Cunha SS. No epidemiological evidence for infant vaccinations to cause allergic disease Vaccine 2005; 23(30): 3875.

30 Bernsen RM. van der Wouden JC. Re: no epidemiological evidence for infant vaccinations to cause allergic disease. Vaccine 2005; 23(12): 1427.

31 Nakajima K et al. Is childhood immunisation associated with atopic disease from age 7 to 32 years? Thorax 2007; 62:270-275.

32 McKeever TM. Lewis SA. Smith C. Hubbard R. Vaccination and allergic disease: a birth cohort study. American Journal of Public Health 2004; 94(6): 985-9.

33 Hurwitz EL. Morgenstern H. Vaccination and risk of allergic disease. American Journal of Public Health; 95(1): 6.

34 Benke G. Abramson M. Raven J. Thien FC. Walters EH. Asthma and vaccination history in a young adult cohort. Australian & New Zealand Journal of Public Health 2004; 28(4): 336-8.

35 McDonald KL. Huq SI. Lix LM. Becker AB. Kozyrskyj AL. Delay in diphtheria, pertussis, tetanus vaccination is associated with a reduced risk of childhood asthma. Journal of Allergy & Clinical Immunology 2008; 121(3):626-31.

36 Bremner SA. Carey IM. DeWilde S. Richards N. Maier WC. Hilton SR. Strachan DP. Cook DG. Timing of routine immunisations and subsequent hay fever risk. Archives of Disease in Childhood 2005; 90(6):567-73.

37 Hivid A. Stellfeld M. Wohlfahrt J. Melbye M. Childhood vaccination and type 1 diabetes. New England Journal of Medicine 2004; 350(14): 1398-404.

38 Anonymous. Infections and vaccinations as risk factors for childhood type 1 (insulin-dependent) diabetes mellitus: a multicentre case-control investigation. EURODIAB Substudy 2 Study Group.

Diabetologia 2000; 43(1): 47-53.

39 DeStefano F et al. Vaccine Safety Datalink Team. Childhood vaccinations, vaccination timing, and risk of type 1 diabetes mellitus. Pediatrics 2001; 108(6): E112.

40 Jefferson T. Demicheli V. No evidence that vaccines cause insulin dependent diabetes mellitus. Journal of Epidemiology & Community Health 1998; 52(10): 674-5.

41 Classen JB. Classen DC. Clustering of cases of type 1 diabetes mellitus occurring 2-4 years after vaccination is consistent with clustering after infections and progression to type 1 diabetes mellitus in autoantibody positive individuals. Journal of Pediatric Endocrinology 2003; 16(4): 495-508.

42 Classen JB. Risk of vaccine induced diabetes in children with a family history of type 1 diabetes. The Open Pediatric Journal 2008; 2: 7-10.

43 Molina V. Shoenfeld Y. Infection, vaccines and other environmental triggers of autoimmunity. Autoimmunity 2005; 38(3): 235-45.

44 Hernán MA. Jick SS. Olek MJ. Jick H. Recombinant hepatitis B vaccine and the risk of multiple sclerosis: a prospective study. Neurology 2004; 63(5): 838-42.

45 Riikonen R. The role of infection and vaccination in the genesis of optic neuritis and multiple sclerosis in children. Acta Neurologica Scandinavica 1989; 80(5): 425-31.

46 MMR vaccine and Idiopathic Thrombocytopenic Purpura. Current Problems in Pharmacovigilance 2001; 27:15.

47 Black C. Kaye JA. Jick H. MMR vaccine and idiopathic thrombocytopaenic purpura. British Journal of Clinical Pharmacology 2003; 55(1): 107-11.

48 Woo EJ et al. Thrombocytopenia after vaccination: Case reports to the US Vaccine Adverse Event Reporting System, 1990-2008. Vaccine 2011; 29: 1313-1323

49 Tsumiyama K, Miyazaki Y, Shiozawa S. Self-Organized criticality theory of auto-immunity. PLoS ONE 2009; 4(12): e8382

50 Esposito S, Di Pietro CM, Madini B, Mastrolia MV, Rigante D. A spectrum of inflammation and demyelination in acute disseminated encephalomyelitis (ADEM) of children. Autoimmunity Reviews 2015; 14: 923-929

51 Li JC, Silverberg JI. Varicella infection is not associated with increasing prevalence of eczema: a U.S. population-based study. British Journal of Dermatology 2015; 173(5): 1169-74

52 Zerbo Q, Qian Y, Yoshida C et al. Association between influenza infection and vaccination during pregnancy and risk of autistic spectrum disorder. JAMA Pediatrics 2016.doi: 10.1001/jamapediatrics.2016.3609. Published online November 28, 2016. Available at http://jamanetwork.com/journals/jamapediatrics/fullarticle/2587559

2 One of the Greatest Scandals in Medicine: Mercury

1 Winship KA. Organic mercury compounds and their

toxicity. Adverse Drug Reactions & Acute Poisoning Reviews 1986; 5(3): 141-80.

2 Memo from an internationally renowned vaccinologist, to the president of Merck's vaccine division in March 1991. Source: Los Angeles Times February 8, 2005 & available at putchildrenfirst.org/media/1.10.pdf. Accessed April 14, 2006.

3 New York Times November 19, 2002

4 Email from Dr. Peter Patriarca, Director, Division of Viral Products, Food and Drug Administration, to Martin Meyers, Acting Director, National Vaccine Program Office, Centers for Disease Control and Prevention.(June 29, 1999). Source: Mercury in Medicine – Taking Unnecessary Risks – A Report Prepared by the Staff of the Subcommittee on Human Rights and Wellness, Committee on government Reform, U.S. House of Representatives, May 2003.

5 Internal email at the Food and drug Administration (FDA). July 2, 1999. Available at putchildrenfirst.org. Accessed April 14, 2006.

6 Grandjean P. et al. Cognitive deficit in 7-year-old children with prenatal exposure to methylmercury. Neurotoxicology & Teratology 1997; 19(6): 417-28, 1997.

7 Bernard S. Enayati A. Redwood L. Roger H. Binstock T. Autism: a novel form of mercury poisoning. Medical Hypotheses 2001; 56(4): 462-71.

8 Cinca I. Dumitrescu I. Onaca P. Serbanescu A. Nestorescu B. Accidental ethyl mercury poisoning with nervous system, skeletal muscle, and myocardium injury. Journal of Neurology, Neurosurgery & Psychiatry 1980; 43(2): 143-9.

9 Mercury in Medicine – Taking Unnecessary Risks – A Report Prepared by the Staff of the Subcommittee on Human Rights and Wellness, Committee on government Reform, U.S. House of Representatives, May 2003.

10 Statement on a survey of mercury in fish and shellfish. Committee on Toxicity of Chemicals in Food, Consumer Products and the Environment. Food Standards Agency. February 17, 2003. Available at food.gov.uk/multimedia/pdfs/COTmercurystatement.PDF (accessed December 15, 2005)

11 Updated COT Statement on a survey of mercury in fish and shellfish. Committee on Toxicity of Chemicals in Food, Consumer Products and the Environment. Food Standards Agency. March 24 2003. Available at food.gov.uk/multimedia/pdfs/cotstatementmercury-fish.PDF (accessed December 15, 2005)

12 I have calculated these doses from average weights of babies at 2 months when they receive their first vaccines in the UK and the known content of mercury in the vaccine used in the UK until 2004.

13 Halsey N.A. Limiting infant exposure to thimerosal in vaccines and other sources of mercury. JAMA 1999; 282(18): 1763-6.

14 Thiomersal and vaccines. NHS Immunisation information. Available at immunisation.nhs.uk/files/thiomersalfsht.pdf Sourced on December 16, 2005.

15 Aschner M. Walker SJ. The neuropathogenesis of mercury toxicity. Molecular Psychiatry 2002; 7 Suppl 2: S40-1.

16 Holmes AS. Blaxill MF. Haley BE. Reduced levels of mercury in first baby haircuts of autistic children. International Journal of Toxicology 2003; 22(4): 277-85, 2003.

17 Bernard S. Enayati A. Roger H. Binstock T. Redwood L. The role of mercury in the pathogenesis of autism. Molecular Psychiatry 2002; 7 Suppl 2:S42-3.

18 Bradstreet J et al. A case-control study of mercury burden in children with autistic spectrum disorders. Journal of American Physicians and Surgeons 2003; 8: 76-9.

19 Geier D. Geier MR. Neurodevelopmental disorders following thimerosal-containing childhood immunisations: a follow-up analysis. International Journal of Toxicology 2004; 23(6): 369-76.

20 Bernard S. Association between thimerosal-containing vaccine and autism. JAMA 2004; 291(2):180.

21 Rimland B. Association between thimerosal-containing vaccine and autism. JAMA 2004; 291(2):180; author reply 180-1, 2004 Jan 14.

22 Geier MR, Geier DA and other online letters available at http://pediatrics.aappublications.org/cgi/eletters/114/3/584 Accessed December 15, 2005.

23 Andrews N. Miller E. Grant A. Stowe J. Osborne V. Taylor B. Thimerosal exposure in infants and developmental disorders: a retrospective cohort study in the United Kingdom does not support a causal association. Pediatrics 2004; 114(3): 584-91.

24 Heron J. Golding J. ALSPAC Study Team. Thimerosal exposure in infants and developmental disorders: a prospective cohort study in the United Kingdom does not support a causal association. Pediatrics 2003; 114(3): 577-83.

25 EMEA Public statement on thiomersal containing medicinal products. Doc. Ref: EMEA/20962/99. London, July 8, 1999. Available at emea.eu.int/pdfs/human/press/pus/2096299EN.pdf Accessed December 15, 2005.

26 Immunization Safety Review: Thimerosal-Containing Vaccines and Neurodevelopmental Disorders. Institute of Medicine. The National Academies Press 2001.

27 Levin M. Taking it to Vaccine Court. Los Angeles Times August 7, 2004. Available at virginiainterfaithcenter.org/pages/ACT/2006VaSession/Mercury/geier/LATimes0807041.pdf Accessed December 15, 2005.

28 Verstraeten T. et al. Vaccine Safety Datalink Team. Safety of thimerosal-containing vaccines: a two-phased study of computerised health maintenance organization databases. Pediatrics 2003; 112(5): 1039-

29 Available at safeminds.org/Generation%20Zero%20Pres.pdf Accessed 15 December, 2005.

30 Thimerosal VSD study Phase 1. February 29, 2000.

Available at safeminds.org/research/library/20010229.pdf Accessed 15 December, 2005.

31 Simpsonwood Minutes. Available at safeminds.org/legislation/foia/Simpsonwood_Transcript .pdf Accessed December 15, 2005

32 Miller FH. Miller WW Jr. Lessons to be learned from Harvard Pilgrim HMO's fiscal roller coaster ride. Journal of Law, Medicine & Ethics 2000; 28(3): 287-304.

33 Data available from fightingautism.org/idea/autism-prevalence-report.php

34 Verstraeten T. Thimerosal, the Centers for Disease Control and Prevention, and GlaxoSmithKline. [Letter] Pediatrics, 2004; 113(4): 932.

35 Geier DA, Geier MR. Early downward trends in Neurodevelopmental disorders following removal of Thimerosal-containing vaccines. Journal of American Physicians and Surgeons 2006; 11: 8-13.

36 Granstrom M. Email to Dr. Diane Simpson, Deputy Director of the US National Immunization Program. June 22, 2001. Available at putchildrenfirst.org. Accessed April 14, 2006.

37 Freed GL. Andreae MC. Cowan AE. Katz SL. Vaccine safety policy analysis in three European countries: the case of thimerosal. Health Policy 2002; 62(3): 291-307.

38 Schechter R. Grether RS. Continuing increases in Autism Reported to California's Developmental Services System. Archives of General Psychiatry 2008; 65:19-24.

39 Geier DA, Hooker BS, Kern JK, King PG, Sykes LK, Geier MR. A dose-response relationship between organic mercury exposure from thimerosal-containing vaccines and neurodevelopmental disorders. International Journal of Environmental Research and Public Health 2014; 11: 9156-9170.

40 Geier DA, King PG, Hooker BS, Dorea JG, Kern JK, Sykes LK, Geier MR. Thimerosal: clinical, epidemiologic and biochemical studies. International Journal of Clinical Chemistry 2015; 444: 212-20.

41 Gallagher CM, Goodman MS. Hepatitis B vaccination of male neonates and autism diagnosis, NHIS 1997-2002. Journal of Toxicology and Environmental Health, Part A 2010; 73: 1665-1677

3 'Mix It With Orange': Aluminium

1 Subgroup Report on the Lowermoor Water Pollution Incident. Committee on Toxicity of Chemicals in Food. DoH 2005. Available at dh.gov.uk/Consultations/ClosedConsultations/Closed ConsultationsArticle/fs/en?CONTENT_ID=4112044& chk=az8fHH

2 Daily Telegraph: August 15, 2001. Available at telegraph.co.uk/news/main.jhtml?xml=/news/2001/08 /15/ncam115.xml

3 Owen PJ. Miles DP. A review of hospital discharge rates in a population around Camelford in North Cornwall up to the fifth anniversary of an episode of aluminium sulphate absorption. Journal of Public Health Medicine 1995; 17(2): 200-4.

4 Altmann P et al. Disturbance of cerebral function in people exposed to drinking water contaminated with aluminium sulphate: retrospective study of the Camelford water incident. BMJ 1999; 319(7213): 807-11.

5 Exley C, Esiri MM. Severe cerebral congophilic angiopathy coincident with increased brain aluminium in a resident of Camelford, Cornwall, UK. Journal of Neurology, Neurosurgery, and Psychiatry 2006; doi:10.1136/jnnp.2005.086553

6 Jefferson T. Rudin M. Di Pietrantonj C. Adverse events after immunisation with aluminium-containing DTP vaccines: systematic review of the evidence. The Lancet Infectious Diseases 2004; 4(2): 84-90.

7 Exley C. Aluminium-containing DTP vaccines[letter]. The Lancet Infectious Diseases 2004; 4(6): 324.

8 Exley C. Aluminium-adsorbed vaccines [letter]. The Lancet Infectious Diseases 2006; 6: 189.

9 Ganrot PO. Metabolism and possible health effects of aluminum. Environmental Health Perspectives 1986; 65: 363-441.

10 Exley C [Editor]. Aluminium and Alzheimer's Disease: The Science that Describes the Link. Elsevier Science 2001.

11 Yokel RA. Brain uptake, retention, and efflux of aluminum and manganese. Environmental Health Perspectives 2002; 110 Suppl 5: 699-704.

12 Cooke K. Gould MH. The health effects of aluminium – a review. Journal of the Royal Society of Health 1991; 111(5): 163-8.

13 Howard JM. Clinical import of small increases in serum aluminum. [Letter] Clinical Chemistry 1984; 30(10): 1722-3.

14 Rees EL. Aluminum Toxicity as Indicated by Hair Analysis. Orthomolecular Psychiatry 1979; 8(1): 37-43.

15 Flack R, Elmore D. Aluminium-26 as a Biological Tracer Using Accelerator Mass Spectrometry. In Zatta PF, Alfrey AC [Eds.]. Aluminium Toxicity in Infants' Health and Disease. World Scientific 1998.

16 DeVoto E. Yokel RA. The biological speciation and tox-icokinetics of aluminum. Environmental Health Perspectives 1994; 102(11): 940-51.

17 Powell JJ. Thompson RP. The chemistry of aluminium in the gastrointestinal lumen and its uptake and absorption. Proceedings of the Nutrition Society 1993; 52(1): 241-53.

18 Greger JL. Baier MJ. Excretion and retention of low or moderate levels of aluminium by human subjects. Food & Chemical Toxicology 1983; 21(4): 473-7.

19 Joint FAO/WHO Expert Committee on Food Additives. Sixty-seventh meeting. Rome, 20-29 June 2006. Summary and Conclusions. Available at ftp://ftp.fao.org/ag/agn/jecfa/jecfa67_final.pdf. Accessed June 9, 2007.

20 Haley BE. In vitro studies of thimerosal toxicity. Presentation to Immunization Safety Review Committee. Institute of Medicine: July 16, 2001.

Available at iom.edu/Object.File/Master/8/176/Transcript7-16.pdf

21 Bishop NJ. Morley R. Day JP. Lucas A. Aluminum neurotoxicity in preterm infants receiving intravenous-feeding solutions. New England Journal of Medicine 1997; 336(22): 1557-61.

22 Bergfors E. Trollfors B. Inerot A. Unexpectedly high incidence of persistent itching nodules and delayed hypersensitivity to aluminium in children after the use of adsorbed vaccines from a single manufacturer. Vaccine 2003; 22(1): 64-9.

23 Bergfors E. Bjorkelund C. Trollfors B. Nineteen cases of persistent pruritic nodules and contact allergy to aluminium after injection of commonly used aluminium-adsorbed vaccines. European Journal of Pediatrics 2005; 164(11): 691-7.

24 Gherardi RK et al. Macrophagic myofasciitis: an emerging entity. Groupe d'Études et Recherche sur les Maladies Musculaires Acquises et Dysimmunitaires (GERMMAD) de l'Association Française contre les Myopathies (AFM). Lancet 1998; 352(9125): 347-52.

25 Gherardi RK et al. Macrophagic myofasciitis lesions assess long-term persistence of vaccine-derived aluminium hydroxide in muscle. Brain 2001; 124(Pt 9): 1821-31.

26 Authier FJ et al. Central nervous system disease in patients with macrophagic myofasciitis. Brain 2001; 124(Pt 5): 974-83.

27 Mark A. Bjorksten B. Granstrom M. Immunoglobulin E responses to diphtheria and tetanus toxoids after booster with aluminium-adsorbed and fluid DT-vaccines. Vaccine 1995; 13(7): 669-73.

28 Cogné M. Ballet JJ. Schmitt C. Bizzini B. Total and IgE antibody levels following booster immunization with aluminum absorbed and nonabsorbed tetanus toxoid in humans. Annals of Allergy 1985; 54(2): 148-51.

29 Exley C et al. Elevated urinary excretion of aluminium and iron in multiple sclerosis. Multiple Sclerosis 2006; 12: 10.1191/135248506ms1312oa

30 van Rensburg SJ et al. Serum concentrations of some metals and steroids in patients with chronic fatigue syndrome with reference to neurological and cognitive abnormalities. Brain Research Bulletin 2001; 55(2): 319-25.

31 Guis S et al. Identical twins with macrophagic myofasciitis: genetic susceptibility and triggering by aluminic vaccine adjuvants? Arthritis & Rheumatism 2002; 47(5): 543-5.

32 Di Muzio A et al. Macrophagic myofasciitis: an infantile Italian case. Neuromuscular Disorders 2004; 14(2): 175-7.

33 Trollfors B, Bergofrs E, Inerot A. Vaccine related itching nodules and hypersensitivity to aluminium [letter]. Vaccine 2005; 23: 975-6.

34 Sedman AB. Wilkening GN. Warady BA. Lum GM. Alfrey AC. Encephalopathy in childhood secondary to aluminum toxicity. Journal of Pediatrics 1984;. 105(5):836-8.

35 Exley C, Swarbrick L, Gherardi RK, Authier FJ. A role for the body burden of aluminium in vaccine-associated macrophagic myofasciitis and chronic fatigue syndrome. Medical Hypotheses. 20009; 72: 135-9.

36 Gherardi RK, Authier FJ. Macrophagic myofasciitis: characterization and pathophysiology. Lupus 2011; 21:184-189

37 Tomljenovic L, Shaw CA. Do aluminium vaccine adjuvants contribute to the rising prevalence of autism? Journal of Inorganic Biochemistry 2011; 105: 1489-1499

38 Aguilar F et al. Safety of aluminium from dietary intake. Scientific opinion of the panel on food additives, flavourings, processing aids and food contact materials (AFC). The European Food Safety Authority Journal 2008; 754: 1-34.

39 Esposito S et al. Autoimmune/inflammatory syndrome induced by adjuvants (ASIA): clues and pitfalls in the pediatric background. Immunologic Research. 2014; 60(2-3): 366-75.

40 Bergfors E, Hermansson G, Nystrom Kronander U, Falk L, Valter L, Trollfors B. How common are long-lasting, intensely itching granulomas and contact allergy to aluminium currently used in pediatric vaccines? A prospective cohort study. European Journal of Pediatrics 2014; 173(10): 1297-307

4 Vaccination Riots: Smallpox and Scarlet Fever

1 Spier RE. Perception of risk of vaccine adverse events: a historical perspective. Vaccine 2002; 20: S78-S84

2 Swales JD. The Leicester anti-vaccination movement. Lancet 1992; 340(8826): 1019-21.

3 Howard CR. The impact on public health of the 19th century anti-vaccination movement. Microbiology Today 2003; 30: 22-4

4 Dick G. Smallpox: A Reconsideration of Public Health Policies. Progress in Medical Virology 1966: 8: 1-29

5 Dixon GW. Immunization against Smallpox. The British Journal of General Practice 1963; 17: 641-8

6 Wynne-Griffith G. From Proceedings of a Symposium on Immunization in Childhood. Cannon DA. E&S Livingstone 1960.

7 Dick GWA. A Symposium on Immunology. The British Journal of Clinical Practice 1963; 17: 620-9

8 Galbraith NS, Forbes P, Mayon-White RT. Changing patterns of communicable disease in England and Wales. Part II — Disappearing and declining diseases. British Medical Journal 1980: 489-492

9 Dick G. Smallpox: A Reconsideration of Public Health Policies. Progress in Medical Virology 1966: 8: 1-29

10 Hopkins, Jack W. 1989. The Eradication of Smallpox: Organizational Learning and Innovation in International Health. Boulder, CO: Westview Press.

11 Brilliant, Lawrence B. 1985. The Management of Smallpox Eradication in India. Ann Arbor, MI: University of Michigan Press.

12 Fenner, F., D. A. Henderon, I. Arita, Z. Jezek, and I. D.

Ladnyi. 1988. Smallpox and Its Eradication. Geneva: World Health Organization.

13 Arita I. Nakane M. Fenner F. Public health. Is polio eradication realistic? Science 2006; 312(5775): 852-4.

5 The Strangler: Diphtheria

1 Martin WJ. The recent trend of Diphtheria in England and Wales. Monthly Bulletin of the Ministry of Health and PHLS 1948: 232-236

2 Bradford Hill A, Knowelden J. Inoculation and poliomyelitis. A statistical investigation in England and Wales in 1949. British Medical Journal 1950; 4669: 1-6

3 Stanley Banks H, Beale AJ. Poliomyelitis and Immunization against Whooping Cough and Diphtheria. British Medical Journal 1950: 251-2

4 Poliomyelitis and Prophylactic Inoculation. Report of the Medical Research Council Committee on Inoculation procedures and Neurological lesions. The Lancet 1956: 1223-1231

5 Memorandum on Vaccination. Monthly Bulletin of the Ministry of Health and PHLS 1952: 77

6 Logan WPD. Recent Trends of Diphtheria. Monthly Bulletin of the Ministry of Health and PHLS 1952: 50-56

7 Martin WJ. The Recent Trend of Diphtheria in England and Wales. Monthly Bulletin of the Ministry of Health and PHLS 1948: 232-236

8 Christie AB. Emergencies in General Practice: Diphtheria. British Medical Journal 1955: 669-671

9 Bloss JFE. Diphtheria in England and Wales in 1954. Monthly Bulletin of the Ministry of Health and PHLS 1955: 194-200

10 Minutes of the Joint Committee on Vaccination and Immunisation. April 21, 1989.

11 The Russian epidemic is covered in great detail in The Journal of Infectious Diseases 2000; supplement I: SI-S248

12 Bergamini M et al. Evidence of increased carriage of Corynebacterium spp. in healthy individuals with low antibody titres against diphtheria toxoid. Epidemiology and Infection 2000; 125: 105-112

13 Pappenheimer AM, Murphy JR. Studies on the molecular epidemiology of diphtheria. The Lancet 1983; 923-5

14 Fanning J. Outbreak of diphtheria in highly immunised community, British Medical Journal. 1947: 371-3

15 Karzon DT, Edwards KM. Diphtheria outbreaks in immunised populations. New England Journal of Medicine 1988; 318: 41-3

16 Santos LS et al. Diphtheria outbreak in Maranhao, Brazil: microbiological, clinical and epidemiological aspects. Epidemiology and Infection 2015; 143(4): 791-8

17 Masterton RG, Tettmar RE, Pile RL, Jones J, Croft KF. Immunity to diphtheria in young British adults. Journal of Infection 1987; 15: 27-32

18 Maple PA, Efstratiou A, George RC, Andrews NJ, Sesardic D. Diphtheria Immunity in UK blood-donors. The Lancet 1995; 345: 963-5

19 Miller E, Rush M, Morgan-Capner P, Hutchinson D, Hindle L. Immunity to diphtheria in adults in England [letter]. British Medical Journal 1994; 308: 598

6. The Captain of Death: TB

1 Pirmohamed M et al. Adverse drug reactions as cause of admission to hospital: prospective analysis of 18 820 patients. BMJ 2004; 329(7456): 15-9.

2 Starfield B. Is US Health Really the Best in the World? JAMA. 2000; 284:483-485.

3 Daniel TM. The impact of tuberculosis on civilization. Infectious Disease Clinics of North America 2004; 18(1): 157-65.

4 Pitman R. Jarman B. Coker R. Tuberculosis transmission and the impact of intervention on the incidence of infection. International Journal of Tuberculosis & Lung Disease 2002; 6(6): 485-91.

5 Maes RF. Tuberculosis II: the failure of the BCG vaccine. Medical Hypotheses 1999; 53(1): 32-9.

6 Heaf F. B.C.G. vaccination against tuberculosis. Monthly Bulletin of the Ministry of Health 1947: 184-93.

7 Anonymous. B.C.G. AND vole bacillus vaccines in the prevention of tuberculosis in adolescents; first (progress) report to the Medical Research Council by their Tuberculosis Vaccines Clinical Trials Committee. British Medical Journal 1956; (4964): 413-27.

8 McKeown T. The Role of Medicine: dream, mirage or nemesis. Nuffield Provincial Hospitals Trust1 976: p.87.

9 Watson JM. Moss F. TB in Leicester: out of control, or just one of those things? BMJ 2001; 322(7295): 1133-4.

10 Minutes of the Joint Committee on Vaccination and Immunisation: November 2, 2001.

11 Minutes of the Joint Committee on Vaccination and Immunisation: October 9, 2000.

12 Minutes of the Joint Committee on Vaccination and Immunisation: November 1, 2002.

13 Minutes of the Joint Committee on Vaccination and Immunisation: June 4, 2004.

14 BBC News. The irresistible rise of 'Tony's crony'. November 17, 2005. Available at http://news.bbc.co.uk/1/hi/business/4446978.stm. Accessed February 28, 2006.

15 Minutes of the Joint Committee on Vaccination and Immunisation. BCG Subgroup: April 7, 2005.

16 ten Dam HG. Hitze KL. Does BCG vaccination protect the newborn and young infants? Bulletin of the World Health Organization 1980; 58(1): 37-41.

17 Rodrigues LC. Noel Gill O. Smith PG. BCG vaccination in the first year of life protects children of Indian subcontinent ethnic origin against tuberculosis in England. Journal of Epidemiology & Community Health 1991; 45(1): 78-80.

18 Packe GE. Innes JA. Protective effect of BCG vaccination in infant Asians: a case-control study. Archives of Disease in Childhood 1988; 63(3): 277-81.

19 Teo SS. Smeulders N. Shingadia DV. BCG vaccine-associated suppurative lymphadenitis. Vaccine 2005; 23(20): 2676-9.

20 Lotte A et al. Second IUATLD study on complications induced by intradermal BCG-vaccination. Bulletin of the International Union Against Tuberculosis & Lung Disease 1988; 63(2): 47-59.

21 Deeks SL et al. Serious adverse events associated with bacille Calmette-Guérin vaccine in Canada. Pediatric Infectious Disease Journal 2005; 24(6): 538-41.

22 Trevenen CL. Pagtakhan RD. Disseminated tuberculoid lesions in infants following BCG vaccination. Canadian Medical Association Journal 1982; 127(6): 502-4.

23 Clark M. Cameron DW. The benefits and risks of bacille Calmette-Guerin vaccination among infants at high risk for both tuberculosis and severe combined immunodeficiency: assessment by Markov model. BMC Pediatrics 2006; 6:5.

24 Gibbons B. Cabinet Written Statement. National Public Health Service Report into an adverse reaction to a BCG immunisation in Aberystwyth. January 18, 2005. Available at wales.gov.uk/organicabinet/content/statements/2005/180105-bcg-e.doc. Accessed February 28, 2006.

25 BBC News. Vaccine 'not faulty' says trust. January 25, 2005. Available at http://news.bbc.co.uk/1/hi/wales/mid/4203349.stm. Accessed 28 February, 2006.

26 Roy A et al. Effect of BCG vaccination against Mycobacterium tuberculosis infection in children: systematic review and meta-analysis. BMJ 2014; 349: g4643

7 A Middle-Class Disease: Polio

1 Bradford Hill A, Knowelden J. Inoculation and Poliomyelitis: a statistical investigation in England and Wales in 1949. British Medical Journal 1950; 4669: 1-6

2 Poliomyelitis and Prophylactic Inoculation: Report of the Medical Research Council Committee on inoculation procedures and neurological lesions. The Lancet 1956: 1223-1231.

3 Francis T et al. An Evaluation of the 1954 poliomyelitis vaccine trials. American Journal of Public Health 1955; 45: 1-63

4 Nathanson N. Langmuir AD. The Cutter incident. Poliomyelitis following formaldehyde-inactivated poliovirus vaccination in the United States during the Spring of 1955. II. Relationship of poliomyelitis to Cutter vaccine. 1963. American Journal of Epidemiology 1995; 142(2): 109-40

5 SV40 Contamination of Polio Vaccine and Cancer. Immunization Safety Review. Institute of Medicine. The National Academies Press 2003.

6 Minutes of Joint Committee on Vaccination and Immunisation. 1 May 1998.

7 Innis MD. Oncogenesis and poliomyelitis vaccine. Nature 1968; 219(157): 972-3.

8 Roberts L. Epidemiology. Minnesota polio case stumps experts. Science 2005; 310(5746): 213.

9 Kew OM. Sutter RW. de Gourville EM. Dowdle WR. Pallansch MA. Vaccine-derived polioviruses and the endgame strategy for global polio eradication. Annual Review of Microbiology 2005; 59: 587-635.

10 Friedrich F, Filippis AM, Schatzmayr HG. Temporal association between the isolation of Sabin-related poliovirus vaccine strains and the Guillain-Barré syndrome. Revista do Instituto de Medicina Tropical de Sao Paulo 1996; 38(1): 55-8.

11 Kinnunen E. Farkkila M. Hovi T. Juntunen J. Weckstrom P. Incidence of Guillain-Barré syndrome during a nationwide oral poliovirus vaccine campaign. Neurology 1989; 39(8): 1034-6.

12 Anlar O. Tombul T. Arslan S. Akdeniz H. Caksen H. Gundem A. Akbayram S. Report of five children with Guillain-Barré syndrome following a nationwide oral polio vaccine campaign in Turkey. Neurology India 2003; 51(4): 544-5.

13 Ehrengut W. Relationship of oral polio vaccine administration to Guillain-Barré syndrome. [Letter] Acta Paediatrica Japonica 1996; 38(4): 423.

14 Friedrich F. Rare adverse events associated with oral poliovirus vaccine in Brazil. Brazilian Journal of Medical & Biological Research 1997; 30(6): 695-703.

15 Böttiger M. The elimination of polio in the Scandinavian countries. Public Health Reviews 1993-94; 21: 27-33

16 Chamberlain R. Poliomyelitis vaccination. British Medical Journal 1987; 295: 158-9

17 Beale AJ. Polio vaccines: time for a change in immunisation policy? Lancet 1990; 335(8693): 839-42.

18 Anonymous. Polio reconsidered. [Editorial] Lancet 1984; 2(8415): 1309-10.

19 HMSO. Immunisation against Infectious Disease ('The Green Book') 1996.

20 VCJD is Variant Creutzfeldt-Jakob disease, the human form of Bovine Spongiform Encephalopathy (BSE) or 'mad cow disease'.

21 CMO report into withdrawal of OPV and CSM Review of TSE and human vaccines. The Stationary Office 2002.

22 WHO Position Statement on recall of Evans/Medeva Polio Vaccine in UK. Statement WHO/8. 20 October 2000. Available at who.int/inf-pr-2000/en/state2000-08.html (downloaded 11 December 2005)

23 OPV and BSE. Report to the Joint Committee on Vaccination and Immunisation 2001: JCVI(01)13.

24 Payne D. More than 4000 out of date vaccines given to children in Ireland. BMJ 2001; 322: 636.

25 Minutes of Joint Committee on Vaccination and Immunisation 25 January 2002

8 When is Polio not called Polio? WHO

1 Andrus JK. de Quadros C. Olive JM. Hull HF. Screening of cases of acute flaccid paralysis for poliomyelitis eradication: ways to improve specificity. Bulletin of the World Health Organization 1992; 70(5): 591-6

2 Goldman AS. Schmalstieg EJ. Freeman DH Jr. Goldman DA. Schmalstieg FC Jr. What was the cause of Franklin Delano Roosevelt's paralytic illness? Journal of Medical

Biography 2003; 11(4): 232-40.

3 Friedrich F, Filippis AM, Schatzmayr HG. Temporal association between the isolation of Sabin-related poliovirus vaccine strains and the Guillain-Barré syndrome. Revista do Instituto de Medicina Tropical de Sao Paulo 1996; 38(1): 55-8.

4 Kinnunen E. Farkkila M. Hovi T. Juntunen J. Weckstrom P. Incidence of Guillain-Barré syndrome during a nationwide oral poliovirus vaccine campaign. Neurology 1989; 39(8): 1034-6.

5 Anlar O. Tombul T. Arslan S. Akdeniz H. Caksen H. Gundem A. Akbayram S. Report of five children with Guillain-Barré syndrome following a nationwide oral polio vaccine campaign in Turkey. Neurology India 2003; 51(4): 544-5.

6 Andrus JK. de Quadros C. Olive JM. Hull HF. Screening of cases of acute flaccid paralysis for poliomyelitis eradication: ways to improve specificity. Bulletin of the World Health Organization 1992; 70(5): 591-6

7 Neogi SB. Polio declining but AFP on the rise. [Letter] Indian Pediatrics 2006; 43(2): 185-6.

8 McKhann et al. Clinical and electrophysiological aspects of acute paralytic disease of children and young adults in northern China. The Lancet 1991; 338: 593-597.

9 Gordon N. Chinese paralytic syndrome or acute motor axonal neuropathy. Archives of Disease in Childhood 1994; 70: 64-65.

10 Shen Y. Xia G. What causes Chinese paralytic syndrome? [Letter] Lancet 1994; 344(8928): 1026,

11 Sample I. WHO aims to wipe out polio within four years. The Guardian, November 17, 2006.

12 Mudur G. Doctors question India's polio strategy after surge in number of cases. BMJ 2006; 333(7568): 568.

13 Paul Y. Evaluation of OPV efficacy is required for polio eradication in India. Vaccine 2005 [letter]; 23: 3097-3098.

14 Aylward RB. Heymann DL. Can we capitalize on the virtues of vaccines? Insights from the polio eradication initiative. American Journal of Public Health 2005; 95(5): 773-7.

15 For the latest figures visit the Global Polio Eradication Initiative website at polioeradication.org/content/general/casecount.pdf

16 John TJ. A developing country perspective on vaccine-associated paralytic poliomyelitis. Bulletin of the World Health Organization 2004; 82(1): 53-7.

17 Paul Y, Priya. Polio eradication in India: some observations. Vaccine 2004; 22: 4144-4148.

18 Patriarca PA. Sutter RW. Oostvogel PM. Outbreaks of paralytic poliomyelitis, 1976-1995. Journal of Infectious Diseases 1997; 175 Suppl 1: S165-72.

19 Walsh D. Polio cases jump in Pakistan as clerics declare vaccination an American plot. The Guardian. February 15, 2007.

20 Sidley P. Seven die in polio outbreak in Namibia. BMJ 2006; 332(7555): 1408.

21 Kew OM. Wright PF. Agol VI. Delpeyroux F. Shimizu H.
Nathanson N. Pallansch MA. Circulating vaccine-derived polioviruses: current state of knowledge. Bulletin of the World Health Organization 2004; 82(1): 16-23.

22 Cochi SL, Kew O. Polio Today. Are we on the verge of global eradication? JAMA 2008; 300 (7):839-841.

9 A Country Affair: Tetanus

1 Luisto M. Iivanainen M. Tetanus of Immunised Children. Developmental Medicine and Child Neurology 1993; 35: 346-358

2 Shimoni Z. Dobrousin A. Cohen J. Pitlik S. Tetanus in an immunised patient. British Medical Journal 1999; 319: 1049

3 Crone NE. Reder AT. Severe tetanus in immunised patients with high anti-tetanus titres. Neurology 1992; 42: 761-4

4 Immunisation against Infectious Disease -- The Green Book. Department of Health 2006. Available at dh.gov.uk/PolicyAndGuidance/HealthAndSocialCareTo pics/GreenBook/fs/en. Accessed March 11, 2007.

5 Bracebridge S. Crowcroft N. White J. Tetanus immunisation policy in England and Wales -- an overview of the literature. Communicable Disease and Public Health 2004; 7: 283-6

6 Moughty A, O Donnell J, Nugent M. Who needs a shot...a review of tetanus immunity in the West of Ireland. Emergency Medicine Journal 2013; 30: 1009-1011

7 Anonymous. Active immunisation against tetanus. Lancet 1967; 2(7517): 662-3.

8 Quast U. Hennessen W. Widmark RM. Mono- and Polyneuritis after Tetanus Vaccination (1970-1977). International Symposium on Immunization: Benefit Versus Risk Factors, Brussels 1978. Developments in Biological Standardization 1979; 43: 25-32

9 Pritchard J. Mukherjee R. Hughes RAC. Risk of relapse of Guillain-Barré syndrome or chronic inflammatory demyelinating polyradiculoneuropathy following immunisation. Journal of Neurology, Neurosurgery and Psychiatry 2002; 73: 348-9

10 Schwarz G. Lanzer G. List WE. Acute midbrain syndrome as an adverse reaction to tetanus immunization. Intensive Care Medicine 1988; 15: 53-54

10 The 'Killer' Disease: Measles

1 Jerome K Jerome. The Idle Thoughts of an Idle Fellow. 1891.

2 Radio National Transcripts. The Health Report. Monday 2nd December, 1996. Available at abc.net.au/rn/talks/8.30/helthrpt/hstories/hr021296.h tm. Downloaded December 29, 2005.

3 The numbers are based on cases reported by doctors. GPs are notoriously bad at reporting all cases, especially mild ones, so I've assumed half of all measles cases were reported. It could be far less, but is unlikely to be more

4 The rates for complications listed below come form a

national survey in 1963. [Miller DL. Frequency of Complications of Measles, 1963. Report On A National Inquiry By The Public Health Laboratory Service In Collaboration With The Society Of Medical Officers Of Health. *British Medical Journal* 1964; 5401: 75-8.] They refer only to notified cases. As under-reporting was common, notified cases are likely to be more serious. Thus the risks of complications below may over-estimate the risk.

5 Anonymous. Control of measles. *Lancet* 1930; 218: 814-816.

6 Ayers GM. England's First State Hospitals p183. London. Wellcome Institute of History of Medicine.

7 Bautista D. Alfonso JL. Corella D. Saiz C. Influence of social factors on avoidable mortality: a hospital-based case-control study. Public Health Reports 2005; 120(1): 55-62.

8 Snell WE. Measles and its complications 50 years ago. Public Health 1976; 90(5): 211-7.

9 Chandra RK. Reduced secretory antibody response to live attenuated measles and poliovirus vaccines in malnourished children. *British Medical Journal* 1975; 2(5971): 583-5.

10 Burstrom B. Diderichsen F. Smedman L. Child mortality in Stockholm during 1885-1910: the impact of household size and number of children in the family on the risk of death from measles. American Journal of Epidemiology 1999; 149(12): 1134-41.

11 Freis Ed. Deaths from Measles in England and Wales in 1961. A Report from The Epidemiological Research Laboratory, Colindale, London, N.W.9. Monthly Bulletin of the Ministry of Health & the PHLS 1963; 22: 167-75.

12 Caiger FF. The treatment of measles. *Lancet* 1923; 204: 864-865.

13 EUvac.net. Measles surveillance annual reports 200102004. Available at ssi.dk/euvac/annual_reports.html. Accessed January 12, 2005.

14 Increase in measles cases in 2006, in England and Wales. CDR Weekly 2006; 16. March 23, 2006. Available at hpa.org.uk/cdr/archives/2006/cdr1206.pdf. Accessed April 18, 2006.

15 Goffe AP et al. Vaccination against measles in general practice. *British Medical Journal* 1963; 5322: 26-8.

16 Anonymous. Vaccination against measles. Clinical trial of live measles vaccine given alone and live vaccine preceded by killed vaccine. Third report to the Medical Research Council by the Measles Vaccines Committee. Practitioner 1971; 206(234): 458-66.

17 Vuorinen P. Vaccination against Measles. *British Medical Journal* 1963; 5360: 759-60.

18 Dick G. Measles again. [Letter] *British Medical Journal* 1980; 280(6224): 1186.

19 PHLS surveillance of reactions to measles vaccines. Available at dh.gov.uk/PublicationsAndStatistics/FreedomOfInform ation/EreadingRoom/EreadingRoomArticle/fs/en?CO NTENT_ID=4140335&chk=Jcczzt. Accessed December 29, 2006.

20 Smith H. Measles again. *British Medical Journal* 1980; 280(6216): 766-7.

21 de Swart RL et al. Prevention of measles in Sudan: a prospective study on vaccination, diagnosis and epidemiology. Vaccine 2001; 19(17-19): 2254-7.

22 Mupere E et al. Measles vaccination effectiveness among children under 5 years of age in Kampala, Uganda. Vaccine 2006; 24: 4111-4115.

23 Kotb MM. Khella AK. Allam MF. Evaluation of the effectiveness of routine measles vaccination: case-control study. Journal of the Egyptian Public Health Association 1999; 74(1-2): 59-68.

24 I place much emphasis on deaths because these are more reliable than most health statistics. The often-quoted numbers of children getting an illness such as measles depend on doctors' notifications, which give notoriously inaccurate figures, primarily from under-reporting.

25 Okuno Y et al. Incidence of subacute sclerosing panencephalitis following measles and measles vaccination in Japan. International Journal of Epidemiology 1989; 18(3): 684-9.

26 Takasu T et al. A continuing high incidence of subacute sclerosing panencephalitis (SSPE) in the Eastern Highlands of Papua New Guinea. Epidemiology & Infection 2003; 131(2): 887-98.

27 Payne FE. Baublis JV. Itabashi HH. Isolation of measles virus from cell cultures of brain from a patient with subacute sclerosing panencephalitis. New England Journal of Medicine 1969; 81(11): 585-9.

28 Miller DL et al. Report of the National Childhood Encephalopathy Study. HMSO 1980.

29 Virus Measles. Adverse drug reactions online information tracking drug analysis print. Medicines and Healthcare products registration Agency (MHRA). DoH. November 21, 2005.

30 Minutes of the Joint Committee on Vaccination and Immunisation. October 15, 1973.

31 Allerdist H. Neurological complications following measles vaccination. Developments in Biological Standardization 1979; 43: 259-64.

32 Monafo WJ et al. Disseminated measles infection after vaccination in a child with a congenital immunodeficiency. Journal of Pediatrics 1994; 124(2): 273-6.

33 Elliman D, Bedford H. The looming measles threat – what can GPs do about it? Pulse: January 8, 2005.

34 Matson DO. Byington C. Canfield M. Albrecht P. Feigin RD. Investigation of a measles outbreak in a fully vaccinated school population including serum studies before and after revaccination. Pediatric Infectious Disease Journal 1993; 12(4): 292-9.

35 Landen MG. Beller M. Funk E. Rolka HR. Middaugh J. Measles outbreak in Juneau, Alaska, 1996: implications for future outbreak control strategies. Pediatrics 1998; 102(6): E71.

36 Paunio M et al. Explosive school-based measles outbreak: intense exposure may have resulted in high risk, even among revaccinees. American Journal of Epidemiology 1998; 148(11): 1103-10.

37 Gustafson TL et al. Measles outbreak in a fully immunised secondary-school population. New England Journal of Medicine 1987; 316(13): 771-4.

38 Anonymous. Measles and Indians. British Medical Journal Clinical Research Ed. 1982; 85(6357): 1762-3.

39 Paunio M et al. Explosive school-based measles outbreak: intense exposure may have resulted in high risk, even among revaccinees. American Journal of Epidemiology 1998; 148(11): 1103-10.

40 MacKenzie D. Monster in the making. New Scientist: April 14, 2001.

41 Pedersen IR. Mordhorst CH. Glikmann G. von Magnus H. Subclinical measles infection in vaccinated seropositive individuals in arctic Greenland. Vaccine 1989; 7(4): 345-8.

42 Muller CP. Measles elimination: old and new challenges? Vaccine 2001; 19(17-19): 2258-61.

43 Mudur G. Indian scientists warn of 'mutant measles' virus. BMJ 2001; 322: 693.

44 Outlaw MC. Pringle CR. Sequence variation within an outbreak of measles virus in the Coventry area during spring/summer 1993. Virus Research 1995; 39(1): 3-11.

45 Anthroposophy is a spiritual philosophy taught by Rudolph Steiner that is, in general, opposed to vaccination.

46 Duffell E. Attitudes of parents towards measles and immunisation after a measles outbreak in an anthroposophical community. Journal of Epidemiology & Community Health 2001; 55(9):685-6.

47 Flöistrup H et al. Allergic disease and sensitization in Steiner school children. Journal of Allergy and Clinical Immunology 2006; 17: 59-66.

48 Kondo N et al. Improvement of food-sensitive atopic dermatitis accompanied by reduced lymphocyte responses to food antigen following natural measles virus infection. Clinical & Experimental Allergy 1993; 23(1): 44-50.

49 Bodner C. Anderson WJ. Reid TS. Godden DJ. Childhood exposure to infection and risk of adult onset wheeze and atopy. Thorax 2000; 55(5): 383-7.

50 Shaheen SO et al. Measles and atopy in Guinea-Bissau. Lancet 1996; 347(9018): 1792-6.

51 Rumbelow H. Measles epidemic ruled out despite fall in MMR jabs. The Times: January 11, 2002.

52 Comerford C. Doctor: January 24, 2002.

53 Rosenlund H et al. Allergic disease and atopic sensitization in children in relation to measles vaccination and measles infection. Pediatrics 2009; 123 (3): 771-8.

54 Leuridan E., et al. Early waning of maternal antibodies in era of measles elimination: longitudinal study. BMJ 2010; 340: c1626 doi:10.1136/BMJ.c1626

55 Uzicanin A., Zimmerman L. Field effectiveness of live attenuated measles-containing vaccines: a review of the published literature. Journal of Infectious Diseases 2011: 204: S133-148

56 De Serres G et al. Higher risk of measles when the first dose of a 2-dose schedule of measles vaccine is given at 12-14 months versus 15 months of age. Clinical Infectious Diseases 2012; 55(3): 394-402

II A Campaign of Terror: Whooping Cough

1 Jenkinson D. Natural course of 500 consecutive cases of whooping cough: a general practice population study. British Medical Journal 1995; 310: 299-302

2 Medical Research Council. The prevention of whooping cough by vaccination. British Medical Journal 1951; 1: 1463-71.

3 Whooping cough, or 'pertussis, is the 'P' of the DTP or DTP-Hib vaccine that was used until 2004. In Britain, it is now the P of the '5-in-1' DTaP/IPV/Hib vaccine and the DTaP/Hib pre-school booster.

4 Madsen T. Vaccination against Whooping Cough. American Medical Association Journal 1933; 101: 187-8

5 Brody M, Sorley RG. Neurologic complications following the administration of pertussis vaccine. New York State Journal of Medicine 1947; 47: 1016

6 Berg JM. Neurological Complications of Pertussis Immunization. British Medical Journal 1958; 24-7

7 Ström J. Is Universal Vaccination against Pertussis Always Justified? British Medical Journal 1960; 1215.

8 Cockburn C. Pertussis Vaccination. The Practitioner 1959; 183: 265-8

9 Ungar J, Pertussis Immunization. The British Journal of General Practice 1963; 17: 673-680

10 Malmgren B, Vahlquist B, Zetterström R. Complications of Immunization [letter] British Medical Journal 1960; 1800-1

11 Payne D. Parents demand names of children given faulty vaccine. BMJ 1999; 318:626.

12 Payne D. Irish children may have been given animal vaccine for whooping cough. BMJ 2001; 323: 128.

13 Barnett A, McVeigh T. Baby deaths may be linked to toxic vaccine. Observer: July 8, 2001.

14 Kulenkampff M, Schwartzman JS, Wilson J. Neurological complications of pertussis inoculation. Archives of Diseases in Childhood 1974; 49: 46-9

15 Minutes of Joint Committee on Vaccination and Immunisation 11 December 1974.

16 Barrie H. Campaign of Terror. American Journal of Diseases of Children 1983; 137: 922-3

17 Crombie DL. Whooping cough: what proportion of cases is notified in an epidemic. [Letter] British Medical Journal 1983; 287(6394): 760-1.

18 Stewart GT. Re: Whooping cough and the whooping cough vaccine [letter]. American Journal of Epidemiology 1984; 119: 135-7

19 Palmer SR. Vaccine efficacy and control measures in pertussis. Archives of Disease in Childhood 1991; 66(7): 854-7.

20 Crowcroft NS, Britto J. Whooping cough — a continuing problem. British Medical Journal 2002; 324: 1537-8

21 Pollock TM, Miller E, Lobb J. Severity of whooping cough in England before and after the decline in pertussis immunisation. Archives of Disease in Childhood 1984; 59: 162-5

22 Miller E, Jacombs B, Pollock TM. Whooping-Cough Notifications [letter]. The Lancet 1980; 718.

23 Do the Right Thing. NHS Magazine March 2001.

24 Thomson D. Monthly Bulletin of the Ministry of Health and PHLS 1953: 92-102

25 Geier D, Geier M. The True Story of Pertussis Vaccination: A Sordid Legacy? Journal of the History of Medicine 2002; 57: 249-284.

26 Minutes of the Joint Committee on Vaccination and Immunisation. 29th March 1977

27 The collection of data relating to adverse reactions to pertussis vaccine. Report of the Advisory Panel. HMSO. 1980

28 Miller DL et al. Report of the National Childhood Encephalopathy Study. HMSO 1980.

29 Miller DL et al. Pertussis Immunisation and serious acute neurological illness in children. British Medical Journal 1993; 307: 1171-6

30 Gale JL. Thapa PB. Wassilak SG. Bobo JK. Mendelman PM. Foy HM. Risk of serious acute neurological illness after immunization with diphtheria-tetanus-pertussis vaccine. A population-based case-control study. JAMA 1994; 271(1): 37-41.

31 Bill Inman. Don't Tell the Patient, Highland Park Publications 1999.

32 Stewart GS. Toxicity of pertussis vaccine: frequency and probability of reactions. Journal of Epidemiology and Community Health 1979; 33: 150-156.

33 DPT Vaccine and Chronic Nervous System Dysfunction: A New Analysis. Institute of Medicine. National Academies Press 1994.

34 Botham SJ, Isaacs D. Incidence of apnoea and bradycardia in preterm infants following triple antigen immunization. Journal of Paediatrics and Child Health 1994; 30: 533-5

35 Slack MH, Schapira D. Severe apnoeas following immunisation in premature infants. Archives of Disease in Childhood 1999; 81: F67-F68

36 BBC: http://news.bbc.co.uk/1/hi/health/3547490.stm

37 Pollock TM, Miller E, Lobb J. Severity of whooping cough in England before and after the decline in pertussis immunisation. Archives of Disease in Childhood 1984; 59: 162-5

38 Barrie H. Pertussis and the wolf. The Practitioner 1986; 230: 391-3.

39 Wilson GS. The Hazards of Immunization. The Athlone Press 1967: 281.

40 Dick G. Convulsive Disorders in Young Children. Proceedings of the Royal Society of Medicine 1974; 67: 371-2

41 Jefferson T, Rudin M, DiPietrantonj C. Systematic review of the effects of pertussis vaccination in children. Vaccine 2003; 21: 2012-23

42 Ditchburn RK. Whooping cough after stopping

pertussis immunisation. British Medical Journal 1979; 1: 1601-3

43 Trollfors B. Bordetella Pertussis Whole Cell Vaccines — Efficacy and Toxicity. Acta Paediatrica Scandinavica 1984; 73(4): 417-25. The rates of vaccine uptake were 95% in France, 40% in Britain and 10% in West Germany.

44 Romanus V, Jonsell R, Berquist S. Pertussis in Sweden after the cessation of general immunization in 1979. The Pediatric Infectious Disease Journal 1987; 6: 364-371

45 Miller E et al. Serological evidence of pertussis in patients presenting with cough in general practice in Birmingham. Communicable Disease and Public Health 2000; 3: 132-4

46 Ranganathan S et al. Pertussis is increasing in unimmunised infants: is a change in policy needed? Archives of Disease in Childhood 1999; 80: 297-9

47 Christie C, Marx ML, Marchant CD, Reising SF. The 1993 Epidemic of Pertussis in Cincinnati — Resurgence of Disease in a Highly Immunised Population of children. The New England Journal of Medicine 1994; 331: 16-21

48 de Melker HE et al. Pertussis in the Netherlands: an Outbreak despite High Levels of Immunization with Whole-Cell Vaccine. Emerging Infectious Diseases 1997; 3: 175-8

49 Jenkinson D. Duration of effectiveness of pertussis vaccine: evidence from a 10 year community study. British Medical Journal 1998; 296: 612-614

50 Hallander HA et al. Pertussis decay after vaccination with DTPa. Response to a first booster dose 3 1/2-6 1/2 years after the third vaccine dose. Vaccine 2005; 23: S359-S364.

51 Harnden A. Grant C. Harrison T. Perera R. Brueggemann AB. Mayon-White R. Mant D. Whooping cough in school age children with persistent cough: prospective cohort study in primary care. BMJ 2006; 333(7560): 174-7.

52 Tan T, Trindade E, Skowronski D. Epidemiology of Pertussis. The Pediatric Infectious Disease Journal 2005; 24: S10-S18

53 Wang K, Fry NK, Campbell H, Amirthalingam G, Harrison TG, Mant D, Harnden A. Whooping cough in school age children presenting with persistent cough in UK primary care after introduction of the preschool booster vaccination: prospective cohort study. BMJ 2014; 348: g3668

54 Klein NP, Bartlett J, Fireman B, Baxter R. Waning Tdap effectiveness in adolescents. Pediatrics 2016; 137(3): e20153326

55 Vilajeliu A et al. Combined tetanus-diphtheria and pertussis vaccine during pregnancy: transfer of maternal pertussis antibodies to the newborn. Vaccine 2015; 33(8): 1056-62

56 Babrera G et al. A case-control study to estimate the effectiveness of maternal pertussis vaccination in protecting newborn infants in England and Wales, 2012-2013. Clinical Infectious Disease 2015; 60(3): 333-7

57 Hardy-Fairbanks AJ et al. Immune response to infants

whose mothers received Tdap vaccine during pregnancy. The Pediatric Disease Journal 2013; 32(11): 1257-1260.

58 Abu Raya et al. The induction of breast milk pertussis specific antibodies following gestational tetanus-diphtheria-acellular pertussis vaccination. Vaccine 2014; 32(43): 5632-7.

59 Raya Abu B, Bamberger E, Almog M, Peri R, Srugo I, Kessel A. Immunization of pregnant women against pertussis: the effect of timing on antibody activity.

60 Kharbanda EO et al. Evaluation of the association of maternal pertussis vaccination with obstetric events and birth outcomes. JAMA 2014; 312(18): 1897-1904.

61 Donegan K, King B, Bryan P. Safety of pertussis vaccination in pregnant women in UK: observational study. BMJ 2014; 349: g4219

62 McGirr A, Fisman DN. Duration of pertussis immunity after DTaP immunization: a meta-analysis. Pediatrics 2015; 135(2): 331-342.

63 Ladhani SN, Andrews NJ, Southern J et al. Antibody response after primary immunization in infants born to women receiving a pertussis-containing vaccine during pregnancy: single arm observational study with a historical comparator. Clinical Infectious Diseases 2015; 61(11): 1637-44.

64 Matthias J, Pritchard PS, Martin SW, Dusek C, Cathey E, D'Alessio R, Kirsch M. Sustained transmission of pertussis in vaccinated 1-5 year old children in a Preschool, Florida, USA. Emerging Infectious Diseases 2016; 22(2): 242-6

12 Good Sense: Rubella

1 Cooper LZ. The history and medical consequences of rubella. Reviews of Infectious Diseases 19985; 7 Suppl 1: S2-10.

2 Sheridan MD. Final Report of a Prospective Study of Children whose Mothers had Rubella in early Pregnancy. British Medical Journal 1964; 5408: 536-9.

3 Miller E. Cradock-Watson JE. Pollock TM. Consequences of confirmed maternal rubella at successive stages of pregnancy. Lancet 1982; 2(8302): 781-4.

4 Manson MM, Logan WDD, Loy RM. Rubella and other virus infections during pregnancy. Reports on Public Health and Medical Subjects 1960, no. 101, Ministry of Health, London.

5 Minutes of the Joint Committee on Vaccination and Immunisations. April 25, 1986.

13 Who wanted the MMR?: MMR/Mumps

1 Philip RN. Reinhard KR. Lackman DB. Observations on a mumps epidemic in a 'virgin' population. 1958. American Journal of Epidemiology 1995; 142(3): 233-53.

2 These are the parotid salivary glands.

3 Anonymous. A retrospective survey of the complications of mumps. Journal of the Royal College of General Practitioners 1974; 24(145): 552-6.

4 Anonymous. The incidence and complications of

mumps. Journal of the Royal College of General Practitioners 1974; 24(145): 545-51.

5 Noah ND. Mumps — worthy of elimination? Current Topics in Clinical Virology. Public Health Laboratory Service 1991: 47-60.

6 Galbraith NS. Young SE. Pusey JJ. Crombie DL. Sparks JP. Mumps surveillance in England and Wales 1962-81. Lancet 1984; 1(8368): 91-4.

7 Anonymous. Vaccine against mumps. British Medical Journal 1967; 2(555):779-80.

8 Dick G. Immunisation. Update Books 1978: p3.

9 Minutes of the Joint Committee on Vaccination and Immunisation. December 11, 1974.

10 Mumps — general information. Health Protection Agency. Available at hpa.org.uk/infections/topics_az/mumps/gen_info.htm. Downloaded December 31, 2005.

11 Beard CM. Benson RC Jr. Kelalis PP. Elveback LR. Kurland LT. The incidence and outcome of mumps orchitis in Rochester, Minnesota, 1935 to 1974. Mayo Clinic Proceedings 1977; 52(1):3-7.

12 Anonymous. Prevention of mumps. British Medical Journal 1980; 281(6250): 1231-2.

13 Cheek JE. Baron R. Atlas H. Wilson DL. Crider RD Jr. Mumps outbreak in a highly vaccinated school population. Evidence for large-scale vaccination failure. Archives of Pediatrics & Adolescent Medicine 1995; 149(7): 774-8.

14 Briss PA et al. Sustained transmission of mumps in a highly vaccinated population: assessment of primary vaccine failure and waning vaccine-induced immunity. Journal of Infectious Diseases 1994; 169(1): 77-82.

15 Miller E. Hill A. Morgan-Capner P. Forsey T. Rush M. Antibodies to measles, mumps and rubella in UK children 4 years after vaccination with different MMR vaccines. Vaccine 1995; 13(9): 799-802.

16 Pebody RG et al. Immunogenicity of second dose measles-mumps-rubella (MMR) vaccine and implications for serosurveillance. Vaccine 2002; 20(7-8): 1134-40.

23

17 Gay N et al. Mumps surveillance in England and Wales supports introduction of two dose vaccination schedule. Communicable Disease Report 1997; CDR Review. 7(2): R21-6.

18 Pugh RN et al. An outbreak of mumps in the metropolitan area of Walsall, UK. International Journal of Infectious Diseases 2002; 6(4): 283-7.

19 Hyde N. Jab fears lead to mumps outbreak. Daily Express, August 6, 2001.

20 Mumps. Communication from Dr David Salisbury, Principal Medical Officer, Department of Health. CEM/CMO/2004/4: 21st May 2004.

]21 UK students at risk of mumps. BMJ 2004; 329: 1062.

22 Mumps Outbreak at a Summer Camp — New York, 2005. MMWR 2006; 55(07): 175-177.

23 Crowley B. Afzal MA. Mumps virus reinfection — clinical findings and serological vagaries. Communicable

Disease & Public Health 2002; 5(4): 311-3.

24 Harling R, White JM, Ramsay ME, Macsween KF, van den Bosch C. The effectiveness of the mumps component of the MMR vaccine: a case control study. Vaccine 2005; 23[31]: 4070-4.

25 Hersh S et al. Mumps outbreak in a highly vaccinated population. The Journal of Pediatrics 1991; 119:187-193

26 Pulse; May 28th 2005.

27 Braeye T, Linina I, DeRoy R, Hutse V, Wauters M, Cox P, Mak R. Mumps increase in Flanders, Belgium, 201202013: Results from temporary mandatory notification and a cohort study among university students. Vaccine 2014; 32: 4393-4398.

29 Yung C-F, Andrews N, Bukasa A, Brown KE, Ramsay ME. Mumps complications and effects of mumps vaccination, England and Wales, 2002-2006. Emerging Infectious Diseases 2011; 17[4]: 661-7.

30 Vygen S, Fischer A, Meurice L et al. Waning immunity against mumps in vaccinated young adults, France 2013. Eurosurveillance 2016; 21(10):pii=30156

14 A Bold Plan: MMR / Measles

1 Jefferson T, Price D, et al. Unintended events following immunization with the MMR: a systematic review. Vaccine 2003; 21: 3954-3960

2 Wakefield AJ, Montgomery SM. Measles, mumps, rubella vaccine: through a glass darkly. Adverse Drug Reactions and Toxicological Reviews 2000; 19: 265-83

3 Fletcher AP, (Referee 3) for Wakefield AJ, Montgomery SM. Measles, mumps, rubella vaccine: through a glass darkly. Adverse Drug Reactions and Toxicological Reviews 2000; 19: 265-83

4 Jefferson T, Price D, Demicheli V, Bianco E. Unintended events following immunization with MMR: a systematic review. Vaccine 2003; 21: 3954-3960

5 Demicheli V, Jefferson T, Rivetti A, Price D. Vaccines for measles, mumps and rubella in children. The Cochrane Collaboration 2005.

6 McDonald JC. Moore DL. Quennec P. Clinical and epidemiologic features of mumps meningoencephalitis and possible vaccine-related disease. Pediatric Infectious Disease Journal 1989; 8[11]: 751-5.

7 Brown EG. Furesz J. Dimock K. Yarosh W. Contreras G. Nucleotide sequence analysis of Urabe mumps vaccine strain that caused meningitis in vaccine recipients. Vaccine 1991; 9[11]: 840-2.

8 Fujinaga T. Motegi Y. Tamura H. Kuroume T. A prefecture-wide survey of mumps meningitis associated with measles, mumps and rubella vaccine. Pediatric Infectious Disease Journal 1991; 10[3]: 204-9.

9 Sugiura A. Yamada A. Aseptic meningitis as a complication of mumps vaccination. Pediatric Infectious Disease Journal 1991; 10[3]: 209-13.

10 New South Wales Legislative Hansard, 27th November, 1992: 10289-10295.

11 Minutes of Joint Sub-Committee on Adverse Reactions to Vaccination and Immunisation. March 8, 1988.

12 Joint Committee on Vaccination and Immunisation;

Minutes of the Meeting held on Friday 6 November 1992.

13 Joint Committee on Vaccination and Immunisation; Minutes of the Meeting held on 5 November 1993.

14 Crowley S, Al-Jawad ST, Kovar IZ, Mumps, measles, and rubella vaccination and encephalitis. BMJ 1989; 299: 660

15 Campbell AGM. Mumps, measles, and rubella vaccination and encephalitis. BMJ 1989; 299:916.

16 Begg NT, Noah ND. Mumps, measles, and rubella vaccination and encephalitis. BMJ 1989; 299:978.

17 Nalin DR. Mumps, measles, and rubella vaccination and encephalitis. BMJ 1989; 299:1219.

18 Gray JA. Burns SM. Mumps meningitis following measles, mumps, and rubella immunisation.[Letter] Lancet 1989; 2[8654]: 98.

19 Murray MW. Lewis MJ. Mumps meningitis after measles, mumps, and rubella vaccination.[Letter] Lancet 1989; 2[8664]: 677.

20 Colville A. Pugh S. Mumps meningitis and measles, mumps, and rubella vaccine.[Letter] Lancet 1992; 340[8822]: 786.

21 Joint Committee on Vaccination and Immunisation; Minutes of the Meeting held on Friday 4 May 1990.

22 Minutes of Joint Sub-Committee on Adverse Reactions to Vaccination and Immunisation. September 17, 1990.

23 From the Chief Medical Officer. Changes in supply of vaccine. DoH PL/CMO/(92)11. September 14, 1992.

24 You & Yours, Radio 4, 11 Aug 2000

25 Evans NJB, Cunliffe PW, Study of Control of Medicines. HMSO 1987

26 Joint Committee on Vaccination and Immunisation; Minutes of the Meeting held on Friday 7 November 1986.

27 Mills H. MMR: the story so far. Private Eye Special Report. May 2002.

28 Prentice T. Triple vaccine for all children. The Times. October 3, 1988.

29 Prentice T. Government boost for vaccine drive. The Times. October 4, 1988.

30 The BSE Enquiry, www.bseinquiry.gov.uk 2000

31 Measles/Rubella: Information for health professionals. Department of Health 1994; 152595M9/94.

32 Is your measles jab really necessary? Bulletin of Medical Ethics 1994; 102: 3-5.

33 Rylance G. Bowen C. Rylance J. Measles and rubella immunisation: information and consent in children. BMJ 1995; 311[7010]: 923-4.

34 Measles/Rubella: Information for health professionals. Department of Health 1994; 152595M9/94.

35 Joint Committee on Vaccination and Immunisation; Minutes of the Meeting held on 5 May 1995.

36 Miller E. The new measles campaign. [Editorial] BMJ 1994; 309[6962]: 1102-3.

37 Vyse AJ et al. Evolution of Surveillance of Measles, Mumps and Rubella in England and Wales: Providing the Platform for Evidence-based Vaccination Policy.

Epidemiologic Reviews 2002; 24:125-136

38 [Miller E. Was Bulletin wrong on measles campaign? Bulletin of Medical Ethics 1111996; 114: 2

39 [Ramsay M. Gay N. Miller E. Rush M. White J. Morgan-Capner P. Brown D. The epidemiology of measles in England and Wales: rationale for the 1994 national vaccination campaign. Communicable Disease Report. CDR Review 1994; 4(12): R141-6.

40 [Gay NJ, Miller E. Was a measles epidemic imminent? Communicable Disease Report 1995; 5: R204-7

41 Cutts FT. Revaccination against measles and rubella. [Editorial] BMJ 1996; 312(7031): 589-90.

42 From the Chief Medical Officer. Change to the routine pre-school booster immunisation programme. July 16 1996. Available at dh.gov.uk/assetRoot/04/01/33/93/04013393.pdf. Accessed April 27, 2006.

43 Letter from Richard Barr to Professor Rawlins. October 18, 1996.

44 Letter from Professor Rawlins to Richard Barr. April 29, 1996.

45 Joint Committee on Vaccination and Immunisation; Minutes of the Meeting held on Friday 2 May 1997.

46 Joint Committee on Vaccination and Immunisation; Minutes of the Meeting held on Friday 1 May 1998.

15 A Further Mystery: MMR / Rubella

1 Freestone DS. Vaccination against rubella in Britain: benefits and risks. Developments in Biological Standardization 1979; 43: 339-48.

2 Anderson RM. May RM. Vaccination against rubella and measles: quantitative investigations of different policies. Journal of Hygiene 1983; 90(2): 259-325.

3 Miller E et al. The epidemiology of rubella in England and Wales before and after the 1994 measles and rubella vaccination campaign: fourth joint report from the PHLS and the National Congenital Rubella Surveillance Programme. Communicable Disease Report. CDR Review 1997; 7(2): R26-32.

4 Davidkin I. Peltola H. Leinikki P. Valle M. Duration of rubella immunity induced by two-dose measles, mumps and rubella (MMR) vaccination. A 15-year follow-up in Finland. Vaccine 2000; 18(27): 3106-12.

5 Protecting women against rubella. Switch from rubella vaccine to MMR. Letter from the Chief medical Officer, PL CMO (2003)7. September 26, 2003.

6 Lévy-Bruhl D, Six C, Parent I. Rubella control in France. Eurosurveillance Monthly 2004; 9(4): 13-14

7 Progress Toward Elimination of Measles and Prevention of Congenital Rubella Infection — European Region, 1990-2004. MMWR weekly 2005; 54(07): 175-178.

8 Tingle AJ. Allen M. Petty RE. Kettyls GD. Chantler JK. Rubella-associated arthritis. I. Comparative study of joint manifestations associated with natural rubella infection and RA 27/3 rubella immunisation. Annals of the Rheumatic Diseases 1986; 45(2): 110-4.

9 Allen AD. Is RA27/3 rubella immunization a cause of chronic fatigue? Medical Hypotheses 1988; 27(3): 217-20.

10 Losonsky GA. Fishaut JM. Strussenberg J. Ogra PL. Effect of immunization against rubella on lactation products. I. Development and characterization of specific immunologic reactivity in breast milk. Journal of Infectious Diseases 1982; 145(5): 654-60.

11 Santoshkumar A. Transmission of live vaccine viruses from vaccinated persons to others. Indian Pediatrics 2000; 37(7): 794-5.

12 Braun C. Kampa D. Fressle R. Willke E. Stahl M. Haller O. Congenital rubella syndrome despite repeated vaccination of the mother: a coincidence of vaccine failure with failure to vaccinate. Acta Paediatrica 1994; 83(6): 674-7.

16 Dr Andrew Wakefield: MMR Scare

1 Wakefield AJ. Pittilo RM. Sim R. Cosby SL. Stephenson JR. Dhillon AP. Pounder RE. Evidence of persistent measles virus infection in Crohn's disease. Journal of Medical Virology 1993; 39(4): 345-53.

2 Ekbom A. Wakefield AJ. Zack M. Adami HO. Perinatal measles infection and subsequent Crohn's disease. Lancet 1994; 344(8921): 508-10.

3 Ekbom A. Daszak P. Kraaz W. Wakefield AJ. Crohn's disease after in-utero measles virus exposure. Lancet 1996; 348(9026): 515-7.

4 Thompson NP. Montgomery SM. Pounder RE. Wakefield AJ. Is measles vaccination a risk factor for inflammatory bowel disease? Lancet 1995; 345(8957): 1071-4.

5 Mills H. MMR: the story so far. Private Eye Special Report. May 2002.

6 Richard Barr. Personal communication. September 25, 2006.

7 Wakefield AJ et al. Ileal-lymphoid-nodular hyperplasia, non-specific colitis, and pervasive developmental disorder in children. The Lancet 1998; 351:637-41

8 Hall C. Vaccination may trigger disease linked to autism. Daily Telegraph. February 27, 1998.

9 BBC News. Child Vaccine linked to autism. February 27, 19998. Available at http://news.bbc.co.uk/1/hi/uk/60510.stm. Accessed April 27, 2006.

10 BBC News. Government reassurance on MMR vaccine. February 27, 1998. Available at http://news.bbc.co.uk/1/hi/uk/60721.stm. Accessed April 27, 2006.

11 MMR vaccination and autism 1998. British Medical Journal 1998; 316: 715-716

12 Fax from Ralph H Henderson, Assistant Director-General, WHO to Tessa Jowell, Minister of State, DoH. March 10, 1998.

13 MRC. Report of the meeting held on 23 March 1998 to examine evidence relating measles or measles vaccine to gastrointestinal inflammation. D409/893.

14 DoH Press release. MMR Vaccine Is Not Linked To Crohn's Disease Or Autism — Conclusion Of An Expert Scientific Seminar. 98/109. March 24, 1998.

Available at
dh.gov.uk/PublicationsAndStatistics/PressReleases/Press
ReleasesNotices/fs/en?CONTENT_ID=4024615&chk
=Io5uBf. Accessed on April 27, 2006.

15 From the Chief Medical Officer. Measles, Mumps,
Rubella (MMR) Vaccine, Crohn's disease and autism. PL
CMO (1998)2.March 27, 1998. Available at
dh.gov.uk/assetRoot/04/01/33/97/04013397.pdf.
Accessed April 27, 2006.

16 MMR: The Royal Free and the drug company. Private
Eye.

17 Ramsay S. Controversial MMR-autism investigator
resigns from research post. Lancet 2001; 358: 1972.

18 Steele L. 'It is not about the science. It's about belief'.
The Guardian. December 5, 2001. Available at vaccina-
tionnews.com/DailyNews/December2001/NotSciBelief.
htm. Accessed April 30, 2006.

19 Barr R. Experts at Risk. Solicitor's Journal July 14,
2006; 902.

20 Odone C. White, middle-class, loving mums. And
their stupidity could kill your child. The Times: June 19,
2006.

21 Transcript of hearing before Mr Justice Keith. Royal
Courts of Justice. October 14, 2002.

22 Letter from Lovells, solicitors, to Ms Isabella Thomas,
May 7, 2004.

23 Miller CG. Questions on the Independence and
Reliability of Cochrane Reviews, with a Focus on
Measles-Mumps-Rubella Vaccine. Journal of American
Physicians and Surgeons 2006; 11: 111-115.

17 The Science: MMR Studies

1 ILNH, in association with autism in a child, was later
described by Wakefield as 'autistic enterocolitis'.

2 Montgomery SM. Morris DL. Pounder RE. Wakefield
AJ. Paramyxovirus infections in childhood and
subsequent inflammatory bowel disease.
Gastroenterology 1999; 116(4): 796-803.

3 Deykin EY. MacMahon B. Viral exposure and autism.
American Journal of Epidemiology 1979; 109(6): 628-
38.

4 Baron-Cohen S et al. Estimating Autism Spectrum
prevalence in the population: a school based study
from the UK. British Journal Psychiatry: (article in
press).

5 Interview with Professor Elizabeth Miller. 26 September,
2006.

6 Macdonald V. Doctors fight back on suspect vaccine.
Daily Telegraph. April 5, 1998.

7 Health Education Authority. MMR – The Facts. 1998.

8 Report of the working party on MMR vaccine.
Committee on Safety of Medicines; 1999

9 Taylor B, Miller E et al. Autism and measles, mumps,
and rubella vaccine: no epidemiological evidence for a
causal association. The Lancet 1999; 353: 2026-9

10 Lingam R. Simmons A. Andrews N. Miller E. Stowe J.
Taylor B. Prevalence of autism and parentally reported
triggers in a north east London population. Archives

of Disease in Childhood 2003; 88(8): 666-70.

11 This is based on copies of letters in my possession.

12 DoH Press Release. Two new independent studies find
no link between MMR vaccination and autism.
1999/0342. June 10, 1999. Available at
dh.gov.uk/PublicationsAndStatistics/PressReleases/Press
ReleasesNotices/fs/en?CONTENT_ID=4025433&chk
=2%2Bqhau. Accessed April 28 2006.

13 Madsen KM et al. A population-based study of
measles, mumps and rubella vaccination and autism.
The New England Journal of Medicine 2002; 347:
1477-1482

14 Goldman GS, Yazbak FE. An Investigation of the
Association Between MMR Vaccination and Autism in
Denmark. Journal of American Physicians and Surgeons
2004; 9: 70-5

15 Kaye JA et al. Mumps, measles, and rubella vaccine
and the incidence of autism recorded by general practitioners: a time trend analysis. British Medical Journal
2001; 322: 460-463

16 Uhlmann V, Martin CM et al. Potential viral
pathogenic mechanism for a new variant inflammatory
bowel disease. Molecular Pathology 2002; 55: 84-90

17 Sheils O, Smyth P, Martin C, O'Leary JJ. Development
of an 'allelic discrimination' type assay to differentiate
between the strain origins of measles virus detected in
intestinal tissue of children with ileocolonic lymphonodular hyperplasia and concomitant developmental
disorder. Abstract (no. 20) presented at Pathological
Society of Great Britain and Ireland. 2002.

18 S. Walker, K. Hepner, J. Segal, A. Krigsman. Persistent
ileal measles virus in a large cohort of regressive
autistic children with ileocolitis and lymphonodular
hyperplasia: revisitation of an earlier study. Presented at
5th International Meeting for Autism Research in
Montreal, Canada in June 2, 2006.

19 Wakefield AJ, Stott C, Limb K. Gastrointestinal
comorbidity, autistic regression and Measles-containing
vaccines. Medical Veritas 2006; 3 (1): 796-802.

20 Immunization Safety Review: Measles-Mumps-Rubella
Vaccine and Autism. Institute of Medicine, The
National Academies Press 2001

21 Bradstreet JJ et al. Detection of Measles Virus Genome
RNA in Cerebrospinal Fluid of Children with
Regressive Autism: a Report of Three Cases. Journal of
American Physicians and Surgeons 2004; 9: 38-45

22 The saga of how these children managed to get investigated would read like a 'Carry On' film were it not so
sinister. Having tried unsuccessfully for a year to
obtain CSF samples from their children in the UK, the
parents flew to the USA to have the necessary tests.
Despite two attempts by the vaccine manufacturers to
obtain injunctions to prevent the investigations going
ahead, the parents managed to get their children
tested, but not without members of the group being
hauled off the plane for a 30 minute interrogation
before taking off in Detroit and a further questioning
at Schiphol airport in Amsterdam on the return. The

virologist in the party has had many years experience of transporting CSF and other samples across international borders. He told me that he had never before experienced an interrogation like that in Detroit.

23 'Initial autism research findings at Harvard – Massachusetts General' Timothy Bluie MD and others; downloaded from the internet September 16th 2004

24 Torrente F et al. Focal-Enhanced Gastritis in Regressive Autism with features Distinct from Crohn's and Helicobacter Pylori Gastritis. American Journal of Gastroenterology 2004; 99: 598-605

25 Krigsman A et al. Preliminary data presented at Congressional Hearing. 2002

26 Singh VK et al. Abnormal Measles-Mumps-Rubella antibodies and CNS autoimmunity in children with autism. Journal of Biomedical Science 2002; 9: 359-364

27 Singh VK et al. Elevated levels of Measles antibodies in children with autism. Pediatric Neurology 2003; 28: 292-4

28 Deer B. Revealed: MMR research scandal. The *Sunday Times*. February 22, 2004.

29 Wakefield AJ. Autism, inflammatory bowel disease, and MMR vaccine. *Lancet* 1998; 351(9112): 1356.

30 Committee on Safety of Medicines. Annual Report For 2004. Available at mhra.gov.uk/home/idcplg?IdcService=GET_FILE&dID=9181&noSaveAs=1&Rendition=WEB Accessed May 31, 2007.

31 MMR: what they didn't tell you. Channel 4 television, Dispatches: Thursday 18 November 2004, 9pm

32 Wakefield AJ. Autistic enterocolitis: is it a histopathological entity? – a reply. Histopathology 2007; 50: 380-384.

33 Wakefield AJ, Ashwood P, Limb K, Anthony A. The significance of ileo-colonic lymphoid nodular hyperplasia in children with autistic spectrum disorder. European Journal of Gastroenterology and Hepatology 2005; 17: 827-836

34 Kennedy RC, Byers VS, Marchalonis JJ. Measles Virus Infection and Vaccination: Potential Role in Chronic Illness and Associated Adverse Events. Clinical Reviews in Immunology 2004; 24: 129-156

35 Goldman GS, Yazbak FE. An Investigation of the Association between MMR Vaccination and Autism in Denmark. Journal of American Physicians and Surgeons 2004; 9: 70-75

36 John Griffin, former Professional Head of Medicines Division, DoH. Personal communication. November 30, 2004.

37 Krigsman A, Boris M, Goldblatt A, Stott C. Clinical presentation and histologic findings at ileocolonoscopy in children with autistic spectrum disorder and chronic gastrointestinal symptoms. Autism Insights 2010; 2: 1-11

18 'Russian Roulette': MMR, Conclusion

1 HMSO. Immunisation against Infectious Disease ('The Green Book') 1996.

2 Monovalent measles vaccine is withdrawn. GP:
September 11, 1998.

3 Johnston L, Branigan K. Doctors ban parents for refusing MMR jabs. Sunday Express. March 4, 2001.

4 Kelly B. Legal warning as GP strikes off MMR refuseniks. Pulse. October 20, 2001.

5 Heath M. 'MMR refuseniks' GP should have nothing to fear from GMC [letter]. Pulse. November 3, 2001.

6 Wigfield M. GP who struck off MMR refuseniks was following me [letter]. Pulse October 27, 2001.

7 Why I took drastic action on dissenters. Pulse April 23, 2005.

8 Joint Committee on Vaccination and Immunisation; Minutes of the Meeting held on Friday 1 May 1998

9 Templeton S-K. MMR: Will we ever be sure it's safe? Sunday Herald. February 10, 2002.

10 MMR – Why the use of single antigens would be inadvisable. CDR weekly. July 26, 2001. Available at hpa.org.uk/cdr/archives/2001/cdr3001.pdf. Accessed April 30, 2006.

11 Hall C. Scientists clear triple vaccine of link to autism. Daily Telegraph. March 25, 1998.

12 Letter from the Chief Medical Officer. Current Vaccine and Immunisation Issues. PL CMO [2001]1. March 9, 2001. Available at dh.gov.uk/assetRoot/04/01/34/04/04013404.pdf. Accessed April 30, 2006.

13 Moreton J. MMR – safe and seaweed-free. Update. March 22, 2001.

14 Templeton S-K. Health board: of course the MMR is safe...the maker said so. July 2001. Available at vaccinationnews.com/DailyNews/July2001/HealthBrd-MMRSafe,MakerSaidSo.htm. Accessed April 28, 2006.

15 BBC News. Fears grow as mumps cases rise. August, 2001. Available at http://news.bbc.co.uk/1/hi/health/1516706.stm. Accessed April 28, 2006.

16 Health Promotion England. MMR The Facts. NHS. 2001.

17 BBC News. Jail threat for MMR refuseniks. February 14, 2002.

18 Duckworth L. Warning over 'real threat' of measles deaths. Independent. January 10, 2002.

19 BBC News. MMR jab defended. Available at http://news.bbc.co.uk/1/hi/health/1806243.stm. Accessed April 30, 2006.

20 Fraser L. Revealed: more evidence to challenge the safety of MMR. Daily Telegraph. June 16, 2002. Available at telegraph.co.uk/news/main.jhtml?xml=%2Fnews%2F2002%2F06%2F16%2Fnmmr16.xml. Accessed April 30, 2006.

21 Connor S. MMR chief blames the media for jab 'errors'. The Independent February 12, 2002.

22 Flynn M. Ogden J. Predicting uptake of MMR vaccination: a prospective questionnaire study. British Journal of General Practice 2004; 54{504}: 526-30.

23 Joint Committee on Vaccination and Immunisation; Minutes of the Meeting held on Friday 30 October

1998.

24 Pearce A, Law C, Elliman D, Cole TJ, Bedford H, the Millennium Cohort Study Child Health Group. Factors associated with uptake of measles, mumps, and rubella vaccine (MMR) and use of single antigen vaccines in a contemporary UK cohort: prospective cohort study. BMJ 2008; 336: 754-7.

25 Bhattacharya S, Young A. GPs want to see a single measles vaccine on NHS. Pulse. February 17, 2001.

26 MMR — why single vaccines are bad medicine. BMA News. April 7, 2001.

27 Media told it must 'end the anti-MMR campaign now.' Doctor July 4, 2006.

28 Demicheli V, Jefferson T, Rivetti A, Price D. Vaccines for measles, mumps and rubella in children. The Cochrane Collaboration 2005.

29 Harling et al. The effectiveness of the mumps component of the MMR vaccine: a case control study. Vaccine 2005; 23: 4070-4074

30 Hersh S et al. Mumps outbreak in a highly vaccinated population. The Journal of Pediatrics 1991; 119:187-193

31 Briss PA et al. Sustained Transmission of Mumps in a Highly Vaccinated Population: Assessment of Primary Vaccine Failure and Waning Vaccine-Induced Immunity. Journal of Infectious Disease 1994; 169: 77-82

32 Pulse; May 28th 2005.

33 Bitnun A et al. Measles Inclusion-Body Encephalitis caused by the Vaccine strain of the Measles Virus. Clinical Infectious Diseases 1999; 29: 855-61

34 Committee on Safety of Medicines, the body that advises the government on drug and vaccine safety

35 Committee on Safety of Medicines. MMR vaccine and Idiopathic Thrombocytopenic Purpura. Current Problems in Pharmacovigilance 2001; 27: August.

36 Vlacha V. Forman EN. Miron D. Peter G. Recurrent thrombocytopenic purpura after repeated measles-mumps-rubella vaccination. Pediatrics 1996; 97(5): 738-9.

37 Minutes of Joint Committee on Vaccination and Immunisation. November 7, 1997.

38 Minutes of Joint Committee on Vaccination and Immunisation. May 7, 1999.

39 Olesen AB, Juul S, Thestrup-Pedersen K. Atopic Dermatitis is increased following Vaccination for Measles, Mumps and Rubella or Measles infection. Acta Derm Venereol. 2003; 83: 445-450.

40 McKeever TM et al. Vaccination and Allergic Disease: a Birth Cohort Study. American Journal of Public Health 2004; 94: 985-9.

41 Arshi S et al. The first rapid onset optic neuritis after measles-rubella vaccination: case report. Vaccine 2004; 22:3240-3242

42 Hansen LF, Nordling MM, Mortensen HB. Acute pancreatitis associated with MMR vaccination. Ugeskrift for Laeger 2003; 165: 2305-6

43 Mühlebach-Sponer M, Zbinden R, da Silva VA, Gnehm HE. Intrathecal rubella antibodies in an adolescent with Guillain-Barré syndrome after mumps-measles-rubella vaccination. European Journal of

Pediatrics 1995; 154: 166

44 Plesner A-M et al. Gait disturbance interpreted as cerebellar ataxia after MMR vaccination at 15 months of age: a follow-up study. Acta Paediatrica 2000; 89: 58-63

45 LeBaron CW, Bi D, Sullivan BJ, Beck C, Gargiullo P. Evaluation of Potentially Common Adverse Events Associated With the First and Second Doses of Measles-Mumps-Rubella Vaccine. Pediatrics 2006; 118 [4]: 1422-1430.

46 Joint Committee on Vaccination and Immunisation; Minutes of the Meeting held on Friday 1 May 1987.

47 Miller C et al. Surveillance of symptoms following MMR vaccine in children. Practitioner 1989; 233: 69-74

48 Vestergaard M et al. MMR Vaccination and Febrile Seizures. Evaluation of Susceptible Subgroups and Long-term Prognosis. Journal of the American Medical Association 2004; 292: 351-357

49 Nagaraj A. Does qualitative synthesis of anecdotal evidence with that from scientific research help in understanding public health issues: a review of low MMR uptake. European Journal of Public Health 2006; 16(1): 85-88, doi: 101093/eurpub/cki058.

50 Smith A, McCann R, McKinlay I. Second dose of MMR vaccine: health professionals' level of confidence in the vaccine and attitudes towards the second dose. Communicable Disease and Public Health 2001; 4: 273-7

51 Petrovic M, Roberts R, Ramsay M. Second dose of measles, mumps, and rubella vaccine: questionnaire survey of health professionals. British Medical Journal 2001; 322: 82-5

52 Henderson R et al. General Practitioners' concerns about childhood immunisation and suggestions for improving professional support and vaccine uptake. Communicable Disease and Public Health 2004; 7: 260-6

53 DoH. Health Professionals 2003. Childhood Immunisation Survey Report. Available at immunisation.nhs.uk/files/HPSurveyreport.pdf. Accessed May 1, 2006.

54 Hairon N. GPs are more confident on MMR but doubts linger. Pulse. May 14, 2005.

55 Casiday R et al. A survey of UL parental attitudes to the MMR vaccine and trust in medical authority. Vaccine 2006; 24: 177-184.

56 Wakefield AJ. Enterocolitis, autism and measles virus. Molecular Psychiatry 2002; 7 Suppl 2: S44-6.

57 Murch SH, Anthony A, Casson DH, Malik M, Berelowitz M, Dhillon AP, Thomson MA, Valentine A, Davies SE, Walker-Smith JA. Retraction of an interpretation. Lancet 2004; 363(9411):750.

58 Barr R. Experts at Risk. Solicitor's Journal July 14, 2006; 902.

59 Valenzise M, Cascio A, Wasniewska M, Zirilli G, Catena MA, Arasi S. Post vaccine acute disseminated encephalomyelitis as the first manifestation of chromosome 22q11.2 deletion syndrome in a 15-month

old baby: a case report. Vaccine 2014; 32[43]: 5552-4

60 http://apps.who.int/gho/data/node.main.A826. Accessed 23 November 2015

61 Murti M, Krajden M, Petric M, Hiebert J, Hemming F, Hefford B, Bigham M, Van Buynder P. Case of vaccine-associated measles five weeks post-immunisation, British Columbia, Canada. Eurosurveillance 2013; 18[49]. Pii: 20649

62 Millson DS. Brother-to-sister transmission of measles after measles, mumps and rubella immunization. Lancet 1989; 1[8632]: 271

63 Hooker BS. Measles-mumps-rubella vaccination timing and autism among young African American boys: a reanalysis of CDC data. Translational neurodegeneration 2014 3:16 DOI: 10.1186/2047-9158-3-16

19 A Spectacular Retreat: Hib

1 Takala AK. Clements DA. Socioeconomic risk factors for invasive Haemophilus influenzae type b disease. Journal of Infectious Diseases 1992; 165 Suppl 1: S11-5.

2 Anderson EC et al. Epidemiology of invasive Haemophilus influenzae infections in England and Wales in pre-vaccination era (1990-2). Epidemiology & Infection 1995; 115[1]: 89-100.

3 Booy R et al. Efficacy of Haemophilus influenzae type b conjugate vaccine PRP-T. Lancet 1994; 344[8919]: 362-6.

4 Eskola J et al. A randomised, prospective field trial of a conjugate vaccine in the protection of infants and young children against invasive Haemophilus influenzae type b disease. New England Journal of Medicine 1990; 323[20]: 1381-7.

5 Booy R. Heath PT. Slack MP. Begg N. Moxon ER. Vaccine failures after primary immunisation with Haemophilus influenzae type-b conjugate vaccine without booster. Lancet 1997; 349[9060]: 1197-202.

6 JCVI Statement: Haemophilus influenzae type b (Hib) Disease and Hib Vaccine.

Available at advisorybodies.doh.gov.uk/jcvi/hib.pdf [downloaded 8th December 2005)

7 Moxon ER. Heath PT. Booy R. Azzopardi HJ. Slack MP. Ramsay ME. 4th European conference on vaccinology: societal value of vaccination. The impact of Hib conjugate vaccines in preventing invasive H. influenzae diseases in the UK. Vaccine 1999; 17 Suppl 3:S11-3, 1999 Oct 29.

8 Ramsay ME. McVernon J. Andrews NJ. Heath PT. Slack MP. Estimating Haemophilus influenzae type b vaccine effectiveness in England and Wales by use of the screening method. Journal of Infectious Diseases 2003; 188[4]: 481-5.

9 Minutes of Joint Committee on Vaccination and Immunisation, 1 November 2002.

10 It has also been suggested that the introduction of the Meningitis C vaccine in 1999 could have decreased the effectiveness of the Hib vaccine, given at the same time.

11 Olowokure B. Hawker J. Blair I. Spencer N. Decrease in effectiveness of routine surveillance of Haemophilus influenzae disease after introduction of conjugate vaccine: comparison of routine reporting with active surveillance system. BMJ 2000; 321[7263]: 731-2.

12 CMO Update 40. A communication to all doctors from the Chief Medical Officer (December 2004)

13 Minutes of Joint Committee on Vaccination and Immunisation. 7 February 2003.

14 Minutes of Joint Committee on Vaccination and Immunisation. 23 February 2005.

15 Haemophilus influenzae type b conjugate vaccines: a review of efficacy data. Heath PT. Pediatric Infectious Disease Journal 1998; 17: S117-22.

16 Baer M. Vuento R. Vesikari T. Increase in bacteraemic pneumococcal infections in children. Lancet [letter] 1995; 345[8950]: 661.

17 Swingler G. Fransman D. Hussey G. Conjugate vaccines for preventing Haemophilus influenzae type b infections. Cochrane Database of Systematic Reviews 2003: [4]:CD001729.

18 Wahlberg J. Fredriksson J. Vaarala O. Ludvigsson J. Abis Study Group. Vaccinations may induce diabetes-related autoantibodies in one-year-old children. Annals of the New York Academy of Sciences 2003; 1005: 404-8.

19 Classen JB. Classen DC. Clustering of cases of insulin dependent diabetes (IDDM) occurring three years after hemophilus influenza B (HiB) immunization support causal relationship between immunization and IDDM. Autoimmunity 2002; 35[4]: 247-53.

20 DeStefano F et al. Vaccine Safety Datalink Team. Childhood vaccinations, vaccination timing, and risk of type 1 diabetes mellitus. Pediatrics 2001; 108[6]: E112.

21 DeStefano F. et al. Vaccine Safety Datalink Research Group. Childhood vaccinations and risk of asthma. Pediatric Infectious Disease Journal 2002; 21[6]: 498-504.

22 D'Cruz OF et al. Acute inflammatory demyelinating polyradiculoneuropathy (Guillain-Barré syndrome) after immunization with Haemophilus influenzae type b conjugate vaccine. Journal of Pediatrics 1989; 115[5 Pt 1]: 743-6.

23 Gervaix A. Caflisch M. Suter S. Haenggeli CA. Guillain-Barré syndrome following immunisation with Haemophilus influenzae type b conjugate vaccine. European Journal of Pediatrics 1993; 152[7]: 613-4.

24 Nazareth B. Slack MP. Howard AJ. Waight PA. Begg NT. A survey of invasive Haemophilus influenzae infections. Communicable Disease Report. CDR Review 1992; 2[2]: R13-6.

25 Minutes of Joint Committee on Vaccination and Immunisation, 1 November 1991.

26 McVernon J. Trotter CL. Slack MP. Ramsay ME. Trends in Haemophilus influenzae type b infections in adults in England and Wales: surveillance study. BMJ 2004; 329[7467]: 655-8.

27 Barbour ML et al. The impact of conjugate vaccine on carriage of Haemophilus influenzae type b. Journal of Infectious Diseases 1995; 171[1]: 93-8.

28 McVernon J. Howard AJ. Slack MP. Ramsay ME. Long-term impact of vaccination on Haemophilus influenzae type b (Hib) carriage in the United Kingdom. Epidemiology & Infection 2004; 132[4]: 765-7.

29 Low N, Redmind SM, Rutjes AWS, Martínez-González NA, Egger M, di Nisio M, Scott P. Comparing Haemophilus influenza type B conjugate vaccine schedules. The Pediatric Infectious Disease Journal 2013; 32[11]: 1245-56.

30 Guifrè M, Daprai L, Cardines R, Bernaschi P et al. Carriage of Haemophilus influenza in the oropharynx of young children and molecular epidemiology of the isolates after fifteen years of H.influenzae type b vaccination in Italy. Vaccine 2015; 33: 6227-6234

20 A Nation of Guinea Pigs: Meningitis C

1 Letter from the Chief Medical Officer: Introduction of immunisation against Group C meningococcal infections. PL CMO [1999]2.

2 Salisbury D. Introduction of a conjugate meningococcal type C vaccine programme in the UK. Journal of Paediatrics & Child Health 2001; 37[5]: S34-6.

3 Miller E. Salisbury D. Ramsay M. Planning, registration, and implementation of an immunisation campaign against meningococcal serogroup C disease in the UK: a success story. Vaccine 2001; 20 Suppl 1: S58-67.

4 Minutes of the Joint Committee on Vaccination and Immunisation, May 7, 1999.

5 Lakshman R et al. Safety of a new conjugate meningococcal C vaccine in infants. Archives of Disease in Childhood 2001; 85[5]: 391-7.

6 Ruggeberg J. Heath PT. Safety and efficacy of meningococcal group C conjugate vaccines. Expert Opinion on Drug Safety 2003; 2[1]: 7-19.

7 Dr [now Professor] Elizabeth Miller, head of vaccination at the government's Health Protection Agency, quoted in Wise J. UK introduces new meningitis C vaccine. BMJ 1999; 319[7205]: 278.

8 Press release: New Meningitis C Vaccine For Schoolchildren And Young Babies. 1999/0645, November 1, 1999. Available at dh.gov.uk/PublicationsAndStatistics/PressReleases/Press ReleasesNotices/fs/en?CONTENT_ID=4025878&chk =gfK7OY. Downloaded December 22, 2005.

9 Ramsay ME. Andrews N. Kaczmarski EB. Miller E. Efficacy of meningococcal serogroup C conjugate vaccine in teenagers and toddlers in England. [Letter] Lancet 2001; 357[9251]: 195-6.

10 Trotter CL. Andrews NJ. Kaczmarski EB. Miller E. Ramsay ME. Effectiveness of meningococcal serogroup C conjugate vaccine 4 years after introduction. Lancet 2004; 364[9431]: 365-7.

11 De Wals P, Trottier P, Pépin J. Relative efficacy of different immunization schedules for the prevention of serogroup C meningococcal diseases: A model-based evaluation. Vaccine 2006; 24: 3500-3504.

12 Kyaw MH. Christie P, Jones IG. Campbell H. The changing epidemiology of bacterial meningitis and invasive non-meningitic bacterial disease in Scotland during the period 1983-99. Scandinavian Journal of Infectious Diseases 2002; 34[4]: 289-98.

13 Jolly K. Stewart G. Epidemiology and diagnosis of meningitis: results of a five-year prospective, population-based study. Communicable Disease & Public Health 2001; 4[2]: 124-9.

14 Minutes of the Joint Committee on Vaccination and Immunisation, May 2, 1997.

15 Davison KL et al. Estimating the burden of serogroup C meningococcal disease in England and Wales. Communicable Disease & Public Health 2002; 5[3]: 213-9.

16 Doctors are asked to report suspected 'adverse drug reactions' [side-effects] by filling in yellow forms and sending these to the DoH. These forms can also be completed electronically. For the first time, nurses were also allowed to complete 'yellow card' reports for the Meningitis C campaign. Drug and vaccine side-effects are notoriously under-reported; it has been estimated that less than 10% of side-effects normally reported.

17 Committee on Safety of Medicines; subcommittee on pharmacovigilance. Conjugated Meningococcal Vaccine: safety review; 2000. SCOP 00/3rd meeting.

18 Update on safety profile of Meningococcal C conjugate vaccine. Joint Committee on Vaccination and Immunisation; 2000: JCVI[00]33

19 Committee on Safety of Medicines, sub group on meningitis C vaccine safety. Meningococcal C conjugate vaccine. 10/01st meeting.

20 Meningococcal GP C conjugate. Adverse drug reactions online information tracking drug analysis print. Medicines and Healthcare products registration Agency [MHRA]. DoH. November 21, 2005.

21 Courtney PA. Patterson RN. Lee RJ. Henoch-Schönlein purpura following meningitis C vaccination. [Letter] Rheumatology 2001; 40[3]: 345-6, 2001 Mar.

22 Abeyagunawardena AS. Goldblatt D. Andrews N. Trompeter RS. Risk of relapse after meningococcal C conjugate vaccine in nephrotic syndrome. Lancet 2003; 362[9382]: 449-50.

23 GSK. Menitorix Summary of Product Characteristics. Obtained from the manufacturer. March 2, 2006.

24 Cartwright KA. Stuart JM. Jones DM. Noah ND. The Stonehouse survey: nasopharyngeal carriage of meningococci and Neisseria lactamica. Epidemiology & Infection 1987; 99[3]: 591-601.

25 Greiner O. Berger C. Day PJ. Meier G. Tang CM. Nadal D. Rates of detection of Neisseria meningitidis in tonsils differ in relation to local incidence of invasive disease. Journal of Clinical Microbiology 2002; 40[11]: 3917-21.

26 Peltola H. Meningococcal vaccines. Current status and future possibilities. Drugs 1998; 55[3]: 347-66.

27 MacLennan JM et al. Safety, immunogenicity, and induction of immunologic memory by a serogroup C meningococcal conjugate vaccine in infants: A randomised controlled trial. JAMA 2000; 283[21]:

2795-801.

21 Less and less choice: The 5-in-1& 6-in-1

1 Hall C. Sweeping changes to baby vaccines. The Daily Telegraph: August 7, 2004.

2 Improvements to childhood immunisation programme. DoH Press release, 2004,0302: August 9, 2004. Available at dh.gov.uk/PublicationsAndStatistics/PressReleases/Press ReleasesNotices/fs/en?CONTENT_ID=4087239&chk=%2Be4dSH

3 Five-in-one baby jab unveiled. BBC News: August 9, 2004. Available at http://news.bbc.co.uk/1/hi/health/3547490.stm

4 Porter A. Five-in-one jab adviser linked to vaccine firm. The *Sunday Times*: August 15th 2004.

5 Baines E. DoH blamed for vaccine launch fiasco. GP: August 16, 2004.

6 New vaccinations for the childhood immunisation programme. Letter from the Chief Medical Officer, DoH; PL CMO (2004)3.

7 Childhood Immunisation Programme. From the Chief Medical Officer. HSS(MD)24/2004 August 4, 2004.

8 Berrington JE et al. Reduced anti-PRP antibody response to Hib immunisation in preterm (<32 weeks) UK infants who receive inactivated polio (eIPV). Vaccine 2007; 25: 8206-8.

9 New combination vaccines still need a boost. Archives of Disease in Childhood 2007; 92(1): 1-2.

10 Scheifele D. Halperin S. Haemophilus influenzae type B disease control using PENTACEL, Canada, 1998-1999. Canada Communicable Disease Report 2000; 26(11): 93-6.

11 Olin P, Rasmussen F, Gottfarb. Schedules and Protection, Simultaneous Vaccination and Safety: Experiences from Recent Controlled Trials. International Journal of Infectious Diseases 1997; 1: 143-7.

12 Demicheli V, Jefferson T. The First International Symposium on Vaccine Safety. Editorial. Vaccine 2004; 22: 2042-2043.

134 Mills E et al. Safety and immunogenicity of a combined five-component pertussis-diphtheria-tetanus-inactivated poliomyelitis-Haemophilus B conjugate vaccine administered to infants at two, four and six months of age. Vaccine 1998; 16(6): 576-85.

14 Pfister RE. Aeschbach V. Niksic-Stuber V. Martin BC. Siegrist CA. Safety of DTaP-based combined immunization in very-low-birth-weight premature infants: frequent but mostly benign cardiorespiratory events. Journal of Pediatrics 2004; 145(1): 58-66.

15 Lee J, Robinson JL, Spady DW. Frequency of apnea, bradycardia, and desaturations following first diphtheria-tetanus-pertussis-inactivated polio-Haemophilus influenzae type B immunization in hospitalised preterm infants. BMC Pediatrics 2006; 6:20. doi:10.1186/1471-2431-6-20.

16 Kitchin N et al. A randomised controlled study of the

reactogenicity of an acellular pertussis-containing pentavalent infant vaccine compared to a quadrivalent whole cell pertussis-containing vaccine and oral poliomyelitis vaccine, when given concurrently with meningococcal group C conjugate vaccine to healthy UK infants at 2, 3 and 4 months of age. Vaccine 2006; 24: 3964-3970.

17 Tickner S, Leman PJ, Woodcock A. 'It's just the normal thing to do': Exploring parental decision-making about the 'five-in-one' vaccine. Vaccine 2007: 7399-7409.

18 Fagnan LG, Shipman SA, Gaudino JA, Mahler J, Sussman AL, Holub J. To give or not to give: approaches to early childhood immunization delivery in Oregon rural primary care practices. The Journal of Rural Health 2011; 27: 385-393

19 Bar-On ES, Goldberg EF, Vidal L, Hellmann S, Leibovici L. Combined DTP-HBV-HIB vaccine versus separately administered DTP-HBV and HIB vaccines for primary prevention of diphtheria, tetanus, pertussis, hepatitis B and Haemophilus influenza B (HIB). Cochrane database systematic review 2009; doi: 10.1002/14651858.CD005530.pub2

20 Lackman GM. Comparative investigation of the safety of hexavalent vaccines for primary scheduled infant immunizations in Germany over a time period of 2 years. Medical Science Monitor 2004; 10(9): 196-8

21 Six-component vaccines. Prescrire 2004; [70]: 50-53

22 von Kries R et al. Sudden and unexpected deaths after the administration of hexavalent vaccines (diphtheria, tetanus, pertussis, poliomyelitis, hepatitis B, Haemophilus influenzae type b); is there a signal? European Journal of Pediatrics 2005; 164(2): 61-9

23 Zinka B, Rauch E, Buettner A, Penning R, Ruëff F. Unexplained cases of sudden infant death shortly after hexavalent vaccination. Vaccine 2006; 24(31-32): 5779-80

24 von Kries R et al. Sudden and unexpected deaths after the administration of hexavalent vaccines (diphtheria, tetanus, pertussis, poliomyelitis, hepatitis B, Haemophilus influenzae type b); is there a signal? European Journal of Paediatrics 2005; 164(2): 61-9

25 Schmitt HJ. A 'signal' requires urgent action. [Editorial] European Journal of Paediatrics 2005; 164(2): 59-60

26 EMEA update on hexavalent vaccines: Hexavac and Infanrix Hexa. European Agency for the evaluation of Medical Products. EMEA/CPMP/5889/03. December 1, 2003. Available at https://lakemedelsverket.se/upload/halso-och-sjukvard/EMEAhexavalentvaccines%5B1%5D.pdf. Accessed March 9th 2006 & November 7th 2016.

27 European Medicines Agency recommends suspension of Hexavac. European Medicines Agency 20 September 2005. Available at ema.europa.eu/ema/index.jsp?curl=pages/news_and_ev ents/news/2009/12/news_detail_000855.jsp&mid=W C0b01ac058004d5cl Accessed Mach 9, 2006 & November 7, 2016

28 Schmitt HJ, Siegrist CA, Salmaso S, Law B, Booy R. B.

Zinka et al., Unexplained cases of sudden infant death shortly after hexavalent vaccination [letter]. Vaccine. 2006; 24{31-32}: 5781-2.

29 von Kries R. Comment on B. Zinka et al., Unexplained cases of sudden infant death shortly after hexavalent vaccination [letter]. Vaccine 2006; 24{31-32}: 5783-4.

30 Maurer W. Death following hexavalent vaccination [letter]. Vaccine 2006; 23: 5461-3.

31 Zinka B. Unexpected cases of sudden infant death shortly after hexavalent vaccination. Vaccine 2006; 24: 5785-6.

32 Vennemann MMT et al. Sudden infant death syndrome: No increased risk after immunisation. Vaccine 2007; 25: 336-340.

33 GlaxoSmithKline. Infanrix hexa Summary Bridging Report. 16 December 2011. Available at https://autismo-evaccini.files.wordpress.com/2012/12/vaccin-dc3a9cc3a8s.pdf. Accessed 10 November 2016

34 Verger P, Collange F, Fressard L, Bocquier A, Gautier A, Pulcini C, Raude J, Peretti-Waterl P. Prevalence and correlates of vaccine hesitancy among General Practitioners: a cross-sectional telephone survey in France, April to July 2014. Eurosurveillance 2016; 21 [47]: 4.

22 Ever More Optimism: Pneumococcus

1 Watson L. Wilson BJ. Waugh N. Pneumococcal polysaccharide vaccine: a systematic review of clinical effectiveness in adults. Vaccine 2002; 20{17-18}: 2166-73.

2 French N. Use of pneumococcal polysaccharide vaccines: no simple answers. Journal of Infection 2003; 46{2}: 78-86.

3 Minutes of the Joint Committee on Vaccination and Immunisation, February 6, 2004.

4 Finch R. Pneumococcal vaccine is delayed by MMR hysteria. Pulse. June 23, 2003

5 Pelton SI. Klein JO. The future of pneumococcal conjugate vaccines for prevention of pneumococcal diseases in infants and children. Pediatrics 2002; 110{4}: 805-14.

6 Musher DM. Pneumococcal vaccine — direct and indirect ('herd') effects. [Editorial] New England Journal of Medicine 2006; 354{14}: 1522-4.

7 Kyaw MH et al. Active Bacterial Core Surveillance of the Emerging Infections Program Network. Effect of introduction of the pneumococcal conjugate vaccine on drug-resistant Streptococcus pneumoniae. New England Journal of Medicine 2006; 354{14}: 1455-63.

8 Minutes of the Joint Committee on Vaccination and Immunisation, October 1, 2004.

9 Hughes G. Drug giant linked to immunisation campaign. The Age: December 22, 2003. Available at theage.com.au/articles/2003/12/21/1071941610958.htm l. Accessed June 10, 2007.

10 Simonite T. GP. February 17, 2006.

11 JCVI. Proposed changes to the routine childhood immunisation schedule. Available at advisorybodies.doh.gov.uk/jcvi/minutes.htm. Accessed

May 20, 2006.

12 Kimman TG et al. Developing a vaccination evaluation model to support evidence-based decision making on national immunization programs. Vaccine 2006; 24: 4769-4778.

13 Available from the Health Protection Agency at hpa.org.uk/infections/topics_az/pneumococcal/eng_w al_age.htm. Accessed January 10, 2006. [no longer available]

14 HPA. Current Epidemiology of Invasive Pneumococcal Disease. Available at hpa.org.uk/infections/topics_az/pneumococcal/Agesp ecificlabcasesIPD.htm. Accessed March 5, 2007.

15 Ispahani P. Slack RC. Donald FE. Weston VC. Rutter N. Twenty year surveillance of invasive pneumococcal disease in Nottingham: serogroups responsible and implications for immunisation. Archives of Disease in Childhood 2004; 89{8}: 757-62.

16 Jones IR. Urwin G. Feldman RA. Banatvala N. Social deprivation and bacterial meningitis in North East Thames region: three year study using small area statistics. BMJ 1997; 314{7083}: 794-5.

17 Melegaro A, Edmunds WJ, Pebody R, Miller E, George R. The current burden of pneumococcal disease in England and Wales. Journal of Infection 2006; 52{1}: 37-48.

18 McIntosh ED. Booy R. Invasive pneumococcal disease in England and Wales: what is the true burden and what is the potential for prevention using 7 valent pneumococcal conjugate vaccine? Archives of Disease in Childhood 2002; 86{6}: 403-6.

19 New campaign to tell parents about new vaccine against pneumococcal disease. DoH. Available at gnn.gov.uk/environment/fullDetail.asp?ReleaseID=22318 98&NewsAreaID=2&NavigatedFromDepartment=False. Accessed 29th August 2006.

20 Jefferson T. Ferroni E. Curtale F. Giorgi Rossi P. Borgia P. Streptococcus pneumoniae in western Europe: serotype distribution and incidence in children less than 2 years old. The Lancet Infectious Diseases 2006; 6{7}: 405-10.

21 CDC cdc.gov/pneumococcal/surveillance.html accessed 14 December 2015

22 Lucero MG et al. Pneumococcal conjugate vaccines for preventing vaccine-type invasive pneumococcal disease and pneumonia with consolidation on x-ray in children under two years of age. The Cochrane Library, Issue 2, 2005

23 Whitney CG et al. Effectiveness of seven-valent pneumococcal conjugate vaccine against invasive pneumococcal disease: a matched case-control study. Lancet 2006; 368: 1495-1502.

24 Lexau CA et al. Active Bacterial Core Surveillance Team. Changing epidemiology of invasive pneumococcal disease among older adults in the era of pediatric pneumococcal conjugate vaccine. JAMA

25 Buttery JP et al. Immunogenicity and safety of a

combination pneumococcal-meningococcal vaccine in infants: a randomised controlled trial. JAMA 2005; 293(14): 1751-8.

26 Tichmann-Schumann I et al. Immunogenicity and reactogenicity of four doses of diphtheria-tetanus-three-component acellular pertussis-hepatitis B-inactivated polio virus-Haemophilus influenzae type b vaccine coadministered with 7-valent pneumococcal conjugate Vaccine. Pediatric Infectious Disease Journal 2005; 24(1): 70-7.

27 Schmitt HJ, Faber J, Lorenz I, Schmole-Thoma B, Ahlers N. The safety, reactogenicity and immunogenicity of a 7-valent pneumococcal conjugate vaccine (7VPnC) concurrently administered with a combination DTaP-IPV-Hib vaccine. Vaccine 2003; 21(25-26): 3653-62.

28 Knuf M, Habermehl P, Cimino C, Petersen G, Schmitt HJ. Immunogenicity, reactogenicity and safety of a 7-valent pneumococcal conjugate vaccine (PCV7) concurrently administered with a DTPa-HBV-IPV/Hib combination vaccine in healthy infants. Vaccine 2006; 24: 4727-4736.

29 Oosterhuis-Kafeja F, Beutels P, Van Damme P. Immunogenicity, efficacy, safety and effectiveness of pneumococcal conjugate vaccines (1998-2006). Vaccine 2007; 25(12): 2194-212.

30 Minutes of the Joint Committee on Vaccination and Immunisation, January 25, 2002.

31 O'Brien KL et al. Efficacy and safety of seven-valent conjugate pneumococcal vaccine in American Indian children: group randomised trial. Lancet 2003; 362(9381): 355-61.

32 Klugman KP et al. Vaccine Trialists Group. A trial of a 9-valent pneumococcal conjugate vaccine in children with and those without HIV infection. New England Journal of Medicine 2003l; 349(14): 1341-8.

33 Wise RP et al. Postlicensure safety surveillance for 7-valent pneumococcal conjugate vaccine. JAMA 2004; 292(14): 1702-10.

34 Andrews N et al. Using the indirect cohort design to estimate the effectiveness of the seven valent pneumococcal conjugate vaccine in England and Wales. PLoS ONE 2011; 6: e1-7.

35 Hsu HE et al. Effect of pneumococcal conjugate vaccine on pneumococcal meningitis. NEJM 2009; 360(3): 244-256.

36 O'Brien KL et al. Effect of pneumococcal conjugate vaccine on nasopharyngeal colonization among immunized and unimmunized children in a community-randomized trial. The Journal of Infectious Diseases 2007; 196(8): 1211-2.

37 Spijkerman J et al. Immunogenicity of 13-valent pneumococcal conjugate vaccine administration according to 4 different primary immunization schedules. JAMA 2013; 310(9): 930-937.

38 Kwak BO, Choung JT, Park YM. The association between asthma and invasive pneumococcal disease: a nationwide study in Korea. Journal of Korean Medical Science 2015; 30(1): 60-5.

39 Schillberg E, Isaac M, Deng X, Peirano G et al. Outbreak of invasive Streptococcus pneumoniae serotype 12F among a marginalized inner city population in Winnipeg, Canada, 2009-2011. Clinical Infectious Diseases 2014; 59(5): 651-7.

40 Nicholls TR, Leach AJ, Morris PS. The short-term impact of each primary dose of pneumococcal vaccine on nasopharyngeal carriage: Systematic review and meta-analysis of randomised controlled trials. Vaccine 2016; 34: 703-713

23 A Vaccine too Soon? HPV

1 Östor AG. Natural history of cervical intraepithelial neoplasia: a critical review. International Journal of Gynecological Pathology 1993; 12(2): 186-92.

2 Cancer statistics registrations. Registrations of cancer diagnosed in 2010 England. National statistics. Available at ons.gov.uk/ons/rel/vsob1/cancer-statistics-registra-tions-england-series-mb1-/no-41-2010/cancer-statistics-registrations-england-series-mb1—no-41-2010-statistical-bulletin.html.pdf Accessed October 19, 2012

3 Mortality statistics DH2 2005. National Statistics. Available at statistics.gov.uk/statbase/Product.asp?vlnk=618. Accessed March 25, 2009.

4 Gardasil – The first cancer vaccine that can prevent Cervical Cancer, Cervical pre-cancer, Vulval pre-cancer and Genital Warts is now approved for use in the European Union. Merck News Release. September 22, 2006.

5 Future II Study Group. Quadrivalent vaccine against human papillomavirus to prevent high-grade cervical lesions. New England Journal of Medicine 2007;. 356(19):1915-27.

6 Sawaya GF. Smith-McCune K. HPV vaccination – more answers, more questions. New England Journal of Medicine 2007;. 356(19):1991-3.

7 Future II Study Group. Effect of prophylactic human papillomavirus L1 virus-like particle vaccine on risk of cervical intraepithelial neoplasia grade 2, grade 3, and adenocarcinoma in situ: a combined analysis of four randomised clinical trials. Lancet 2007; 369: 1861-8.

8 Paavonen J.et al. HPV PATRICIA study group. Efficacy of a prophylactic adjuvanted bivalent L1 virus-like-particle vaccine against infection with human papillomavirus types 16 and 18 in young women: an interim analysis of a phase III double-blind, randomised controlled trial. Lancet 2007; 369(9580): 2161-70.

9 Kahn JA. Burk RD. Papillomavirus vaccines in perspective. Lancet 2007; 369(9580): 2135-7.

10 Karlsson R. Jonsson M. Edlund K. Evander M. Gustavsson A. Boden E. Rylander E. Wadell G. Lifetime number of partners as the only independent risk factor for human papillomavirus infection: a population-based study. Sexually Transmitted Diseases 1995; 22(2): 119-27.

11 Shin HR et al. Prevalence of human papillomavirus infection in women in Busan, South Korea. International Journal of Cancer 2003; 103(3): 413-21.

12 Block SL et al. Protocol 016 Study Group. Comparison of the immunogenicity and reactogenicity of a prophylactic quadrivalent human papillomavirus (types 6, 11, 16, and 18) L1 virus-like particle vaccine in male and female adolescents and young adult women. Pediatrics 2006; 118(5): 2135-45.

13 Scientific Discussion. EMEA. Available at emea.europa.eu/humandocs/PDFs/EPAR/gardasil/070306en6.pdf. Accessed February 16, 2007.

14 Foggo D, Cardy P. Mystery illness paralyses girl given cervical cancer jab. Sunday Times. 14 December 2008.

15. Joint Committee on Vaccination and Immunisation. Minutes of Meeting held on Wednesday 17 October 207.

16. Keam SJ. Harper DM. Human papillomavirus types 16 and 18 vaccine (recombinant, AS04 adjuvanted, adsorbed) [Cervarix]. Drugs 2008; 68(3): 359-72.

17.Cervarix European Public Assessment Report. Scientific Discussion. EMEA. Available at emea.europa.eu/humandocs/PDFs/EPAR/cervarix/H-721-en6.pdf Accessed 25 March 2009.

18

19 The FUTURE I/II Study Group. Four year efficacy of prophylactic human papillomavirus quadrivalent vaccine against low grade cervical, vulvar, and vaginal intraepithelial neoplasia and anogenital warts: randomised controlled trial. BMJ 2010; 340: c3493

20 Brinth LS, Pors K, Theibel AC, Mehlsen J. Orthostatic intolerance and postural tachycardia syndrome as suspected adverse effects of vaccination against human papilloma virus. Vaccine 2015; 33: 2602-5.

21 Wacholder S et al. Risk of miscarriage with bivalent vaccine against human papillomavirus (HPV) types 16 and 18: pooled analysis of two randomised controlled trials. BMJ 2010; 340: c712

22 Crowe E et al. Effectiveness of quadrivalent human papillomavirus vaccine for the prevention of cervical abnormalities: case-control study nested within a population based screening programme in Australia. BMJ 2014; 348: g1458

23 Söderlund-Strand A, Uhnoo I, Dillner J. Change in population prevalences of human papillomavirus after initiation of vaccination: the high-throughput HPV monitoring study. Cancer Epidemiology, Biomarkers and Prevention 2014; 23(12): 2757-64

24 Tomljenovic L, Shaw CA. Death after Quadrivalent Human Papillomavirus (HPV) Vaccination: Cause or Coincidence? Pharmaceutical Regulatory Affairs 2012; S12 – 001.

25 Lee SH. An open-letter of complaint to the Director-General of the World health Organization, Dr Margaret Chan. Available at http://sanevax.org/wp-content/uploads/2016/01/Allegations-of-Scientific-Misconduct-by-GACVS.pdf

26 Liu XC, Bell CA, Simmonds KA, Svenson LW, Russell ML. Adverse events following HPV vaccination. Alberta 2006-2014. Vaccine 2016; 34: 1800-1805

24 A vaccine to save the NHS money: Rotavirus

1 Tam CC, Rodrigues LC, Viviani L et al. Longitudinal study of infectious intestinal disease in the UK (IID2 study): incidence in the community and presenting to general practice. Gut 2012; 61: 69-77

2 Harris JP, Jit M, Cooper D, Edmunds WJ. Evaluating rotavirus vaccination in England and Wales Part I: Estimating the burden of disease. Vaccine 2007; 25: 3962-3970

3 Samad L, Marven S, El Bashir H, Sutcliffe AG, Cameron JC, Lynn R, Taylor B. Prospective surveillance study of the management of intussusception in UK and Irish infants. British Journal of Surgery 2012; 99(3): 411-5

4 Kaiser AD, Applegate KE, Ladd AP. Current success in the treatment of intussusception in children. Surgery 2007; 142(4) 469-75

5 Jit M, Peabody R, Chen M, Andrews N, Edmunds WJ. Estimating the number of deaths with rotavirus as a cause in England and Wales. Human Vaccines 2007; 3(1): 23-6.

6 Plenge-Bönig A, Solo-Ramirez N, Karmaus W, Petersen G, Davis S, Forster J. Breastfeeding protects against acute gastroenteritis due to rotavirus in infants. European Journal of Paediatrics 2010; 169(12): 1471-6

7 Marlow R, Muir P, Vipond B, Lyttle M, Trotter C, Finn A. Assessing the impacts of the first year of rotavirus vaccination in the United Kingdom. Eurosurveillance 2015; 20(48): pii=30077

8 Soares-Weiser K, MacLehose H, Bergman H, Ben-Aharon I, Nagpal S, Goldberg E, Pitan F, Cunliffe N. Vaccines for preventing rotavirus diarrhea: vaccines in use. Cochrane Database Systematic Review 2012; 11:CD008521

9 Clark A, Jit M, Andrews N, Atchison C, Edmunds WJ, Sanderson C. Evaluating the potential risks and benefits of infant rotavirus vaccination in England. Vaccine 2014; 32: 3604-3610

10 Contopoulos-Ioannidis DG, Halpern MS, Maldonado Y. Trends in Hospitalization for Intussusception in California in relationship to the introduction of New Rotavirus Vaccines, Pediatric Infectious Disease Journal 2015; 34(7): 712-7.

11 Rosillon D, Buyse H, Friedland L, Ng S-P, Velazquez FR, Breuer T. Risk of intussusception after rotavirus vaccination: meta-analysis of post-licensure studies. Pediatric Infectious Disease Journal 2015; 34(7): 763-8.

12 Donato CM, Ch'ng LS, Boniface KF, Crawford NW, Buttery JP, Lyon M, Bishop RF, Kirkwood CD. Identification of strains of RotaTeq rotavirus vaccine in infants with gastroenteritis following routine vaccination. Journal of Infectious Disease 2012; 206(3): 377-83

25 'The Influence': Influenza (Flu)

1 Ghendon Y. Introduction to pandemic influenza through history. European Journal of Epidemiology 1994; 10(4): 451-3.

2 A pandemic is an epidemic, or outbreak, that covers a

large part of the globe

3 Potter CW. A history of influenza. Journal of Applied Microbiology 2001; 91(4): 572-9.

4 The Lancet; January 22, 1892: 204-5.

5 Willis. Lancet; July 18, 1891.

6 Thornton P. The Lancet; January 30, 1892: 279.

7 Waring JI. A history of medicine in South Carolina 1900-70. p33. South Carolina Medical Association: 1971.

8 Langford C. The age pattern of mortality in the 1918-19 influenza pandemic: an attempted explanation based on data for England and Wales. Medical History 2002; 46(1): 1-20.

9 Cohen D. WHO and the pandemic flu 'conspiracies'. BMJ 2010;340:c2912

10 Chan KNK, O'Neill S, Mandeville KL. OP78 Scientists, competing interests and the media: a content analysis of newspaper reporting in H1N1 influenza. Journal of Epidemiology and Community Health 2012; 66: A31-A31

11 Käll A. The Pandemrix — narcolepsy tragedy: how it started and what we know today. Acta Paediatrica 2013; 102(1): 2-4

12 Beck F, Butters D, Matsumoto G, Whitehouse M. Queries about vaccines containing squalene. Immunology and Cell Biology: doi: 10.1038/icb.2010.10

13 Sachedina N, Donaldson LJ. Paediatric mortality related to pandemic influenza A H1N1 infection in England: an observational population-based study. Lancet 2010. DOI:10.1016/S0140-6736(10)61195-6.

14 Christu CN. Influenza. Journal — Lancet 1959; 79(3): 118-20.

15 Graham Davies E et al. Manual of Childhood Infections. Royal Colleges of Paediatrics and Child Health. 2001.

16 Loughlin J, Poulios N, Napalkov P, Wegmuller Y. Monto AS. A study of influenza and influenza-related complications among children in a large US health insurance plan database. Pharmacoeconomics 2003; 21(4): 273-83.

17 Immunisation Against Infectious Disease 1996 — 'The Green Book'. HMSO. Available at dh.gov.uk/PolicyAndGuidance/HealthAndSocialCareTopics/GreenBook/GreenBookGeneralInformation/GreenBookGeneralArticle/fs/en?CONTENT_ID=4097254&chk=isTfGX

18 Chambers C, Skowronski D, Sabaiduc S, Winter A, Dickinson J, De Serres G, Gubbay J, Drews S, Martineau C, Eshaghi A, Krajden M, Bastien N, Li Y. Interim estimates of 2015/16 vaccine effectiveness against influenza A(H1N1)pdm09, Canada, February 2016. Euro Surveill. 2016;21(11):pii=30168. DOI: http://dx.doi.org/10.2807/1560-7917.ES.2016.21.11.30168

19 Bueving HJ et al. Influenza vaccination in children with asthma: randomized double-blind placebo-controlled trial. American Journal of Respiratory & Critical Care Medicine 2004; 169(4): 488-93, 2004.

20 Cates CJ, Jefferson TO, Bara AI, Rowe BH. Vaccines for preventing influenza in people with asthma. The Cochrane Library, issue 4; 2003.

21 Christy C. Aligne CA. Auinger P. Pulcino T. Weitzman M. Effectiveness of influenza vaccine for the prevention of asthma exacerbations. Archives of Disease in Childhood 2004; 89(8): 734-5.

22 Tan A, Bhalla P, Smyth R. Vaccines for preventing influenza in people with cystic fibrosis. The Cochrane Library, issue 4:2003.

23 Yoshi AY, Iyer VN, Hartz MF, Patel AM, Li JT. Effectiveness of trivalent inactivated influenza vaccine in influenza-related hospitalization in children: A case-control study. Allergy and Asthma Proceedings 2012; 33(2): e23-27

24 Hardelid P. Pebody R. Andrews N. Mortality caused by influenza and respiratory syncytial virus by age group in England and Wales 1999-2010. Influenza and other respiratory viruses 2012: DOI: 10.1111/j.1750-2659.2012.00345.x

25 Li-Kim-Moy J et al. Systematic review of fever, febrile convulsions and serious adverse events following administration of inactivated trivalent influenza vaccines in children. European Communicable Disease Bulletin 2015; 20(25). pii: 21164

26 Collignon P J, Doshi P, Jefferson T. Re: Adverse events following influenza vaccination in Australia — should we be surprised? BMJ Rapid response. 11 March 2011

27 Peabody R. et al. Effectiveness of seasonal influenza vaccine in preventing laboratory-confirmed influenza in primary care in the United Kingdom: 2014/15 end of season results. EuroSurveillance 2015; 20(36):PII=30013.

28 Ahrens K, Louik C, Kerr S, Mitchell AA, Werler MM. Seasonal influenza vaccination during pregnancy and the risks of preterm delivery and small for gestational age birth. Paediatric and Perinatal Epidemiology 2014; 24: 498-509

29 From Mortality Statistics. Office for National Statistics. HMSO.

30 Cooke MK et al. Influenza and other respiratory viruses surveillance in the United Kingdom: October 2003 to May 2004. CDR Supplement. Available at hpa.org.uk/cdr/archives/2005/flu2004_5.pdf

31 Hardelid P, Peabody R, Andrews N, Mortality caused by influenza and respiratory syncytial virus by age group in England and Wales 1999-2010. Influenza and other Respiratory Viruses 2013; 1: 35-45

32 Minutes of the Joint Committee on Vaccination and Immunisation Influenza Subgroup meeting, December 8, 1976.

33 Smith S et al. Vaccines for preventing influenza in healthy children. The Cochrane Database of Systematic Reviews 2006, Issue 1.

34 Jefferson T. Smith S. Demicheli V. Harnden A. Rivetti A. Safety of influenza vaccines in children. [Letter] Lancet 2005; 366(9488): 803-4.

35 Zhou W. Pool V. DeStefano F. Iskander JK. Haber P. Chen RT. VAERS Working Group. A potential signal of Bell's palsy after parenteral inactivated influenza vaccines: reports to the Vaccine Adverse Event Reporting System (VAERS) — United States, 1991-2001.

Pharmacoepidemiology & Drug Safety 2004; 13(8): 505-10.

36 Mutsch M. Zhou W. Rhodes P. Bopp M. Chen RT. Linder T. Spyr C. Steffen R. Use of the inactivated intranasal influenza vaccine and the risk of Bell's palsy in Switzerland. New England Journal of Medicine 2004; 350(9): 896-903.

37 Crawford C, Grazko MB, Raymond WR, Rivers BA, Munson PD. Reversible blindness in bilateral optic neuritis associated with nasal flu vaccine. Binocular Vision & Strabology Quarterly, Simms-Romano's 2012; 27(3): 171-3.

38 Kelso JM. Safety of Influenza vaccines. Current Opinion in Allergy and Clinical Immunology 2012; 12(4): 383-8

39 Tarabichi Y, Li K, Nguyen C, Wang X et al. The administration of intranasal live attenuated influenza vaccine induces changes in the nasal microbiota and nasal epithelium gene expression profiles. Microbiome 2015; 3: 74

40 Safranek TJ et al. Reassessment of the association between Guillain-Barré syndrome and receipt of swine influenza vaccine in 1976-1977: results of a two-state study. Expert Neurology Group. American Journal of Epidemiology 1991; 133(9): 940-51.

41 Schonberger LB et al. Guillain-Barré syndrome following vaccination in the National Influenza Immunization Program, United States, 1976-1977. American Journal of Epidemiology 1979; 110(2): 105-23.

42 Haber P. DeStefano F. Angulo FJ. Iskander J. Shadomy SV. Weintraub E. Chen RT. Guillain-Barré syndrome following influenza vaccination. JAMA 2004; 292(20): 2478-81.

43 Zerbo Q, Qian Y, Yoshida C et al. Association between influenza infection and vaccination during pregnancy and risk of autistic spectrum disorder. JAMA Pediatrics 2016.doi: 10.1001/jamapediatrics.2016.3609. Published online November 28, 2016. Available at http://jamanetwork.com/journals/jamapediatrics/fullarticle/2587559

26 Lobbying achieves a U-turn: Meningitis B

1 JCVI interim position statement on use of Bexsero meningococcal B vaccine in the UK. July 2013. Available at https://www.gov.uk/government/publications/jcvi-interim-position-statement-on-the-use-of-bexsero-meningococcal-b-vaccine-in-the-uk . Accessed 29 July 2016

2 JCVI position statement on use of Bexsero meningococcal B vaccine in the UK. March 2014. Available at https://www.gov.uk/government/publications/meningococcal-b-vaccine-jcvi-position-statement. Accessed 29 July 2016

3 Pace D, Pollard AJ. Meningococcal disease: clinical presentation and sequelae. Vaccine 2012; 30S: B3-B9

4 Ladhani SN, Flood JS, Ramsay ME, Campbell H, Gray SJ, Kaczmarski EB, Mallard RH, Guiver M, Newbold LS, Borrow R. Invasive meningococcal disease in England

and Wales: implications for the introduction of new vaccines. Vaccine 2012; 30: 3710-3716

5 Vesikari T, Esposito S, Prymula R, Ypma E, Kohl I, Toneatto D, Dull P, Kamura A for the EU Meningococcal B Infant Vaccine Study Group. Immunogenicity and safety of an investigational multi-component, recombinant, meningococcal serogroup B vaccine (4CMenB) administered concomitantly with routine infant and child vaccinations: results of two randomised trials. Lancet 2013; 381(19669): 825-35

6 Vogel U, Taha M-K, Vazquez JA, Findlow J et al. Predicted strain coverage of a meningococcal multi-component vaccine (4CMenB) in Europe: a qualitative and quantitative assessment. Lancet Infectious Diseases 2013; 13(5): 416-25

7 Ladhani SN, Giuliani MM, Biolchi K et al. Effectiveness of meningococcal B vaccine against endemic hypervirulent Neisseria meningitides W strain, England. Emerging Infectious Diseases 2016; 22(2): 309-11.

8 Tenenbaum T, Niessen J, Schroten H. Severe upper extremity dysfunction after 4CMenB vaccination in a young infant. The Pediatric Infectious Disease Journal 2016; 35: 94-96.

27 Another vaccine we just don't need: Hepatitis B

1 Carnall D. Shire Hall communications and the case for hepatitis B immunisation. BMJ 1996; 313: 825.

2 The British Liver Trust receives funding from several pharmaceutical companies including GlaxoSmithKline, the manufacturer of the Hepatitis B vaccine. See britishlivertrust.org.uk/content/helping/acknowledgements.asp. Accessed January 17th 2006.

3 Hepatitis B: Out of the Shadows, 2004. The British Liver Trust. Available at britishlivertrust.org.uk/content/diseases/hepatitis_b_overview_associated_docs/Out%20of%20the%20Shadows%20report.pdf

4 BMA calls for universal childhood immunization against hepatitis B, Press release: May 10, 2005. Available at bma.org.uk/pressrel.nsf/wlu/SGOY-6C8D8L?OpenDocument&vw=wfmms. Accessed June 3, 2005.

5 Board of Science and education. Hepatitis B vaccination in childhood. May 2005. Available at bma.org.uk/ap.nsf/Content/Hepbchildhood?OpenDocument&Highlight=2,hepatitis,b. Accessed June 3, 2005.

6 Vaccine bid backed. BMA News: May 21, 2005.

7 Mangtani P. Hall AJ. Normand CE. Hepatitis B vaccination: the cost effectiveness of alternative strategies in England and Wales. Journal of Epidemiology & Community Health 1995; 49(3): 238-44.

8 Minutes of the Joint Committee on Vaccination and Immunisation, May 2, 1997.

9 Minutes of the Joint Committee on Vaccination and Immunisation, October 9, 2000.

10 Graham Davies E et al. Manual of Childhood

Infections. Royal Colleges of Paediatrics and Child Health. 2001.

11 Aggarwal R. Ranjan P. Preventing and treating hepatitis B infection. *BMJ* 2004; 329(7474): 1080-6.

12 Hahné S. Ramsay M. Balogun K. Edmunds WJ. Mortimer P. Incidence and routes of transmission of hepatitis B virus in England and Wales, 1995-2000: implications for immunisation policy. Journal of Clinical Virology 2004; 29(4): 211-20.

13 Powell E. Duke M. Cooksley WG. Hepatitis B transmission within families: potential importance of saliva as a vehicle of spread. Australian & New Zealand Journal of Medicine 1985; 15(6): 717-20.

14 Villarejos VM. Visona KA. Gutierrez A. Rodriguez A. Role of saliva, urine and feces in the transmission of type B hepatitis. New England Journal of Medicine 1974; 291(26): 1375-8.

15 Shapiro ED. Lack of transmission of hepatitis B in a day care center. Journal of Pediatrics 1987; 110(1): 90-2.

16 Niermeijer P. Gips CH. Natural history of acute hepatitis B in previously healthy patients: A prospective study. Acta Hepato-Gastroenterologica 1977; 24(5): 317-25.

17 Perrillo RP. Hepatitis B: transmission and natural history. Gut 1993; 34(2 Suppl): S48-9.

18 Fattovich G. Natural history and prognosis of hepatitis B. Seminars in Liver Disease 2003; 23(1): 47-58.

19 Immunization Practices Advisory Committee. Hepatitis B Virus: A Comprehensive Strategy for eliminating Transmission in the United States through Universal Immunization Childhood Vaccination: Recommendations of the Immunization Practices Advisory Committee [ACIP]. MMWR 1991; 40(RR-13): 1-19.

20 Boxall EH. Sira J. Standish RA. Davies P. Sleight E. Dhillon AP. Scheuer PJ. Kelly DA. Natural history of hepatitis B in perinatally infected carriers. Archives of Disease in Childhood Fetal & Neonatal Edition 2004; 89(5): F456-60.

21 Bazin H. A brief history of the prevention of infectious diseases by immunisations. Comparative Immunology, Microbiology & Infectious Diseases 2003; 26(5-6): 293-308.

22 Hadler SC et al. Long-term immunogenicity and efficacy of hepatitis B vaccine in homosexual men. New England Journal of Medicine 1986; 315(4) :209-14.

23 Coursaget P et al. Twelve-year follow-up study of hepatitis B immunization of Senegalese infants. Journal of Hepatology 1994; 21(2): 250-4.

24 Whittle H. Jaffar S. Wansbrough M. Mendy M. Dumpis U. Collinson A. Hall A. Observational study of vaccine efficacy 14 years after trial of hepatitis B vaccination in Gambian children. *BMJ* 2002; 325(7364): 569.

25 West DJ. Calandra GB. Vaccine induced immunologic memory for hepatitis B surface antigen: implications for policy on booster vaccination. Vaccine 1996; 14(11): 1019-27.

26 Girard M. Autoimmune hazards of hepatitis B vaccine. Autoimmunity Reviews 2005; 4(2): 96-100.

27 Duclos P. Adverse events after hepatitis B vaccination. CMAJ Canadian Medical Association Journal. 147(7):1023-6, 1992 Oct 1.

28 Shaw FE Jr. et al. Postmarketing surveillance for neurologic adverse events reported after hepatitis B vaccination. Experience of the first three years. American Journal of Epidemiology 1988; 127(2): 337-52.

29 Fourrier A et al. Hepatitis B vaccine and first episodes of central nervous system demyelinating disorders: a comparison between reported and expected number of cases. [Letter] British Journal of Clinical Pharmacology 2001; 51(5): 489-90.

30 France suspends hepatitis B immunisation for adolescents in schools. Eurosurveillance weekly 1998; 2:41. Available at eurosurveillance.org / ew/1998/981008.asp#2. Accessed January 17, 2006.

31 Touzé E. Gout O. Verdier-Taillefer MH. Lyon-Caen O. Alperovitch A. [The first episode of central nervous system demyelinization and hepatitis B virus vaccination]. [French] Revue Neurologique 2000; 156(3): 242-6.

32 Touzé E et al. Hepatitis B vaccination and first central nervous system demyelinating event: a case-control study. Neuroepidemiology 2002; 21(4): 180-6.

33 Ascherio A et al. Hepatitis B vaccination and the risk of multiple sclerosis. New England Journal of Medicine 2001; 344(5): 327-32.

34 Confavreux C. Suissa S. Saddier P. Bourdes V. Vukusic S. Vaccinations and the risk of relapse in multiple sclerosis. Vaccines in Multiple Sclerosis Study Group. New England Journal of Medicine 2001; 344(5): 319-26.

35 Hanslik T. Viboud C. Flahault A. Vaccinations and multiple sclerosis.[letter] New England Journal of Medicine 2001; 344(23): 1793-4.

36 Gout O. Vaccinations and multiple sclerosis.[letter] New England Journal of Medicine 2001; 344(23): 1794.

37 Sturkenboom MC. Fourrier A. Vaccinations and multiple sclerosis.[letter]. New England Journal of Medicine 2001; 344(23): 1794.

38 Hernán MA. Jick SS. Olek MJ. Jick H. Recombinant hepatitis B vaccine and the risk of multiple sclerosis: a prospective study. Neurology 2004; 63(5): 838-42.

39 Langer-Gould, Qian L, Tartof SY et al. Vaccines and the risk of multiple sclerosis and other central ervous system denyelinating diseases. JAMA Neurology 2014; 71(12): 1506-13.

40 There is no national register of people with MS in the UK. This estimate is taken from the Multiple Sclerosis Trust. See https://www.mstrust.org.uk/a-z/prevalence-and-incidence-multiple-sclerosis Accessed April 25, 2017.

41 Cogan FM. Hep B coincided with my first MS attack [letter]. Pulse: March 5, 2005.

42 Pozzilli P et al. Hepatitis B vaccine associated with an

increased type 1 diabetes in Italy. Presented at the Annual meeting of the American Diabetes Association, San Antonio, TX. June 13, 2000.

43 Geier DA. Geier MR. A case-control study of serious autoimmune adverse events following hepatitis B immunization. Autoimmunity 2005; 38(4):295-301.

44 Pope JE. Stevens A. Howson W. Bell DA. The development of rheumatoid arthritis after recombinant hepatitis B vaccination. Journal of Rheumatology 1998; 25(9): 1687-93.

45 Agmon-Levin N, Zafrir Y, Paz Z et al. Ten cases of systemic lupus erythematosus related to hepatitis B vaccine. Lupus 2009; 18: 1192-1197.

46 Calista D. Morri M. Lichen planus induced by hepatitis B vaccination: a new case and review of the literature. International Journal of Dermatology 2004; 43(8): 562-4.

47 Shepherd C. Is CFS linked to immunisations? The CFS Research Review, Winter 2001. Available at cfids.org/archives/2001rr/2001-rr1-article03.asp. Accessed January 17, 2006.

48 De Carvalho JF, shoenfeld Y. Status epilepticus and lymphocytic pneumonitis following hepatitis B vaccination. European Journal of Internal Medicine 2008: 19(5): 383-385.

49 Zafrir Y, Sgmon-Levin N, Paz Z, Shilton T, Shoenfeld Y. Autoimmunity following Hepatitis B vaccine as part of the spectrum of 'Autoimmune (AutoOinflammatory) Syndrome induced by Adjuvants' (ASIA): analysis of 93 cases. Lupus 2012; 21: 146-152.

50 Garly ML. Jensen H. Martins CL. Bale C. Balde MA. Lisse IM. Aaby P. Hepatitis B vaccination associated with higher female than male mortality in Guinea-Bissau: an observational study. Pediatric Infectious Disease Journal 2004; 23(12): 1086-92.

51 Girard M. World Health Organization Vaccine Recommendations: Scientific Flaws or Criminal Misconduct? Journal of American Physicians and Surgeons 2006; 11(1): 22-23

28 Profit ahead of the Public Good: Vaccines and Big Pharma

1 Marwick C. British firm halts vaccine manufacture, research. JAMA 1990; 264(18):2370.

2 Rosenthal E. Drug makers' push leads to cancer vaccines' fast rise. The New York Times: 20 August 2008.

3 Bosely S. Vaccination campaign funded by drug firm. Guardian: March 26th 2007.

4 Cassels A. Lock up your daughters Gardasil is on the loose. Available at commonground.ca/iss/0709194/cg194_cassels.shtml. Downloaded November 27th 2008.

5 Kudjawu Y. Levy-Bruhl D. Celentano LP. O'Flanagan D. Salmaso S. Lopalco P. Mullins N. Bacci S. VENICE working group. The current status of HPV and rotavirus vaccines in national immunisation schedules in the EU-preliminary results of a VENICE survey.

Euro Surveillance2007; 12(4):E070426.1.

6 de Melo-Martin I. The promise of the human papillomavirus vaccine does not confer immunity against ethical reflection. Oncologist 2006; 11(4): 393-6.

7 Raffle AE. Human papillomavirus vaccine policy. Lancet 2007; 369(9559): 367-8.

8 Anonymous. Should HPV vaccines be mandatory for all adolescents?. Lancet 2006; 368(9543):1212.

9 Tanday S. Doubt on HPV jabs for schoolgirls. GP: 4th May 2007.

10 Minutes of Joint Committee on Vaccination and Immunisation. May 2, 1997.

11 For a disturbing exposé of the way Drug Companies practice, read 'The Truth about the Drug Companies' by Marcia Angell, former editor in chief of The New England Journal of Medicine. Random House 2004.

12 Bekelman JE. Li Y. Gross CP. Scope and impact of financial conflicts of interest in biomedical research: a systematic review. JAMA 2003; 289(4): 454-65.

13 abc.net.au/rn/perspective/stories/2007/2108059.htm #transcript. Accessed 28th January 2009

14 These principles were enshrined in the Alma Ata Declaration of 1978.

15 Banerji D. Hidden menace in the Universal Child Immunisation Programme. Journal of the Indian Medical Association 1986; 84(8): 229-32.

16 Mukherjee SB. Radio advertising of varicella vaccine. Indian Pediatrics 2006; 43(6): 556-7.

29 Death by Vaccination: The Developing World

1 Kristensen I. Aaby P. Jensen H. Routine vaccinations and child survival: follow up study in Guinea-Bissau, West Africa. BMJ 2000; 321(7274): 1435-8.

2 WHO, UNICEF. Global Immunization Vision and Strategy 2006-2015. Available at who.int/vaccines/GIVS/. Accessed on May 6, 2006.

3 Mulholland K. Barreto ML. Routine vaccination and child survival in Guinea-Bissau. Lessons can be learnt from this study. [Letter] BMJ 2001; 322(7282): 360.

4 Folb Pl. WHO Global Advisory Committee on Vaccine Safety. Routine vaccination and child survival in Guinea-Bissau. WHO responds to Guinea-Bissau report. [Letter] BMJ 2001; 322(7282): 361.

5 Aaby P. Jensen H. Routine vaccination and child survival in Guinea-Bissau. Author's reply to commentary. [Letter] BMJ 2001; 322(7282): 360.

6 Aaby P. et al. Differences in female-male mortality after high-titre measles vaccine and association with subsequent vaccination with diphtheria-tetanus-pertussis and inactivated poliovirus: reanalysis of West African studies. Lancet 2003; 361(9376): 2183-8.

7 Aaby P. Rodrigues A. Biai S. Martins C. Veirum JE. Benn CS. Jensen H. Oral polio vaccination and low case fatality at the paediatric ward in Bissau, Guinea-Bissau. Vaccine 2004; 22(23-24): 3014-7.

8 Aaby P. Jensen H. Gomes J. Fernandes M. Lisse IM. The introduction of diphtheria-tetanus-pertussis vaccine

and child mortality in rural Guinea-Bissau: an observational study. International Journal of Epidemiology 2004; 33(2): 374-80.

9 Aaby P, Ibrahim SA, Libman M, Jensen H. The sequence of vaccinations and increased female mortality after high-titre measles vaccine: Trials from rural Sudan and Kinshasa. Vaccine 2006; 24: 2764-2771.

10 Aaby P, Jensen H, Walraven G. Age-specific changes in the female-male mortality ratio related to the pattern of vaccination: An observational study from rural Gambia. Vaccine 2006: 24(22): 4701-8.

11 Global Advisory Committee on Vaccine Safety. Weekly Epidemiological Record 2004; 79: 269-272.

12 Garly ML. Jensen H. Martins CL. Bale C. Balde MA. Lisse IM. Aaby P. Hepatitis B vaccination associated with higher female than male mortality in Guinea-Bissau: an observational study. Pediatric Infectious Disease Journal 2004; 23(12): 1086-92.

13 Aaby P, Jensen H, Garly ML. Bale C. Martins C. Lisse I. Routine vaccinations and child survival in a war situation with high mortality: effect of gender. Vaccine 2002; 21(1-2): 15-20.

14 Hall AJ. Vaccination and child mortality. Lancet 2004; 364(9452): 2156-7.

15 Shann F. Non-specific effects of vaccination: vaccines have non-specific (heterologous) effects. [Letter] BMJ 2005; 330(7495): 844.

16 Adegbola RA et al. Elimination of Haemophilus influenzae type b (Hib) disease from The Gambia after the introduction of routine immunisation with a Hib conjugate vaccine: a prospective study. Lancet 2005; 366(9480): 144-50.

17 Babaniyi OA. A 10-year review of morbidity from childhood preventable diseases in Nigeria: how successful is the expanded programme on immunization (EPI)? An update. Journal of Tropical Pediatrics 1990; 36(6): 306-13.

18 Breiman RF. Streatfield PK. Phelan M. Shifa N. Rashid M. Yunus M. Effect of infant immunisation on childhood mortality in rural Bangladesh: analysis of health and demographic surveillance data. Lancet 2004; 364(9452): 2204-11.

19 Dalton C. Unexpected beneficial effects of measles immunisation. Measles vaccination may be marker for other health seeking behaviours. [Letter] BMJ 2000; 320(7239): 938.

20 Emerton D. Unexpected beneficial effects of measles immunization. Socioeconomic confounding may also play a part. [Letter] BMJ 2000; 320(7239): 938.

21 Aaby P, Jensen H. Benn CS. Lisse IM. Non-specific effects of vaccination: survival bias may explain findings. [Letter] BMJ 2005; 330(7495): 844-5.

22 Simonsen L. Kane A. Lloyd J. Zaffran M. Kane M. Unsafe injections in the developing world and transmission of bloodborne pathogens: a review. Bulletin of the World Health Organization 1999; 77(10): 789-800.

23 WHO. The World Health Report 2002. Available at who.int/whr/2002/en/. Accessed March 17, 2006.

24 Kane A. Lloyd J. Zaffran M. Simonsen L. Kane M. Transmission of hepatitis B, hepatitis C and human immunodeficiency viruses through unsafe injections in the developing world: model-based regional estimates. Bulletin of the World Health Organization 1999; 77(10): 801-7.

25 Crabb C. Researchers argue that unsafe injections spread HIV more than unsafe sex. Bulletin of the World Health Organization 2003; 81(4): 307.

26 John TJ. Did India have the world's largest outbreak of poliomyelitis associated with injections of adjuvanted DPT? [Letter] Indian Pediatrics 1998; 35(1): 73-5.

27 Mupere E et al. Measles vaccination effectiveness among children under 5 years of age in Kampala, Uganda. Vaccine 2006; 24: 4111-4115.

28 de Swart RL et al. Prevention of measles in Sudan: a prospective study on vaccination, diagnosis and epidemiology. Vaccine 2001; 19(17-19): 2254-7.

29 Klingele M. Hartter HK. Adu F. Ammerlaan W. Ikusika W. Muller CP. Resistance of recent measles virus wild-type isolates to antibody-mediated neutralization with vaccinees with antibody. Journal of Medical Virology 2000; 62(1): 91-8.

30 Garly ML. Aaby P. The challenge of improving the efficacy of measles vaccine. Acta Tropica 2003; 85(1): 1-17.

31 D'Souza RM, D'Souza R. Vitamin A for treating measles in children (Cochrane Review). The Cochrane Library 2003, issue 4.

32 Edejer TT. Aikins M. Black R. Wolfson L. Hutubessy R. Evans DB. Cost effectiveness analysis of strategies for child health in developing countries. BMJ 2005; 331(7526): 1177.

33 Glasziou PP. Mackerras DE. Vitamin A supplementation in infectious diseases: a meta-analysis. BMJ 1996; 306(6874): 366-70.

34 Glasziou PP. Mackerras DE. Vitamin A supplementation in infectious diseases: a meta-analysis. BMJ 1993; 306(6874): 366-70.

35 Aaby P. Bhuiya A. Nahar L. Knudsen K. de Francisco A. Strong M. The survival benefit of measles immunization may not be explained entirely by the prevention of measles disease: a community study from rural Bangladesh. International Journal of Epidemiology 2003; 32(1): 106-16.

36 Aaby P. Simondon F. Samb B. Cisse B. Jensen H. Lisse IM. Soumare M. Whittle H. Low mortality after mild measles infection compared to uninfected children in rural West Africa. Vaccine 2002; 21(1-2): 120-6.

37 UNICEF. The state of the world's children 2006. Available at unicef.org/sowc06/pdfs/sowc06_fullreport.pdf. Accessed May 21, 2006.

38 UNICEF. Immunization Summary 2006. Available at unicef.org/publications/files/Immunization_Summary_2006.pdf. Accessed May 26, 2006.

39 Rose G. When public health may not be public health. [Letter] BMJ 2000;321(7264): 834-5.

40 From GAVI website at vaccinealliance.org/index.php. Accessed March 17, 2006.

41 Obaro SK. Palmer A. Vaccines for children: policies, politics and poverty. Vaccine. 21(13-14):1423-31, 2003 Mar 28.

42 A Long Way to Go: a critique of GAVI's initial impact. Save the Children UK. March 2002. Available at savethechildren.org.uk/scuk_cache/scuk/cache/cmsattach/721_GAVI_advocacy.pdf. Accessed March 17, 2006.

43 Puliyel JM. Plea to restore public funding for vaccine development. [Letter] *Lancet* 2004; 363(9409): 659.

44 Mansfield P, Phadke A, Kale A. Blanket hepatitis B vaccination is questionable in India. [Letter] *BMJ* 2006; 332: 976.

45 WHO. Immunization maintains strong performance made in last quarter century. Millions more could be saved with new vaccines, stronger health systems. October 4, 2005. Available at who.int/mediacentre/news/releases/2005/pr48/en/index.html. Accessed March 20, 2006.

46 Aaby P et al. Early diphtheria-tetanus-pertussis vaccination associated with higher female mortality and no difference in male mortality in a cohort of low birthweight children: an observational study within a randomised trial. Archives of Diseases in Childhood 2012: 97: 685-691.

47 Médecins sans Frontières (MSF); The Right Shot: extending the reach of affordable and adapted vaccines. 2012. Accessed from msfaccess.org/content/rightshot on 14th March 2016.

48 Benn CS, Netea MG, Selin LK, Aaby P. A small jab — a big effect: nonspecific immunomodulation by vaccines. Trends in Immunology 2013; 34(9): 431-9.

49 Sørup S, Benn CS, Poulsen A, Krause TG, Aaby P, Ravn H. Live vaccine against measles, mumps and rubella and the risk of hospital admissions for nontargeted infections. JAMA 2014; 311(8): 826-835.

50 Faneye AO, Adeniji JA, Olusola BA, Motayo BO, Akintunde GB. Measles virus infection among vaccinated and unvaccinated children in Nigeria. Viral Immunology 2015; 28(6): 304-8.

Informed Consent: Conclusion

1 Karzon DT. Immunization on public trial. [Editorial] New England Journal of Medicine 1977; 297(5): 275-7.

2 General Medical Council, Good Medical Practice. 2013

3 Pollard A. Childhood Immunisation: what is the future? Archives of Disease in Childhood 2007; 92: 426-433.

4 Miller CL. Measles — the present status of vaccination. Practitioner 1967; 199(193): 607-15.

5 Vuorinen P. Vaccination Against Measles. *British Medical Journal* 1963; 5360: 759-60 .

6 Higson N. MMR debate: Quiz the specialists. BBC News. January 17, 2001. Available at http://news.bbc.co.uk/1/hi/talking_point/forum/1111419 1.stm. Accessed March 22, 2006.

7 BBC News. Children infected at 'measles parties'. July 20, 2001. Available at http://news.bbc.co.uk/1/hi/in_depth/health/1448848.stm. Accessed March 22, 2006.

8 Wolfe RM. Vaccine safety activists on the Internet. [Editorial] Expert Review of Vaccines 2002; 1(3): 249-52.

9 NHS immunisation website. immunisation.nhs.uk/. Accessed March 23, 2006.

10 BMA. Childhood immunisation : a guide for healthcare professionals. June 2003. Available at bma.org.uk/ap.nsf/Content/immunisation. Accessed March 24, 2006.

11 Fine PE. Herd immunity: history, theory, practice. Epidemiologic Reviews 1993; 15(2): 265-302.

12 Jack A. Top health agency set to unify vaccination policy. Financial Times. February 28, 2007.

13 King S. Diphtheria Immunization. The Practitioner 1965; 195: 289-291.

14 Metcalfe Brown C. Pertussis Immunization. The Practitioner 1965; 195: 292-295.

15 HMSO. Immunisation against Infectious Disease ('The Green Book') 1996.

16 Immunisation against Infectious Disease — The Green Book. Department of Health, 2006. Available at dh.gov.uk/PolicyAndGuidance/HealthAndSocialCareTopics/GreenBook/fs/en. Accessed March 11, 2007.

17 CDC. Guide to contraindications* and precautions** to commonly used vaccines. February 2005. Available at cdc.gov/nip/recs/contraindications_vacc.htm. Accessed June 20, 2006.

18 Miller DW, Miller CG. On Evidence, Medical and Legal. Journal of American Physicians and Surgeons 2005; 10: 70-75.

19 Hak E. Schonbeck Y. De Melker H. Van Essen GA. Sanders EA. Negative attitude of highly educated parents and health care workers towards future vaccinations in the Dutch childhood vaccination program. Vaccine 2005; 23(24): 3103-7.

20 Panhotra BR. Saxena AK. Negative attitude of health care workers towards childhood vaccination program. [Letter] Vaccine 2005; 23(48-49): 5459-60.

21 Burton-Jeangros C. Golay M. Sudre P. [Compliance and resistance to child vaccination: a study among Swiss mothers]. [French] Revue d'Epidemiologie et de Santé Publique 2005; 53(4): 341-50.

22 Wilson K. Mills EJ. Norman G. Tomlinson G. Changing attitudes towards polio vaccination: a randomised trial of an evidence-based presentation versus a presentation from a polio survivor. Vaccine 2005; 23(23): 3010-5.

23 NHS Immunisation Information, Department of Health. Health Professionals 2003: Childhood Immunisation Survey Report. Available at immunisation.nhs.uk/files/HPSurveyreport.pdf. Accessed March 9, 2006.

Index

Resources

BabyJabs, a children's immunisation service – of which the author is medical director – that offers parents an informed choice of single and small combination vaccinations.
>   BabyJabs@samedaydoctor
>   Pinnacle House
>   23-26 St Dunstan's Hill, London EC3R 8HN
>   Tel: 020 7337 1370
>   www.babyjabs.co.uk

JABS (Justice Awareness and Basic Support), a self-help support group for parents
>   jackie@jabs.org.uk
>   1 Gawsworth Road, Golborne, Warrington, Cheshire WA3 3RF
>   Tel: 01942 713 565 Fax: 01942 201 323
>   www.jabs.org.uk

Department of Health Immunisation website
>   www.immunisation.nhs.uk

Public Health England, a government-funded body. Its website provides information on infectious diseases and immunisations.
>   www.gov.uk / government / organisations / public-health-england